# Mindfulness-Based Play Therapy

*Mindfulness-Based Play Therapy* is a transtheoretical and neurobiologically informed guide rooted in the belief that the therapeutic alliance is essential to play therapy's effectiveness.

In these pages, clinicians will find the tools they need to help children and families use mindfulness to increase attentional focus and enhance sensory processing, emotion regulation, and reflective awareness. Clinicians will also find a variety of non-directive and directive play-based therapeutic experiences to use in sessions as well as a set of evidence-based practices that supports children with anxiety disorders, trauma, and neurodivergence.

**Lynn Louise Wonders** is a licensed professional counselor (LPC), certified professional counselor (CPCS), registered play therapist-supervisor (RPT-S), and a doctoral student at Saybrook University, conducting research about mindfulness and mental health. She has provided child and family therapy services since 2002 and clinical supervision, consultation, and training since 2010.

"Lynn Louise Wonders examines how integrating mindfulness practices in play therapy nurtures and enhances profoundly deep and meaningful connections with children and families. This book underscores the importance of weaving mindfulness into both professional and personal practices to help play therapists attain genuine alignment and attunement. Through practical strategies and a focus on cultural sensitivity and individualized care, this text highlights the transformative impact of focused awareness in fostering therapeutic growth for children."

**Rachel A. Altvater,** *PsyD, RPT-S, owner and psychologist,*
*Creative Psychological Health Services*

"Whether you are a seasoned therapist or new to the field, you will appreciate the masterful savviness that Lynn Louise Wonders shows in weaving psychological theory, scientific research, and clinical wisdom. She passionately integrates the transformative power of mindfulness with the magic of play therapy as she demonstrates how to facilitate healing with therapeutic presence and attunement. This book is a valuable therapeutic resource and an absolute must for every clinician's library!"

**Joelle Harrison,** *LPCC, NCC, RPT-S,*
*author and licensed professional clinical counselor*

"If you want to integrate mindfulness interventions into your play and child therapy practice, then this is the book for you! Supported by the foundations of neuroscience and play therapy theory, Lynn Louise Wonders provides practical mindfulness skills to immediately transfer into clinical practice. A must-have resource."

**Janet A. Courtney,** *PhD, RPT-S,*
*founder of FirstPlay® Therapy*

# Mindfulness-Based Play Therapy

A Transtheoretical and Neurobiological Approach to Psychotherapy with Children and Families

Lynn Louise Wonders

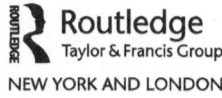
Routledge
Taylor & Francis Group

NEW YORK AND LONDON

Designed cover image: Getty Images

First published 2025
by Routledge
605 Third Avenue, New York, NY 10158

and by Routledge
4 Park Square, Milton Park, Abingdon, Oxon, OX14 4RN

*Routledge is an imprint of the Taylor & Francis Group, an informa business*

© 2025 Lynn Louise Wonders

ISBN: 978-1-032-73404-0 (hbk)
ISBN: 978-1-032-73403-3 (pbk)
ISBN: 978-1-003-46858-5 (ebk)

DOI: 10.4324/9781003468585

Typeset in Adobe Caslon Pro
by KnowledgeWorks Global Ltd.

To the memory of Eric Green, PhD (1974–2024)

Dear Eric, your mentorship through the process of formulating and formalizing Mindfulness-Based Play Therapy® greatly influenced and inspired this work. Your nurturing and wise guidance continues to live in my heart and mind every day. This book is dedicated to you, with honor, love, and gratitude.

# CONTENTS

# FOREWORD

*Rosalind Heiko, PhD, RPT-S*

In Jon J Muth's children's story (2002), a retelling of Count Leo Tolstoy's story of *The Three Questions*, Nikolai brings three questions to his friends Gogol the monkey, Sonya the heron, and Pushkin the dog. Although each of the friends tries their best to answer from their interests and perspectives, Nikolai finally determines that the very best answer should come from Leo the Turtle, who lived long and high in the mountains and was quite wise. These three questions, paraphrased, were as follows:

> *When is the right time to begin?*
> *Who is primary?*
> *What is most essential?*

Soon after Nikolai meets up with Leo the Turtle, a series of events makes it clear to Nikolai that the most significant time and place lands in the very moment in which he finds himself. His primary focus needs to center on the person next to him. The right thing to do is always his best. For in the present moment, each of us can find our meaning, our purpose, and our compassion.

Lynn Louise Wonders has captured the essence of what it means to define and focus on mindful experience within play therapy practice. She embodies an awareness of authentic engagement both personally with many years of experience as a teacher and practitioner of meditation, tai chi, qigong, and yoga and professionally, as a mindfulness expert within the play therapy field, as well as in her counseling and larger therapeutic communities. She is a special human and professional. Years ago, she welcomed me into the world of online play therapy training and invited me to teach with a like-minded professional faculty. I'd never taught on Zoom before. She patiently guided me to slow down and relish reiterating the main points in order to focus participant attention on what was essential. In other words, she guided me to be exquisitely mindful of the impact of my subject. In the years since, her wisdom and compassion shines through every project to which she turns her attention.

In this book, Wonders applies her considerable knowledge and experience in the field of play therapy and her over 30 years of personal and professional mindfulness-based practices to helping therapists effectively engage in mindfulness training in a variety of therapeutic circumstances with children and families, and especially in her work with parents and families. Her commitment to play therapy and counseling brings a rich perspective to the legacy, history, and traditions of mindfulness practice and its intersection with psychotherapy and play therapy in particular. She explores foundational play therapy theories with regard to how these theories can be viewed through a prescriptive, integrative, transtheoretical lens. She beautifully engages therapists to concentrate on the person-of-the-therapist within the relational therapeutic alliance as a means of attending to moment-to-moment mindful exchanges between therapist and client.

### Question: When is the right time to begin?

*Begin right now.*

Wonders understands that concentration on mindfulness allows the therapist to attune to the child's experience in an embodied way through symbolic play and the interpretation of non-verbal cues. Maintaining heightened awareness enhances resonance between therapist and client through her examples of mindful breathing, body scans, present-moment awareness, meditation, and mindful movement activities. She stresses that mindfulness within therapeutic work brings ample benefits for practitioners: lower stress levels, higher levels of job satisfaction, enhanced reflective capacities, greater sensitivity and insight, improved emotional regulation, and connection with clients and peers. The multisensory, embodied aspects of mindfulness practice enhance our therapeutic work with children and families by activating processes involved in neural integration. In her chapter on the neurobiology of mindfulness and child development, Wonders beautifully expands on the interconnectedness of neurobiological mechanisms, child development theories, and how they play a crucial role in play therapy practice.

Reflective practice builds trust and safety within the therapeutic relationship. The emotionally regulated and attuned play therapist is then able to forge a crucial alliance with clients and their families and caregivers. This book emphasizes that therapists who center their mindful practice on self-awareness can develop the capacity for non-judgmental acknowledgment of their own emotions, thoughts, and behaviors. Play therapists can thus expand their conscious awareness of rupture and repair in therapeutic interactions. Wonders guides a greater appreciation of transference and countertransference reactions, in order to increase perspective-taking in an embodied way through daily mindfulness practice.

Wonders shares the necessary nine core attitudes from Kabat-Zinn's foundational curriculum to enhance specific applications of mindfulness in daily life. She emphasizes that maintaining positivity and an appreciation of gratitude and acceptance leads to greater resilience and capacity on the part of both therapist and client. This, in turn, fosters an attitude of engagement and satisfaction with self-growth for clients, their families, and the play therapists themselves.

### Question: Who is primary?

*Set your focus on the person by your side.*

Wonders considers seminal and historical play therapy theories and the intersection with intentional, mindful practice. She explores the basic tenets, phases, and practical, creative applications of mindfulness healing work inherent in Adlerian Play Therapy, Child-Centered Play Therapy, Cognitive Behavioral Play Therapy, Ecosystemic Play Therapy, Gestalt Play Therapy, Jungian Play Therapy, Psychodynamic/Object Relations Play Therapy, Developmental and Attachment-Based Play Therapy.

Wonders also lends a focus on mindfulness within prescriptive play therapy, which includes comprehensive treatment planning, tailored interventions, therapist flexibility and adaptability, and a focus on thorough assessment, family support, and collaboration with caregivers. Wonders delves into how to design a prescriptive treatment plan, inviting self-reflection and mindfulness practices to enhance crucial person-of-the-therapist attunement.

Wonders reminds us that working with children and their caregivers involves navigating a multitude of complex dynamics and developmental needs of all parties, requiring therapists to be consistently attuned, present, and emotionally regulated. Wonders focuses on mindfulness practice for therapists themselves to build emotional capacity, reduce stress, and prevent burnout. Both therapist and client receive the generous benefits of this practice.

She takes us through the ancient roots of mindfulness, as well as Eastern and Western traditions in contemplative practices, weaving connections of parent-child work through models that include Filial Therapy, Theraplay®, FirstPlay® Therapy, and Child-Parent Relationship Therapy (CPRT). Each offers opportunities for mindful play, parenting and caregiver exercises, resources, and reflective, mindful practice.

**Question: What is most essential?**

*It is essential to do your best. The person by your side is counting on you.*

A variety of sensory play and mindful sand and water play activities are playfully addressed. Later in the book, Wonders turns her attention to expanding our reach through mindfulness-based games and activities to enhance breath and body awareness (e.g., conscious breathing and breath awareness games, sensory walks, yoga poses, and mindful storytelling, among many suggested activities), consistently finding ways to engage caregivers.

Wonders weaves together vital information on case conceptualization, assessment, therapy planning, and documentation. In their book *Play Therapy Treatment Planning with Children and Families*, Wonders and Affee (2024) recognize that being prescriptive means the therapist must constantly monitor the quality of the child's connection to the therapist and the treatment and modify the course of action as necessary. "There is a dynamic and fluidly responsive element of prescriptive treatment planning. Being prescriptive involves ongoing observation, reading the client in the therapy room, and watching and listening to the non-verbal and verbal feedback the child provides" (Wonders & Affee, 2024, p. 37). In other words, expanding awareness in mindful practice on the part of the play therapist enables that therapist to choose the best avenue for formulation and integrated therapeutic follow-through for clients and their families.

Wonders includes a chapter that encourages therapists to center attention on practicing cultural humility. She invites play therapists to commit to ongoing learning to recognize our biases and limitations through a cultural competence lens. She believes designing a culturally inclusive playroom is essential to a mindfulness-based therapeutic practice. Wonders concludes the book with a chapter on the importance of ritual and closure activities with children through mindfulness-based interventions to celebrate client growth and achievement from initial sessions through termination.

Our life and professional journeys can only be enhanced by mindful practice and engagement. Lynn Louise Wonders has beautifully amplified our understanding and therapeutic capacity in this work of the heart and mind.

The time is now, the most important one is you, and the right thing to do is soak up all this wisdom and these mindful opportunities for practice.

## References

Muth, J. J. (2002). *The three questions: Based on a story by Leo Tolstoy.* Scholastic Press.
Wonders, L. L., & Affee, M. L. (2024). *Play therapy treatment planning with children and families: A guide for mental health professionals.* Routledge.

# PREFACE: THE INCEPTION AND EVOLUTION OF MINDFULNESS-BASED PLAY THERAPY

## Introduction

The story of Mindfulness-based Play Therapy® (MBPT) begins with my personal journey into mindfulness, which started in 1991, two years after my college graduation. Immersing myself in a mindfulness-based stress management program, I was captivated by the transformative power of meditation, yoga, tai chi, and chi kung (qigong). The benefits were so profound that by 1995, I trained to be an instructor and began teaching these practices, a role I cherished and continued until 2019.

Mindfulness became a lifeline as I balanced the demands of graduate school, parenting two young children, and working part-time as a freelance writer and educational consultant. In 2003, as an associate professional counselor, I introduced a social-emotional literacy program in preschools, integrating mindfulness into the social and emotional learning (SEL) curriculum I created. This experience laid the groundwork for incorporating mindfulness into therapeutic practices with children and families.

After training in play therapy, I began naturally blending mindfulness into my clinical work with children and families. By 2010, I started teaching mental health professionals and supervisees how to utilize mindfulness in play therapy. Over the years, mindfulness became an integral part of all my professional endeavors, featuring the concept and practice in continuing education training since 2010 and through my website blog since 2012. Between 2011 and 2019, I organized and led multiple self-care and training retreats, incorporating mindfulness-based practices.

It wasn't until early 2023, during training in Synergetic Play Therapy® with Lisa Dion, that I had an epiphany. Dion's inclusion of mindfulness in her own work along with her encouragement to step into my most aligned and authentic self, illuminated the potential for me to take all I had been doing for over 30 years and formally unite my experience with mindfulness and play therapy. Thus, MBPT was conceived and debuted officially through professional training events.

MBPT is not a model. It is a transtheoretical and neurobiologically informed *approach* to play therapy that integrates mindfulness-based practices, supported by robust research about the positive effects of mindfulness on mental health, into therapeutic play experiences for children and families. This approach blends readily with historically significant and seminal play therapy theories, including Child-Centered, Jungian, Cognitive Behavioral, Developmental and Attachment-based, Ecosystemic, Psychodynamic and Object Relations, Gestalt, and Adlerian Play Therapy. Peer-reviewed research supports mindfulness-based methods, which help children with anxiety disorders, trauma, sorrow and loss, difficulties adjusting, and children who identify as neurodivergent.

Several play therapy models and all the seminal play therapy theories will be explored in this book, showcasing how mindfulness can enhance therapeutic practices from a wide variety of frameworks. The concept and practice of mindfulness are universally available to anyone and everyone, and it is my intention that MBPT builds upon the recent and historical work of teachers, philosophers, researchers, and authors immersed in the use and practice of mindfulness who have come before me and that this approach to play therapy will be widely embraced by clinicians regardless of theoretical orientation.

## Mindfulness Promotes Attunement and Therapeutic Presence

Mindfulness is particularly beneficial in enhancing a therapist's ability to remain present and attuned during therapy sessions (Siegel, 2010). Play therapy requires therapists to enter the child's world, observing their

non-verbal cues and symbolic play. This deep level of engagement necessitates a high degree of presence and attunement. However, children are
highly intuitive, and if a therapist is not authentically attuned, they will
sense the lack of presence, and this can be problematic for the quality of
the therapeutic experience in the therapy room (Dion, 2018; Erskine,
2019; Geller & Greenberg, 2012). Studies on therapeutic presence indicate that clients who perceive their therapists as fully present report better therapeutic outcomes (Geller & Greenberg, 2012).

Additionally, Richard Erskine (2019) highlights the importance of
developmental attunement in integrative psychotherapy, showing that
a lack of attunement can disrupt the therapeutic process. Lisa Dion
(2018) further underscores this point by explaining that children can
intuitively sense the therapist's internal state, and any incongruence or
lack of authenticity can negatively impact the therapeutic relationship
and outcomes. It is essential that therapists cultivate an ability to attune
to the child in the present moment for the most effective therapeutic
outcomes.

### *Mindfulness Leads to Understanding the Child's World*

Play therapy is a unique form of psychotherapy in that it utilizes the
natural medium of play to help children express their thoughts and feelings (Landreth, 2012; Ray, 2011; Wonders, 2021). Children often communicate through play rather than words, using toys and games as their
way of exploring, experiencing, and expressing their thoughts, feelings,
observations, and desires. To effectively engage with a child during play
therapy, I realized in my own clinical experiences that the therapist must
be deeply attuned to the subtle nuances of a child's play. This means
astutely observing non-verbal cues, including facial expressions, body
language, and the thematic elements of their play. My own mindfulness
practices enhanced my ability to focus intently on these cues, improving
my conceptualization and connection with children in the playroom and
with their caregivers as well. I concluded upon reflection that my many
years of mindfulness practice within the context of play therapy services
had significantly supported the essential need for therapeutic alliance,
non-judgment, acceptance, rapport, trust, and quality of presence in the
relationship between myself and my clients as evidenced by consistently

positive treatment outcomes, caregiver satisfaction, and low client attrition before therapy completion.

### Mindfulness Leads to Maintaining Heightened Awareness

Reflecting on over 20 years as a psychotherapist, I see that my commitment to mindfulness outside of therapy sessions has naturally enhanced my mindfulness within sessions. Being mindful within sessions has helped me maintain a heightened awareness so that I am fully present with my clients in the moment. Bringing this mindful presence into therapy sessions has made it easier to notice and respond to the fleeting and subtle expressions of a child's inner world. In reviewing video recordings of supervisees who utilized mindfulness with their clients, I noticed that the supervisees who regularly practiced mindfulness in their personal lives naturally brought that ability for heightened awareness into the playroom with clients. This high level of presence enables the therapist to tune into the child's emotional state, providing more effective and empathetic interventions.

### Mindfulness Fosters Safety and Trust

The presence cultivated through my personal mindfulness practice has not only been beneficial for my attunement but also felt by the children and families I have worked with. I've realized over the years in my work and in all the play therapy training and supervision I've provided for others that a therapist who is fully present and attuned creates a safe and trusting environment. Children are highly perceptive and can sense when an adult is authentically engaged and attentive (Dion, 2018; Erskine, 2019; Greenberg, 2012). When a child has the experience of being genuinely seen and heard, a secure therapeutic relationship is established, which is foundational for effective play therapy regardless of theoretical orientation.

### The Nine Attitudes of Mindfulness in Play Therapy

MBPT integrates mindfulness principles with the remedial and therapeutic effects of play to help children heal from past trauma, reduce anxiety symptoms, and develop emotional regulation, resilience, and self-awareness. Jon Kabat-Zinn (2003) outlines nine core elements foundational to mindfulness practice he calls "attitudes." Each of these attitudes can be deeply beneficial when applied to play therapy, creating a nurturing environment that supports children's growth and healing.

1. **Non-Judging**

   **Mindfulness Attitude:** Non-judging involves observing without evaluating or labeling experiences as good or bad.

   **Application in Play Therapy:** Therapists who adopt a non-judging stance create a safe space for children, allowing them to express their thoughts and emotions freely without fear of criticism. This fosters trust and encourages children to explore their feelings and behaviors openly during play.

2. **Patience**

   **Mindfulness Attitude:** Patience means allowing things to unfold in their own time, recognizing that growth and change take time.

   **Application in Play Therapy:** By practicing patience, therapists honor the child's unique pace of development and healing. This attitude helps therapists avoid rushing the therapeutic process, providing children with the time they need to process their experiences through play.

3. **Beginner's Mind**

   **Mindfulness Attitude:** Beginner's mind involves approaching situations with a sense of curiosity and openness, as if encountering them for the first time.

   **Application in Play Therapy:** Embracing a beginner's mind allows therapists to see each session and each child as unique. This perspective helps therapists stay open to new insights and creative interventions, enhancing their responsiveness to the child's needs and the dynamics of play.

4. **Trust**

   **Mindfulness Attitude:** Trust involves having confidence in oneself and in the experience of whatever arises in the present moment.

   **Application in Play Therapy:** Building trust is fundamental in play therapy. Therapists need to trust their own skills and intuition, as well as the child's inherent ability to heal and grow. This mutual trust strengthens the therapeutic relationship and supports the child's journey.

5.  **Non-Striving**

    **Mindfulness Attitude:** Non-striving means focusing on the present moment rather than striving for specific outcomes or goals.

    **Application in Play Therapy:** Non-striving helps therapists stay present with the child without imposing expectations or agendas. This attitude encourages a process-oriented approach, where the focus is on the child's immediate experience and expression through play, rather than on achieving predetermined therapeutic milestones. While having a plan for therapy with goals and objectives is essential, during the play therapy session, the therapist can be fully present with the child and postpone any thought process about the treatment plan for another time outside of sessions (Ray, 2011; Wonders, 2024b).

6.  **Acceptance**

    **Mindfulness Attitude:** Acceptance involves acknowledging things as they are without resisting or denying them.

    **Application in Play Therapy:** Acceptance allows therapists to fully embrace the child's current emotional and behavioral state. This attitude fosters an environment of unconditional positive regard, where children feel valued and understood, which is crucial for their emotional healing and growth.

7.  **Letting Go**

    **Mindfulness Attitude:** Letting go means releasing attachment to specific thoughts, feelings, or outcomes.

    **Application in Play Therapy:** In play therapy, letting go enables therapists to adapt to the flow of the child's play and emotions. This flexibility allows therapists to meet children where they are, facilitating spontaneous and meaningful therapeutic interactions.

8.  **Gratitude**

    **Mindfulness Attitude:** Gratitude involves appreciating the positive aspects of life and experiences.

> **Application in Play Therapy:** Cultivating gratitude in play therapy helps therapists focus on the child's strengths and progress, however small. Expressing gratitude for the child's efforts and resilience can enhance their sense of self-worth and motivation to engage in the therapeutic process. Gratitude expressed to caregivers for participating as partners in the child's therapy can enhance therapeutic alliance with caregivers whose buy-in and participation is often essential for positive outcomes.

9. **Generosity**

> **Mindfulness Attitude:** Generosity means giving freely without expecting anything in return.
>
> **Application in Play Therapy:** Generosity in play therapy involves giving children the gift of attention, presence, and empathy. Therapists who practice generosity create a nurturing environment where children feel cared for and supported, which can significantly enhance the therapeutic alliance and the child's overall well-being.

Incorporating the nine attitudes of mindfulness into play therapy enriches the therapeutic experience for both the therapist and the child. These attitudes foster a compassionate, accepting, and flexible approach that honors the child's individual journey and promotes healing through the natural process of play. By embodying these attitudes, therapists can create a safe and supportive space where children can explore, express, and transform their inner worlds.

### *Embarking on a Journey with Mindfulness-based Play Therapy®*

As we transition to the chapters ahead, we will delve deeper into the rich history and evolution of mindfulness as a practice. We will explore how personal mindfulness practice can profoundly benefit therapists, enhancing their presence and attunement in therapeutic settings. Additionally, we will examine the integration of mindfulness into play therapy sessions with children and families, providing both exploration of multiple theoretical foundations and practical examples of interventions. Each chapter is designed to equip you with a comprehensive understanding of how MBPT can be applied to foster healing and growth for children and families. This journey promises to be enlightening, offering insights and tools that can transform your therapeutic practice. Let us now embark on this path, beginning with an exploration of the roots of mindfulness.

-Lynn Louise Wonders

## References

Dion, L. (2018). *Aggression in play therapy: A neurobiological approach for integrating intensity.* WW Norton & Company.

Erskine, R. G. (2019). Developmentally based, relationally focused integrative psychotherapy: Eight essential points. *International Journal of Integrative Psychotherapy, 10,* 1–10.

Geller, S. M., & Greenberg, L. S. (2012). *Therapeutic presence: A mindful approach to effective therapy.* American Psychological Association.

Greenberg, L. S. (2012). Emotions, the great captains of our lives: Their role in the process of change in psychotherapy. *American Psychologist, 67*(8), 697.

Kabat-Zinn, J. (2003). Mindfulness-based interventions in context: Past, present, and future. *Science and Practice, 10*(2), 144–156.

Landreth, G. L. (2012). *Play therapy: The art of the relationship.* Routledge.

Ray, D. C. (2011). *Advanced play therapy: Essential conditions, knowledge, and skills for child practice.* Routledge.

Siegel, D. J. (2010). *The mindful therapist: A clinician's guide to mindsight and neural integration. Norton Series on Interpersonal Neurobiology.* WW Norton & Company.

Wonders, L. L. (2021). Theoretical roots and branches of the evolving field of play therapy. In *Play therapy and telemental health* (pp. 3–24). Routledge.

# ACKNOWLEDGMENTS

This book represents the culmination of years of practice, contemplation, research, and collaboration, and I am deeply grateful to many individuals and institutions for their support and contributions.

First and foremost, I would like to thank my husband, Dennis Wonders, whose unwavering support has been invaluable throughout this journey. His encouragement and patience with the long hours of work have made it possible for this book to be completed.

I am also deeply indebted to my colleagues and professors at the Department of Humanistic Psychology at Saybrook University. The stimulating academic environment and the opportunities for collaboration and discussion provided by my peers and mentors have been instrumental in the development of this work. Special thanks go to Dr. Israel Espinosa, Dr. Eric Willmarth, Dr. Marina Smirnova, Dr. Jenny DeDecker, Dr. Vasiliki Georgoulas-Sherry and Dr. Terri Goslin-Jones for their critical feedback and support in my learning.

My gratitude extends to some of my most revered professional colleagues Dr. Rosalind Heiko, Dr. Janet Courtney, Lisa Dion, Judith Norman, Rose LaPiere, who have inspired me and supported me along the way.

I give special thanks to Dr. Alyssa Caldbeck who supported and helped me with the research for this book.

Last, I am grateful to all of my teachers from whom I have learned about mindfulness practices from over 30 years. I want to specifically acknowledge Dr. Jon Kabat-Zinn from whom I have learned so much about mindfulness in practicality for myself, my students, and my therapy clients over the years.

Thank you all.

# ABOUT THE AUTHOR

Lynn Louise Wonders is licensed and certified as a professional counselor and supervisor in the state of Georgia. She has provided clinical psychotherapy services for children, families, couples, and individual adults since 2001 and has served as a clinical supervisor, professional consultant, and a play therapy continuing education trainer for clinicians worldwide since 2010. She was one of the very first to develop online learning in the field of play therapy. Ms. Wonders taught mindfulness classes, including meditation, yoga, tai chi, and chi kung from 1995 to 2019. She is published in numerous academic and professional books on the topic of play therapy, co-editor and chapter author of *Nature-Based Play Therapy* and *Play Therapy Treatment Planning*. She is the author of *When Parents Are at War: A Child Therapist's Guide to Navigating High Conflict Divorce & Custody Cases*, *The Midlife Self-Discovery Workbook*, the *Miss Piper's Playroom* therapeutic children's book series, and several more children's books. Ms. Wonders has provided clinical supervision training and supervision for the supervisor since 2015. She is working toward her PhD in the Department of Humanistic Psychology at Saybrook University. Ms. Wonders has three young adult children and one grandson. She lives with her husband and their little dog named Bodhi in Florida.

# 1
## THE ORIGINS AND TRUE MEANING OF MINDFULNESS

## Introduction

Understanding the true definition and meaning of mindfulness, along with its rich history, is important for therapists who want to learn about Mindfulness-based Play Therapy® (MBPT). This foundational knowledge allows therapists to fully grasp and appreciate the depth and significance of mindfulness, which goes beyond its common associations with stress reduction and relaxation. Mindfulness, rooted in ancient contemplative traditions such as Buddhism, Hinduism, and Taoism, cultivates present-moment awareness, acceptance, and non-judgmental observation of one's thoughts, emotions, and sensations (Tan & Tan, 2021). This practice has been handed down and expanded into a way of being, living, and showing up in the world for us and our clients.

## Clearing Up Misconceptions about Mindfulness

Mindfulness is often misunderstood, and several misconceptions can eclipse its true nature and benefits. These misunderstandings can arise from oversimplified or misrepresented information, often spread through popular media, social networks, and even well-meaning but misinformed individuals. When mindfulness is portrayed as only a

DOI: 10.4324/9781003468585-1

relaxation technique or a quick fix for stress, it diminishes the depth and richness of this ancient practice rooted in centuries of philosophical traditions. Such false narratives can discourage some people from practicing mindfulness, leading to unrealistic expectations and disappointment when the practice does not deliver instant bliss or complete emotional control. Additionally, commercial interests may exploit these misconceptions, promoting mindfulness products or programs that need more authenticity and depth. This widespread misinformation can obscure the essence of mindfulness, which is about cultivating awareness, acceptance, and presence in the current moment, regardless of whether those moments are pleasant or challenging. By understanding and addressing these misconceptions, we can reconnect with the profound and transformative potential of mindfulness, honoring its true purpose and benefits. Let's examine some common misconceptions about mindfulness.

### *Mindfulness Does Not Equate to an Empty Mind*

One common misconception is that mindfulness involves clearing the mind of all thoughts. Mindfulness is about being more aware of one's thoughts, feelings, and sensations without judgment, rather than eliminating them (Kabat-Zinn, 2015; Morris, 2023; Tan & Tan, 2021). This practice encourages individuals to observe their mental activity with curiosity and acceptance, recognizing that thoughts and feelings naturally arise and pass. Instead of striving for a blank mind, mindfulness teaches us to acknowledge whatever is present in our consciousness at any given moment. This includes recognizing patterns of thinking, emotional reactions, and physical sensations without becoming entangled or overwhelmed. The goal is not to suppress or banish thoughts but to develop a mindful relationship with them, seeing them as transient mental events rather than definitive truths or commands. This perspective allows for greater clarity and insight into one's inner life, fostering a sense of peace and balance. By learning to witness our mental landscape without judgment, we can cultivate a deeper understanding of ourselves and our experiences, ultimately leading to greater emotional resilience and well-being (Rechtschaffen, 2014; Siegel, 2017).

### Mindfulness Does Not Always Lead to Relaxation

Another widespread belief is that mindfulness is solely for relaxation. While it can reduce stress and promote relaxation, its purpose is broader, encompassing the cultivation of a deeper awareness of the present moment, which can enhance clarity, focus, and emotion regulation. Mindfulness involves intentionally directing attention to one's current experiences with openness and curiosity. This heightened awareness helps individuals gain a clearer understanding of their thoughts, emotions, and bodily sensations as they unfold. By practicing mindfulness, people can develop a more refined ability to observe their mental processes without immediate reaction or judgment, allowing for more thoughtful and deliberate responses to life's challenges (Kabat-Zinn, 2015; Morris, 2023; Tan & Tan, 2021). This practice also improves concentration and focus, as individuals learn to anchor their attention on the present moment rather than being distracted by past regrets or future anxieties. Additionally, mindfulness fosters emotion regulation by helping individuals recognize and manage their emotional states more effectively. Rather than merely serving as a tool for relaxation, mindfulness cultivates a comprehensive approach to mental and emotional well-being, promoting a balanced and mindful way of living that transcends mere stress relief.

### Mindfulness Is Not a Religious Practice

There is often a misconception that mindfulness is inherently a religious practice. Although it originated in Buddhist meditation, mindfulness is most often practiced in a secular context and has been adapted for various therapeutic and educational settings (Murphy, 2016; Tan & Tan, 2021). This versatility allows mindfulness to be adapted and accessible to people of all backgrounds, regardless of their spiritual or religious beliefs. It can be naturally integrated into any religious practice, enhancing spiritual awareness and connection, or it can be entirely secular, focusing solely on mental and emotional well-being.

### Mindfulness Is Not a Quick Fix

Some people hope for mindfulness to be a quick fix for their problems. It is, however, a skill that requires consistent practice and patience to experience its full benefits. Developing mindfulness requires regularly dedicating time and effort to cultivate present-moment awareness and non-judgmental acceptance. It is a gradual process that unfolds over time, yielding often profound changes in how individuals relate to their thoughts, emotions, and experiences. By integrating mindfulness into daily life, individuals can achieve lasting improvements in mental clarity, emotional resilience, and overall well-being, demonstrating that mindfulness is far more than a temporary solution, but a universally applicable practice that fosters a balanced and mindful way of living (Laurie & Blandford, 2016).

### Mindfulness Does Not Require Stillness

Many believe that mindfulness requires sitting still, but it can be organically incorporated into everyday activities such as walking, eating, or washing dishes. This informal mindfulness practice integrates mindfulness into the flow of daily life rather than confining it to formal meditation sessions. Walking meditation, for instance, involves focusing on each step, the ground's sensation underfoot, the rhythm of breathing, and the surrounding sights and sounds. Mindful eating emphasizes full attention to the experience of eating, from the colors and textures to the body's signals of hunger and fullness, fostering a healthier relationship with food. Even routine tasks like loading a dishwasher or folding laundry can become meditative by concentrating on the textures, sounds, and movement of the hands and arms. This shift in focus transforms mundane chores into calming, centering activities, reducing stress, and enhancing overall well-being by fostering a deeper connection to daily experiences and surroundings.

### Mindfulness Does Not Guarantee a State of Bliss

Another misconception is that mindfulness is about achieving a state of bliss. Instead, mindfulness involves accepting and being present with whatever one is experiencing, whether it is pleasant or unpleasant (Kabat-Zinn, 2015; Sipe, 2021). The practice is about cultivating an open, non-judgmental awareness of the present moment, acknowledging thoughts, emotions, and sensations as they arise without trying to change, suppress, or escape them. For example, if one feels anxious or stressed, mindfulness encourages observing these feelings with curiosity and compassion rather than resistance or frustration. This approach helps individuals build resilience and emotion regulation by learning to face and endure difficult experiences rather than avoiding them. By fostering an attitude of acceptance and presence, mindfulness enables people to navigate life's ups and downs with greater equanimity, fostering a deeper understanding of themselves and their responses to various situations. This shift from seeking constant positivity to embracing the full spectrum of human experience is a core aspect of mindfulness practice, leading to a more balanced and grounded way of living.

### Mindfulness Is Not Passive

Mindfulness is often seen as a passive activity, but it requires active engagement and conscious effort to maintain awareness and presence. Practicing mindfulness involves deliberately focusing on the present moment, which can be challenging in our fast-paced, distraction-filled world (Kabat-Zinn, 2015; Sipe, 2021, Tan & Tan, 2021). This active engagement means continuously bringing the mind back to the here and now whenever it wanders, which often happens. It also involves a commitment to observe thoughts, feelings, and sensations without judgment, cultivating a sense of curiosity and openness. This process demands regular practice and a willingness to face whatever arises, be it discomfort, boredom, or restlessness. Mindfulness requires setting aside time for formal practice, such as meditation or mindfulness walks, and incorporating mindful awareness into everyday activities. The effort invested in maintaining this state of awareness leads to greater self-awareness, emotion regulation, and overall well-being, demonstrating that mindfulness is far from passive but rather a dynamic and intentional practice (Laurie & Blandford, 2016).

### Mindfulness Is Not Only for Abled and Privileged People

It is a misconception that only certain people can practice mindfulness. Mindfulness is accessible to everyone, regardless of age, race, gender, education, or religion, and can be adapted to suit individual needs and preferences. This universal accessibility means that mindfulness can be practiced by children, adults, and seniors from all walks of life, each finding methods and techniques that resonate with their unique life stages and experiences. Mindfulness transcends cultural boundaries, allowing people from diverse cultural backgrounds to adapt and integrate the practice into their lives in ways that respect and honor their traditions and beliefs (Fuchs et al., 2013; Proulx et al., 2018; Thirumaran et al., 2013).

For individuals who identify as neurodivergent, mindfulness can be particularly beneficial and can be adaptable to meet their individual needs. Techniques can be modified to accommodate different sensory preferences and cognitive styles, ensuring that the practice is effective. For example, mindfulness exercises can be tailored to involve more movement for those who find stillness challenging or to include sensory-friendly materials and environments (Singha & Singha, 2024).

The adaptability of mindfulness also extends to its integration into various lifestyles and routines, making it a flexible practice that can be woven into daily activities. By recognizing and respecting the diverse ways in which people experience and interact with the world, mindfulness can be customized to enhance its accessibility and effectiveness, ensuring that everyone, regardless of their neurodivergence or cultural background, can benefit from its profound impact on mental and emotional well-being. This inclusive approach underscores the fundamental principle that mindfulness is a universally applicable practice capable of enriching the lives of all who engage with it.

### *Mindfulness Does Not Require Formal Meditation Practice*

Mindfulness is often equated with a formal meditation practice. While meditation is indeed one common way to experience and practice, mindfulness can also be cultivated through various activities and techniques beyond formal meditation as mentioned previously in daily activities (Laurie & Blandford, 2016; Mantzios & Giannou, 2019). Engaging in creative arts such as painting, drawing, or sculpting allows individuals to immerse themselves fully in the present moment, focusing on colors, textures, and movement. Mindful listening to music involves paying close attention to the intricacies of a musical piece, including individual instruments, melody, harmony, and rhythm, and noticing the emotional impact of the music. Gardening is another mindful activity, where tending to plants encourages a connection with nature and fosters presence and patience. The body scan technique involves mentally scanning the body from head to toe, paying attention to sensations and tension without judgment, and promoting relaxation and bodily awareness. Practices like tai chi, qigong, or mindful stretching involve slow, deliberate movements synchronizing the mind and body. Mindful cooking transforms meal preparation into a meditative experience by focusing on the process, from chopping vegetables to savoring aromas and presenting the final dish. Journaling, whether through gratitude or reflective writing, helps process emotions and experiences with mindful awareness. Mindful sports such as rock climbing, surfing, or archery require intense concentration and present moment focus on physical sensations and mental strategies. Walking in nature with mindfulness enhances the experience by observing natural sounds, sights, and feelings. Mindful technology use involves engaging with digital content fully present and noticing reactions and feelings to reduce digital overwhelm. These diverse methods demonstrate that mindfulness can be integrated into virtually any activity, allowing individuals to find practices that resonate with their interests and lifestyles.

### *Mindfulness Is Not Merely a Passing Fad*

Some people view mindfulness as a trend or fad, but it has a long history and is supported by a growing body of scientific research demonstrating its benefits for mental and physical health. Originating from ancient Buddhist practices, mindfulness has been a cornerstone of wisdom-based traditions for thousands of years, emphasizing the cultivation of awareness, presence, and compassion. In recent decades, mindfulness has been adapted into a secular practice, making it accessible to people of all backgrounds and beliefs. This modern adaptation has been extensively studied, with robust research validating its efficacy. Many commercial organizations have capitalized on the term mindfulness, and it has become associated with only a few known practices (Purser et al., 2021; Van Dam et al., 2018; Wilson, 2016). However, with ongoing daily practice, mindfulness can become a conscious state of mind, a way of being, that can be observed during any activity.

*Mindfulness Is Not a Frivolous Practice*

Numerous studies have shown that mindfulness can significantly reduce stress, anxiety, and depression while enhancing emotion regulation and resilience (Grossman et al., 2004; Hofmann et al., 2010). It has been found to improve attention, concentration, and cognitive flexibility, leading to better decision-making and problem-solving skills (Jha et al., 2007; Zeidan et al., 2010). Mindfulness has demonstrated positive effects on physical health, including lower blood pressure, improved immune function, and reduced symptoms of chronic pain (Creswell et al., 2019 Kabat-Zinn et al., 1985). These benefits are attributed to the way mindfulness fosters a deeper connection between the mind and body, promoting overall well-being.

Given its rich history and substantial evidence base, mindfulness is far from a passing trend. It represents a profound approach to enhancing quality of life, rooted in ancient wisdom and bolstered by modern science. Resistance to practicing mindfulness may stem from misconceptions or discomfort with change, but it is worth examining more closely. Embracing mindfulness can be a challenge, yet it offers an opportunity for personal growth and meaningful connection to oneself and others. By approaching mindfulness with an open mind and willingness to explore, individuals can experience its transformative potential, leading to a more balanced and fulfilling life.

Mindfulness is a witnessing practice of being fully present in the moment, inviting attuned focus and acceptance of what is observed (Anālayo, 2021). When first learning how to practice, it can be helpful to experience mindfulness through more traditional experiences such as guided mindfulness exercises, breathing activities, or taking a gentle yoga or meditation class. (Once experienced and practiced more formally, the practice can be carried over into the simplest of endeavors in everyday life and into the play therapy room.)

*Therapists Benefit from Mindfulness Practice*

The integration of mindfulness into the daily life of the therapist is not only a beneficial practice (McCollum & Gehart, 2010; Shapiro & Carlson, 2017) but an essential one if the therapist wants to embrace

MBPT with clients. Working with children and their caregivers involves navigating many complex dynamics and developmental needs, requiring therapists to be consistently attuned, present, and emotionally resilient  (Porges, 2011; Schore, 2001; Siegel, 2012). The next chapter in this book underscores the importance of mindfulness as a crucial form of personal self-care for therapists (Christopher & Maris, 2010; Posluns & Gall, 2020), highlighting how it enhances the therapeutic alliance and the overall effectiveness of play therapy for children and families (Dickinson & Daly, 2021; Jennings & Apsche, 2014; Meany-Walen, 2018).

## Ancient Eastern Roots and Traditions of Mindfulness

Though widely popularized, often watered down, and often misunder-stood as a fad in recent years, mindfulness is a practice that has ancient roots in various contemplative traditions, including Buddhism, Hinduism, and Taoism (Brazier, 2013; Khemraj et al., 2023; Vörös, 2016). These tra-ditions all emphasize focusing on the present moment while cultivating non-judgmental and accepting awareness.

Historically, mindfulness has been integral to Eastern spiritual and philosophical practices for centuries (Anālayo, 2021; Ditrich, 2016a; Neves-Pereira et al., 2018). In the tradition of Buddhism, mindfulness (sati) is one of the core aspects of the Eightfold Path, which aims to achieve enlightenment (Ditrich, 2016b). Hinduism includes mindful-ness within its practice of yoga and meditation, emphasizing a focused awareness of the present moment (Sharma & Singh, 2024). Taoism also incorporates mindfulness through practices that harmonize the mind and body with the flow of nature (Cleary, 2000). These traditions have long recognized the benefits of mindfulness in achieving mental clarity, emotional balance, and spiritual growth (Gu et al., 2018).

### Mindfulness Was Brought to the West

The introduction of mindfulness to the West can largely be attributed to the works of several key figures who studied these ancient practices and sought to bring their benefits to a broader audience (Singla, 2011). In the 1960s and 1970s, Western scholars and practitioners began to explore and integrate mindfulness into Western psychology and medicine (Buchholz, 2015; Wang et al., 2021). Several influential figures were instrumental in introducing mindfulness to the West. These pioneers brought valuable insights from the East that would later shape the development of mindfulness in Western contexts.

### Thich Nhat Hanh

A Vietnamese Zen Buddhist monk, Thich Nhat Hanh (2007, 2009), played a significant role in bringing mindfulness to the West. His teachings emphasized the practice of mindful living and advocated for mindfulness in daily activities. His books and retreats reached a wide Western audience, promoting the integration of mindfulness into everyday life.

### Jack Kornfield

An American author and teacher in the Vipassana movement, Jack Kornfield (1993) studied under Buddhist masters in Southeast Asia. He co-founded the Insight Meditation Society (IMS) in Massachusetts, which became a cornerstone for the dissemination of mindfulness and meditation practices in the West.

### Joseph Goldstein

Alongside Jack Kornfield, Joseph Goldstein (1976) co-founded the IMS. He has written extensively on mindfulness and meditation, contributing to the popularization, and understanding of these practices in the West.

### Sharon Salzberg

A co-founder of the IMS in Barre, Massachusetts, in 1975, alongside Jack Kornfield and Joseph Goldstein, Salzberg (1995) has been a leading figure in bringing mindfulness and loving-kindness meditation to the West. Her works have been instrumental in making these practices accessible.

### Pema Chödrön

Pema Chödrön (1991) is an American Buddhist nun in the lineage of Chögyam Trungpa Rinpoche. She is known for her practical and accessible teachings on mindfulness and meditation. Her books, including *When Things Fall Apart* (1997) and *The Places That Scare You* (2001), have helped many Westerners understand and practice mindfulness.

*Tara Brach*

Tara Brach is a well-known meditation teacher, psychologist, and author who has contributed significantly to bringing mindfulness and compassion practices to the West. She founded the Insight Meditation Community of Washington, DC, and her books, such as *Radical Acceptance* (2003) and *Radical Compassion* (2019), have reached a wide audience.

*Jon Kabat-Zinn*

Jon Kabat-Zinn is perhaps the most prominent figure in the secularization and popularization of mindfulness in the West. A molecular biologist by training, Kabat-Zinn studied under Buddhist teachers and was inspired to integrate mindfulness into mainstream medicine. In 1979, he founded the Stress Reduction Clinic at the University of Massachusetts Medical School, where he developed the Mindfulness Based Stress Reduction (MBSR) program.

## Secularization of Mindfulness in the West

The MBSR program was designed to help patients cope with chronic pain, stress, and illness by teaching them mindfulness meditation techniques (Kabat-Zinn, 1990). Jon Kabat-Zinn (1982) carefully removing any religious and cultural connotations from the practice, presenting mindfulness in a way that was accessible and appealing to a secular audience. This approach allowed mindfulness to be widely accepted and integrated into various fields, including healthcare, education, and corporate settings.

### *The Impact of MBSR on the Field of Mental Health*

The success of MBSR marked a turning point in the acceptance and integration of mindfulness into Western psychology and medicine (Bishop, 2002; Buchholz, 2015; Grossman et al., 2004; Zheng, 2022). The program's emphasis on empirical research and clinical outcomes helped to establish the credibility and effectiveness of mindfulness practices.

Numerous studies have since demonstrated the benefits of MBSR and other mindfulness-based interventions, showing significant improvements in reducing stress, anxiety, and depression, and enhancing overall well-being (Choudhary, 2023; Khoury et al., 2015; Zhang et al., 2021).

### Further Expansion and Integration

Following the success of MBSR, other mindfulness-based interventions were developed to address specific psychological and medical conditions. Notable examples include the following.

### Mindfulness-Based Cognitive Therapy (MBCT)

Developed by Zindel Segal, Mark Williams, and John Teasdale (2002), MBCT combines mindfulness practices with cognitive therapy techniques to prevent relapse in individuals with recurrent depression.

### Acceptance and Commitment Therapy (ACT)

Developed by Steven C. Hayes et al. (2011), ACT incorporates mindfulness and acceptance strategies to help individuals develop psychological flexibility and commit to valued actions.

### Dialectical Behavior Therapy (DBT)

Developed by Marsha Linehan (1993), DBT integrates mindfulness practices to help individuals increase awareness of self and others, regulate their emotions, and develop effective interpersonal skills.

## Ongoing Research and Adaptation of Mindfulness for Health and Well-Being

The integration of mindfulness into Western contexts continues to evolve, with ongoing research exploring its applications in various fields (Creswell et al., 2017). Studies consistently support the efficacy of mindfulness practices in improving mental health and overall well-being (Enkema et al., 2020; Huong & Vu, 2023; Nagar & Ahmed, 2023). Additionally, adaptations of mindfulness practices for specific populations, such as children (Byrd et al., 2020; Duraccio & Jensen, 2020), veterans (Colgan et al., 2017; Schure et al., 2018), and individuals with chronic illnesses

(Ahola et al., 2017; Jefferson et al., 2020), have expanded the reach and impact of mindfulness.

By secularizing and popularizing mindfulness, the pioneers of mindfulness-based practice in the West have made it accessible to a broad audience, leading to widespread acceptance and integration into various domains of life (Shapiro & Weisbaum, 2020). The ongoing research and adaptation of mindfulness practices continue to demonstrate their profound impact on mental health and quality of life, ensuring that mindfulness remains a valuable tool for personal and professional growth (Shapiro & Carlson, 2017).

## Neuroimaging Research Supporting Positive Effects of Mindfulness

One notable area of research focuses on the physiological and psychological mechanisms underlying mindfulness. Neuroimaging studies have revealed that regular mindfulness practice can lead to shifts in the brain, specifically in the regions associated with attention, emotion regulation, and self-awareness (Tang et al., 2013; Weder, 2022; Wheeler et al., 2017). For instance, research has shown increased gray matter density in the prefrontal cortex and hippocampus, areas related to memory and learning, as well as decreased activity in the amygdala, which is involved in stress and anxiety responses (Hölzel et al., 2011; Tang et al., 2013). These findings suggest mindfulness may enhance cognitive flexibility, reduce stress reactivity, and promote emotional resilience (Dahl et al., 2020; Sünbül, 2020). Additionally, long-term mindfulness practitioners exhibit stronger connectivity between brain regions involved in self-regulation and introspection (Fox et al., 2014), further supporting the benefits of mindfulness on brain function and overall mental health.

## Mindfulness in the Digital Space

There has been a growing interest in the digital adaptation of mindfulness interventions in recent years (Ellis et al., 2022; Osborne et al., 2022; Wang et al., 2021). Mobile applications and online platforms offer accessible and scalable means to deliver mindfulness training to diverse populations

(Bégin et al, 2022; Mrazek et al., 2018). Preliminary evidence suggests that digital mindfulness interventions can effectively reduce stress and improve well-being (Cavanagh et al., 2018; Champion et al., 2018; Coelhoso et al., 2019; Gao et al., 2022). However, further research is needed to establish their long-term efficacy and optimal design features. Additionally, researchers are exploring the potential of integrating mindfulness with other therapeutic modalities, such as cognitive-behavioral therapy (CBT) and positive psychology, to create comprehensive and individualized treatment approaches.

## Mindfulness Research Continues

The ongoing research and adaptation of mindfulness for health and well-being highlight its versatile and dynamic nature. As the field continues to evolve, it is crucial to maintain rigorous scientific inquiry and innovative application to fully harness mindfulness' potential in promoting holistic health and enhancing the quality of life. This includes exploring new ways to integrate mindfulness into various therapeutic and educational settings, ensuring accessibility for diverse populations, and continuously refining techniques to maximize benefits. By staying committed to evidence-based practice, mindfulness can be a powerful tool for fostering mental, emotional, and physical well-being.

## Expansion into Education: Mindfulness in Schools

Building on the success of mindfulness programs in clinical settings, educators began to recognize the potential benefits of mindfulness for children and adolescents. The Mindfulness in Schools Project (MiSP) was developed to bring mindfulness practices into educational settings, helping students improve their focus, emotion regulation, and overall well-being. MiSP also sought to support the well-being of educators in the classroom (Weare, 2018). Programs like MiSP provide teachers with the training and resources needed to integrate mindfulness into the classroom, fostering a supportive and mindful learning environment (Roeser et al., 2022).

Research (McKeering & Hwang, 2019; Weare, 2023) has shown that mindfulness in schools can improve academic performance, reduce behavioral problems, and enhance social and emotional skills. By teaching mindfulness to children and adolescents, these programs aim to equip them with valuable tools for managing stress and promoting mental health throughout their lives (Chi et al., 2018; Dunning et al., 2019; Eklund et al., 2017).

### *Ongoing Impact and Research on Mindfulness in Schools*

Mindfulness is increasingly being integrated into social and emotional learning (SEL) curricula. In 2022, the Collaborative for Academic, Social, and Emotional Learning (CASEL) conducted a comprehensive review and reported that mindfulness practices are effective components of SEL programs, contributing to improved social skills, empathy, and emotional resilience in students.

Long-term studies are beginning to emerge, showing the sustained benefits of mindfulness education. Davidson and Lutz (2023) tracked students over five years and found that those who participated in mindfulness programs had better mental health outcomes and academic success compared to their peers who did not engage in such practices.

Recent reports also highlight the importance of making mindfulness programs accessible to all students, regardless of socioeconomic background. A 2023 policy brief by the National Education Association (NEA) emphasizes the need for equitable implementation of mindfulness programs to ensure that all students, especially those in under-resourced schools, can benefit from these practices. Innovative approaches to mindfulness in schools include the use of technology. Mitsea et al. (2023) discuss how digital mindfulness apps and virtual reality experiences are being used to engage students in mindfulness practices in more interactive and accessible ways.

## From Historical Origins to Contemporary Applications

From its ancient beginnings in the Buddhist practice of sati, mindfulness has evolved into a significant element in Western applications for mental and physical health with a substantial ongoing body of research. Initially emphasizing awareness and presence within spiritual traditions, mindfulness has been widely adopted in therapeutic contexts. Today, it is utilized in schools to enhance students' well-being and is accessible through various digital platforms. This broad and enduring presence highlights its versatility and profound impact on holistic health, affirming mindfulness as a vital practice for improving quality of life across diverse settings.

Mindfulness has demonstrated its adaptability and relevance through its integration into multiple facets of modern life. Its origins lie in the Buddhist practice of sati, which emphasizes the cultivation of awareness and attention to the present moment. This ancient practice has been meticulously studied and adapted in Western psychology, where it has shown significant benefits for mental and physical health. Research has revealed that mindfulness can reduce stress, anxiety, and depression, while also enhancing emotion regulation, cognitive function, and overall well-being.

The adoption of mindfulness in schools illustrates its potential to support young people in developing emotional intelligence, concentration, and resilience. Programs designed to teach mindfulness to students have been shown to improve behavior, academic performance, and emotional health. Beyond educational settings, the digital age has further expanded the reach of mindfulness, making guided practices and resources available through apps, online courses, and virtual communities. This digital dissemination ensures that mindfulness can be practiced by a wider audience, transcending geographical and cultural barriers.

## Conclusion

As mindfulness continues to be explored and integrated into various aspects of life, it remains crucial to maintain rigorous scientific inquiry and innovative application. This approach ensures that mindfulness can be tailored to meet the needs of diverse populations while preserving its core principles. The enduring presence and purpose of mindfulness in humanity underscore its importance as a practice that promotes holistic health, personal growth, and a deeper connection to the present moment. By embracing mindfulness, individuals can enhance their quality of life, cultivate inner peace, and navigate the complexities of modern living with greater ease and clarity. Now, let us consider the importance of therapists who are interested in MBPT developing their own mindfulness practice.

## References

Ahola Kohut, S., Stinson, J. N., Davies-Chalmers, C., Ruskin, D., & van Wyk, M. (2017). Mindfulness-based interventions in clinical samples of adolescents with chronic illness: A systematic review. *Journal of Alternative and Complementary Medicine*, *23*(8), 581–589. https://doi.org/10.1089/acm.2016.0316

Anālayo, B. (2021). Monitoring and acceptance: Key dimensions in establishing mindfulness. *Mindfulness, 13,* 1901–1906. https://doi.org/10.1007/s12671-021-01770-x

Bishop, S. R. (2002). What do we really know about mindfulness-based stress reduction? *Psychosomatic Medicine, 64,* 71–83. https://doi.org/10.1097/00006842-200201000-00010

Brazier, C. (2013). Roots of mindfulness. *European Journal of Psychotherapy & Counselling, 15,* 127–138. https://doi.org/10.1080/13642537.2013.795336

Buchholz, L. (2015). Exploring the promise of mindfulness as medicine. *JAMA, 314*(13), 1327–1329. https://doi.org/10.1001/jama.2015.7023

Byrd, R. J., Milner, R. J., & Luke, C. (2020). *Mindfulness techniques for working with children and adolescents* (1st ed.). Routledge. https://doi.org/10.4324/9781351133159-20

Cavanagh, K., Churchard, A., O'Hanlon, P., Mundy, T., Votolato, P., Jones, F., Gu, J., & Strauss, C. (2018). A randomized controlled trial of a brief online mindfulness-based intervention in a non-clinical population: Replication and extension. *Mindfulness, 9*(4), 1191–1205. https://doi.org/10.1007/s12671-017-0856-1

Champion, L., Economides, M., & Chandler, C. (2018). The efficacy of a brief app-based mindfulness intervention on psychosocial outcomes in healthy adults: A pilot randomized controlled trial. *PLoS ONE, 13*(12), e0209482. https://doi.org/10.1371/journal.pone.0209482

Chi, X., Bo, A., Liu, T., Zhang, P., & Chi, I. (2018). Effects of mindfulness-based stress reduction on depression in adolescents and young adults: A systematic review and meta-analysis. *Frontiers in Psychology, 9,* 1034. https://doi.org/10.3389/fpsyg.2018.01034

Chödrön, P. (1991). *The wisdom of no escape: And the path of loving-kindness.* Shambhala Publications.

Chödrön, P. (1997). *When things fall apart: Heart advice for difficult times.* Shambhala Publications.

Chödrön, P. (2001). *The places that scare you: A guide to fearlessness in difficult times.* Shambhala Publications.

Choudhary, M. (2023). Mindfulness and well-being: Mindfulness-based interventions for promoting well-being and its impact on cognitive, emotional, and physiological processes. *Lloyd Business Review, 2*(1), 1–18. https://doi.org/10.56595/lbr.v2i1.12

Christopher, J. C., & Maris, J. A. (2010). Integrating mindfulness as self-care into counseling and psychotherapy training. *Counselling and Psychotherapy Research, 10,* 114–125. https://doi.org/10.1080/14733141003750285

Cleary, T. (2000). *Taoist meditation: Methods for cultivating a healthy mind and body.* Shambhala Publications.

Coelhoso, C. C., Tobo, P. R., Lacerda, S. S., Lima, A. H., Barrichello, C. R. C., Amaro, E. Jr., & Kozasa, E. H. (2019). A new mental health mobile app for well-being and stress reduction in working women: Randomized controlled trial. *Journal of Medical Internet Research, 21*(11), e14269. https://doi.org/10.2196/14269

Colgan, D. D., Wahbeh, H., Pleet, M. M., Besler, K., & Christopher, M. (2017). A qualitative study of mindfulness among veterans with posttraumatic stress disorder: Practices differentially affect symptoms, aspects of well-being, and potential mechanisms of action. *Journal of Evidence-Based Complementary & Alternative Medicine, 22*(3), 482–493. https://doi.org/10.1177/2156587216684999

Creswell, J. D., Lindsay, E. K., Villalba, D. K., & Chin, B. (2019). Mindfulness training and physical health: Mechanisms and outcomes. *Psychosomatic Medicine, 81*(3), 224–232.

Dahl, C. J., Wilson-Mendenhall, C. D., & Davidson, R. J. (2020). The plasticity of well-being: A training-based framework for the cultivation of human flourishing. *Proceedings of the National Academy of Sciences, 117*(51), 32197–32206. https://doi.org/10.1073/pnas.2014859117

Davidson, R. J., & Lutz, A. (2023). Longitudinal impact of mindfulness training on mental health and academic performance in students. *Developmental Psychology*, *59*(2), 225–238. https://doi.org/10.1037/dev0001338

Dickinson, R., & Daly, E. (2021). Incorporating mindfulness in Adlerian play therapy. *The Journal of Individual Psychology*, 77, 446–460.

Ditrich, T. (2016a). Buddhism between Asia and Europe: The concept of mindfulness through a historical lens. *Asian Studies*, *4*(1), 197–213. https://doi.org/10.4312/as.2016.4.1.197-213

Ditrich, T. (2016b). Situating the concept of mindfulness in the Theravāda tradition. *Asian Studies*, *4*(2), 13–33. https://doi.org/10.4312/as.2016.4.2.13-33

Dunning, D. L., Griffiths, K., Kuyken, W., Crane, C., Foulkes, L., Parker, J., & Dalgleish, T. (2019). Research review: The effects of mindfulness-based interventions on cognition and mental health in children and adolescents – A meta-analysis of randomized controlled trials. *Journal of Child Psychology and Psychiatry*, *60*(3), 244–258. https://doi.org/10.1111/jcpp.12980

Duraccio, K. M., & Jensen, C. D. (2020). Mindfulness for pediatric health conditions. In P. R. Steffen (Ed.), *Mindfulness for everyday living: Mindfulness in behavioral health*. Springer. https://doi.org/10.1007/978-3-030-51618-5_4

Eklund, K., O'Malley, M., & Meyer, L. (2017). Gauging mindfulness in children and youth: School-based applications. *Psychology in the Schools*, *54*(1), 101–114. https://doi.org/10.1002/pits.21983

Ellis, D. M., Draheim, A. A., & Anderson, P. L. (2022). Culturally adapted digital mental health interventions for ethnic/racial minorities: A systematic review and meta-analysis. *Journal of Consulting and Clinical Psychology*. https://doi.org/10.1037/ccp0000759

Enkema, M. C., McClain, L. M., Bird, E., Halvorson, M. A., & Larimer, M. E. (2020). Associations between mindfulness and mental health outcomes: A systematic review of ecological momentary assessment research. *Mindfulness*, *11*, 2455–2469. https://doi.org/10.1007/s12671-020-01442-2

Fox, K. C., Nijeboer, S., Dixon, M. L., Floman, J. L., Ellamil, M., Rumak, S. P., Sedlmeier, P., & Christoff, K. (2014). Is meditation associated with altered brain structure? A systematic review and meta-analysis of morphometric neuroimaging in meditation practitioners. *Neuroscience and Biobehavioral Reviews*, *43*, 48–73. https://doi.org/10.1016/j.neubiorev.2014.03.016

Fuchs, C., Lee, J. K., Roemer, L., & Orsillo, S. M. (2013). Using mindfulness-and acceptance-based treatments with clients from nondominant cultural and/or marginalized backgrounds: Clinical considerations, meta-analysis findings, and introduction to the special series: Clinical considerations in using acceptance-and mindfulness-based treatments with diverse populations. *Cognitive and Behavioral Practice*, *20*(1), 1–12.

Gao, M., Roy, A., Deluty, A., Sharkey, K. M., Hoge, E. A., Liu, T., & Brewer, J. A. (2022). Targeting anxiety to improve sleep disturbance: A randomized clinical trial of app-based mindfulness training. *Psychosomatic Medicine*, *84*(5), 632–642. https://doi.org/10.1097/PSY.0000000000001083

Goldstein, J. (1976). *The experience of insight: A simple and direct guide to Buddhist meditation*. Shambhala Publications.

Grossman, P., Niemann, L., Schmidt, S., & Walach, H. (2004). Mindfulness-based stress reduction and health benefits: A meta-analysis. *Journal of Psychosomatic Research*, *57*(1), 35–43. https://doi.org/10.1111/j.2042-7166.2003.tb04008.x

Hanh, T. N. (2007). *Planting seeds: Practicing mindfulness with children*. Parallax press.

Hanh, T. N. (2009). *Happiness*. ReadHowYouWant. com.

Hayes, S. C., Strosahl, K. D., & Wilson, K. G. (2011). *Acceptance and commitment therapy: The process and practice of mindful change.* Guilford press.

Hofmann, S. G., Sawyer, A. T., Witt, A. A., & Oh, D. (2010). The effect of mindfulness-based therapy on anxiety and depression: A meta-analytic review. *Journal of Consulting and Clinical Psychology, 78*(2), 169. https://doi.org/10.1037/a0018555

Hölzel, B. K., Carmody, J., Vangel, M., Congleton, C., Yerramsetti, S. M., Gard, T., & Lazar, S. W. (2011). Mindfulness practice leads to increases in regional brain gray matter density. *Psychiatry Research, 191*(1), 36–43. https://doi.org/10.1016/j.pscychresns.2010.08.006

Huong, H., & Vu, X. (2023). Examining the scientific foundation of mindfulness and alternative approaches for improving mental health well-being. *The American Journal of Social Science and Education Innovations.* https://doi.org/10.37547/tajssei/volume05issue11-06

Jefferson, F. A., Shires, A., & McAloon, J. (2020). Parenting self-compassion: A systematic review and meta-analysis. *Mindfulness, 11*(9), 2067–2088.

Jennings, L., & Apsche, J. (2014). The evolution of a fundamentally mindfulness-based treatment methodology: From DBT and ACT to MDT and beyond. *International Journal of Behavioral Consultation and Therapy, 9*(2), 22–28. https://doi.org/10.1037/h0100986

Jha, A. P., Krompinger, J., & Baime, M. J. (2007). Mindfulness training modifies subsystems of attention. *Cognitive, Affective, & Behavioral Neuroscience, 7*(2), 109–119. https://doi.org/10.3758/CABN.7.2.109

Kabat-Zinn, J. (1982). An outpatient program in behavioral medicine for chronic pain patients based on the practice of mindfulness meditation: Theoretical considerations and preliminary results. *General Hospital Psychiatry, 4*(1), 33–47. https://doi.org/10.1016/0163-8343(82)90026-3

Kabat-Zinn, J. (1990). *Full catastrophe living: Using the wisdom of your body and mind to face stress, pain, and illness.* Delta.

Kabat-Zinn, J. (2015). Mindfulness. *Mindfulness, 6*(6), 1481–1483.

Kabat-Zinn, J., Lipworth, L., & Burney, R. (1985). The clinical use of mindfulness meditation for the self-regulation of chronic pain. *Journal of Behavioral Medicine, 8,* 163–190.

Khemraj, S., Pettongma, P. W. C., Thepa, P. C. A., Patnaik, S., Wu, W. Y., & Chi, H. (2023). Implementing mindfulness in the workplace: A new strategy for enhancing both individual and organizational effectiveness. *Journal for ReAttach Therapy and Developmental Diversities, 6*(2s), 408–416.

Khoury, B., Sharma, M. K., Rush, S. E., & Fournier, C. (2015). Mindfulness-based stress reduction for healthy individuals: A meta-analysis. *Journal of Psychosomatic Research, 78*(6), 519–528. https://doi.org/10.1016/j.jpsychores.2015.03.009

Kornfield, J. (1993). *A path with heart: A guide through the perils and promises of spiritual life.* Bantam Books.

Laurie, J., & Blandford, A. (2016). Making time for mindfulness. *International Journal of Medical Informatics, 96,* 38–50.

Linehan, M. M. (1993). *Cognitive-behavioral treatment of borderline personality disorder.* Guilford Press.

Mantzios, M., & Giannou, K. (2019). A real-world application of short mindfulness-based practices: A review and reflection of the literature and a practical proposition for an effortless mindful lifestyle. *American Journal of Lifestyle Medicine, 13*(6), 520–525.

McCollum, E. E., & Gehart, D. R. (2010). Using mindfulness meditation to teach beginning therapists therapeutic presence: A qualitative study. *Journal of Marital and Family Therapy*, *36*(3), 347–360. https://doi.org/10.1111/j.1752-0606. 2010.00214.x

McKeering, P., & Hwang, Y. (2019). A systematic review of mindfulness intervention for individuals with developmental disabilities: Long-term effects and areas for future research. *Journal of Autism and Developmental Disorders*, *49*, 479–496. https://doi. org/10.1007/s10803-018-3752-1

Meany-Walen, K. K. (2018). Exploring mindfulness in play therapy: A qualitative study. *International Journal of Play Therapy*, *27*(1), 21–33. https://doi.org/10.1037/ pla0000056

Mitsea, E., Drigas, A., & Skianis, C. (2023). Digitally assisted mindfulness in training self-regulation skills for sustainable mental health: a systematic review. *Behavioral Sciences*, *13*(12), 1008.

Morris, S. G. (2023). *The scientific history of mindfulness: 1938 to 2020* (Doctoral dissertation), University of Kent.

Mrazek, M. D., Franklin, M. S., Phillips, D. T., Baird, B., & Schooler, J. W. (2018). Mindfulness training improves working memory capacity and GRE performance while reducing mind wandering. *Psychological Science*, *24*(5), 776–781. https://doi. org/10.1177/0956797612459659

Murphy, A. (2016). Mindfulness-based therapy in modern psychology: Convergence and divergence from early Buddhist thought. *Contemporary Buddhism*, *17*(2), 275–325.

Nagar, R., & Ahmed, M. (2023). Examining the intersection of mindfulness, social justice, and community psychology. *Journal of Community Psychology*, *51*(5), 902–918. https://doi.org/10.1002/jcop.22914

Neves-Pereira, M., Mullin, A. P., Elliott, M., & Burkhardt, M. (2018). Mindfulness-based cognitive therapy for treating mood disorders in clinical practice: Evidence from clinical and biological studies. *Biological Psychiatry*, *85*(9), 1051–1061. https://doi. org/10.1016/j.biopsych.2017.08.014

Osborne, D., Jennings, S., & Krieger, D. (2022). The impact of mindfulness-based stress reduction (MBSR) on occupational stress in healthcare professionals: A randomized controlled trial. *Health Psychology*, *41*(7), 515–525. https://doi.org/10.1037/ hea0001062

Porges, S. W. (2011). *The polyvagal theory: Neurophysiological foundations of emotions, attachment, communication, and self-regulation*. Norton.

Posluns, K., & Gall, T. L. (2020). Dear mental health practitioners, take care of yourselves: A literature review on self-care for mental health practitioners. *Professional Psychology: Research and Practice*, *51*(3), 222–230. https://doi.org/10.1037/pro0000306

Proulx, J., Croff, R., Oken, B., Aldwin, C. M., Fleming, C., Bergen-Cico, D., ... Noorani, M. (2018). Considerations for research and development of culturally relevant mindfulness interventions in American minority communities. *Mindfulness*, *9*, 361–370.

Purser, R. E. (2021). McMindfulness: How mindfulness became the new capitalist spirituality. *Journal of Global Buddhism*, *22*(1), 251–258.

Rechtschaffen, D. (2014). *The way of mindful education: Cultivating well-being in teachers and students*. WW Norton & Company.

Roeser, R. W., Schonert-Reichl, K. A., Jha, A. P., Cullen, M., Wallace, L., Wilensky, R., Oberle, E., Thomson, K., Taylor, C., & Harrison, J. (2022). Mindfulness training and reductions in teacher stress and burnout: Results from two randomized, waitlist-control field trials. *Journal of Educational Psychology*, *114*(1), 92–111. https://doi. org/10.1037/edu0000678

Salzberg, S. (1995). *Loving-kindness: The revolutionary art of happiness*. Shambhala Publications.

Schore, A. N. (2001). Effects of a secure attachment relationship on right brain development, affect regulation, and infant mental health. *Infant Mental Health Journal: Official Publication of the World Association for Infant Mental Health*, 22(1–2), 7–66.

Schure, M. B., Christopher, J., & Christopher, S. (2008). Mind–body medicine and the art of self-care: Teaching mindfulness to counseling students through yoga, meditation, and qigong. *Journal of Counseling & Development*, 86(1), 47–56.

Segal, Z. V., Williams, J. M. G., & Teasdale, J. D. (2002). *Mindfulness-based cognitive therapy for depression: A new approach to preventing relapse*. Guilford Press.

Shapiro, S. L., & Carlson, L. E. (2017). *The art and science of mindfulness: Integrating mindfulness into psychology and the helping professions* (2nd ed.). American Psychological Association.

Shapiro, S. L., & Weisbaum, E. (2020). Mindful discipline: A loving approach to setting limits and raising emotionally intelligent children. *Journal of Child Psychology and Psychiatry*, 61(6), 623–631. https://doi.org/10.1111/jcpp.13244

Sharma, P., & Singh, P. (2024). Translating theoretical insights into an emotion regulation flexibility intervention: assessing effectiveness. *Cognition and Emotion*, 1–22. https://doi.org/10.1080/02699931.2024.2413366

Siegel, D. J. (2012). *The mindful brain: Reflection and attunement in the cultivation of well-being*. Norton.

Singha, R., & Singha, S. (2024). Understanding neurodiversity and mindfulness: A holistic approach to addiction in professional preparation programs. In *AIn Autism, Neurodiversity, and Equity in Professional Preparation Programs* (pp. 255–275). IGI Global.

Singla, R. (2011). Mindfulness-based interventions for depression: A systematic review of meta-analyses. *Clinical Psychology Review*, 30(2), 125–134. https://doi.org/10.1016/j.cpr.2009.10.003

Sipe, W. (2021). *Bringing willingness and values to challenging times*. YouTube. https://www.youtube.com/watch?v=RIvuVF3xjmY&t=0s

Sünbül, S. (2020). Understanding the mechanisms of mindfulness: A neurobiological perspective. *Current Opinion in Psychology*, 28, 292–297. https://doi.org/10.1016/j.copsyc.2020.06.007

Tan, C., & Tan, C. (2021). Introduction to mindfulness. *Mindful Education: Insights from Confucian and Christian Traditions*, 51–67. https://link.springer.com/book/10.1007/978-981-16-1405-7

Tang, Y. Y., Hölzel, B. K., & Posner, M. I. (2015). The neuroscience of mindfulness meditation. *Nature Reviews Neuroscience*, 16(4), 213–225. https://doi.org/10.1038/nrn3916

Tang, Y. Y., Tang, R., & Posner, M. I. (2013). Brief meditation training induces smoking reduction. *Proceedings of the National Academy of Sciences*, 110(34), 13971–13975.

Van Dam, N. T., van Vugt, M. K., Vago, D. R., Schmalzl, L., Saron, C. D., Olendzki, A., Meissner, T., Lazar, S. W., Kerr, C. E., Gorchov, J., Fox, K. C. R., Field, B. A., Britton, W. B., Brefczynski-Lewis, J. A., & Meyer, D. E. (2018, Jan). Mind the hype: A critical evaluation and prescriptive agenda for research on mindfulness and meditation. *Perspectives on Psychological Science*, 13(1), 36–61. https://doi.org/10.1177/1745691617709589. Epub 2017 Oct 10. Erratum in: Perspect Psychol Sci. 2020 Sep;15(5):1289–1290. https://doi.org/10.1177/1745691620924057. PMID: 29016274; PMCID: PMC5758421.

Vörös, S. (2016). Buddhism and Cognitive (Neuro) science: An Uneasy Liaison?. Asian Studies, 4(1), 61–80. https://doi.org/10.4312/as.2016.4.1.61-80

Wang, X., Zhao, Z., & Han, S. (2021). The impact of mindfulness-based stress reduction on mental health and well-being: A meta-analysis. *Mindfulness*, 12(7), 1429–1442. https://doi.org/10.1007/s12671-021-01614-8

Weare, K. (2023). Where have we been and where are we going with mindfulness in schools? *Mindfulness*, *14*(2), 293–299. https://doi.org/10.1007/s12671-023-02086-8

Weder, M. (2022). Mindfulness and mental health: An overview. *Journal of Psychiatric Research, 144*, 343–354. https://doi.org/10.1016/j.jpsychires.2022.08.023

Wilson, T. D. (2016). Mindfulness for social change: A new paradigm for engagement. *Social Science and Medicine*, *165*, 157–166. https://doi.org/10.1016/j.socscimed.2016.07.030

Zeidan, F., Johnson, S. K., Diamond, B. J., David, Z., & Goolkasian, P. (2010). Mindfulness meditation improves cognition: Evidence of brief mental training. *Consciousness and Cognition*, *19*(2), 597–605. https://doi.org/10.1016/j.concog.2010.03.014

Zheng, M., Xu, Z., & Qu, Y. (2022, Sep 27). The effect of mindful leadership on employee innovative behavior: Evidence from the healthcare sectors in China. *International Journal of Environmental Research and Public Health*, *19*(19), 12263. https://doi.org/10.3390/ijerph191912263. PMID: 36231559; PMCID: PMC9566192.

# 2

## MINDFULNESS FOR THERAPISTS

### ENHANCING THERAPIST WELL-BEING AND THERAPEUTIC EFFECTIVENESS THROUGH PERSONAL PRACTICE

### Introduction

Mindfulness is more than a therapeutic tool. It is a vital form of ongoing, daily self-care. For psychotherapists, particularly those working with children and families, maintaining personal well-being is crucial (American Psychological Association, 2021). The nature of therapeutic work, especially play therapy, involves navigating often complex family dynamics and addressing the varying developmental needs and vulnerabilities of children and their families (Crenshaw & Stewart, 2014; Wonders & Affee, 2024). This multifaceted role requires therapists to be consistently attuned, present, and emotionally resilient.

Over the years I have noticed that many therapists want to learn and utilize mindfulness-based interventions in the scope of play therapy services without first having a foundation of having personally practiced mindfulness. I have found that when therapists are able to come to the therapy room with their own personal and authentic experience with mindfulness, the implementation of mindfulness-based interventions is far more effective. There are numerous reasons therapists will find Mindfulness-based Play Therapy® to be more effective when they embrace mindfulness as a practice outside of therapy with clients. Self-care for the therapist is ethically essential so that therapists have the capacity to be fully present for clients, and the practice of mindfulness contributes to self-care.

## Mindfulness Fosters Emotional Resilience for the Therapist

The therapeutic work with children and families in providing play therapy services can be taxing due to often complicated family dynamics (Wonders, 2021). When serving the needs of minor children who are embedded in the systems of family, community, school, social relationships, and culture, self-care through mindfulness practices supports therapists in being able to manage the emotional and mental demands of their professional work. The level of emotional engagement required in play therapy can be stressful, and without adequate self-care, therapists may find themselves experiencing compassion fatigue or burnout. By engaging in regular mindfulness exercises, therapists can cultivate emotional balance, reduce stress, and prevent burnout (Dye et al., 2020). Mindfulness-based practices, such as meditation, breathing exercises, and mindful movement, provide therapists with tools to center themselves, process their emotions, and return to a place of regulation and clarity.

Mindfulness practices help therapists to develop a balanced emotional state by increasing awareness of their own emotions and reactions while regulating their nervous systems (Guendelman  et al., 2017; Mohammed et al., 2018; Teper et al., 2017; Wheeler et al., 2017). Through regular mindfulness exercises, therapists learn to observe their thoughts and feelings without immediate judgment or reaction. This non-judgmental awareness allows them to better understand their emotional responses and manage them effectively, preventing the buildup of stress and emotional overload.

## Mindfulness Supports Stress Management

The layered work of play therapy, while most often joyful and fulfilling, can also result in high levels of stress for therapists. Providing play therapy services carries the risk of vicarious trauma and compassion fatigue when working with children who have suffered trauma or are straddled with anxiety, depression, and very difficult life circumstances. Some therapeutic work environments can be more stress-inducing than others for therapists. The nature of challenging cases, differing family dynamics, personalities, and emotionally charged situations can create tension and emotional drain for therapists. Mindfulness practices such as focused breathing, grounding, and different kinds of meditation can activate the body's relaxation response, reducing the production of stress hormones, and promote a regulated state (Bostock et al., 2019; Gamaiunova et al., 2022; Gardi et al., 2022). These practices can be easily integrated into daily routines, providing therapists with effective tools to manage stress.

## Mindfulness Helps Prevent Burnout

Burnout is a common issue among therapists who serve and support children and families due to the emotionally demanding nature of the work. Mindfulness practices help prevent burnout by fostering self-compassion and resilience (Burton et al., 2017; Davis & Hayes, 2011; Grensman et al., 2021; Rudaz et al., 2017; Zuo et al., 2022). By regularly engaging in mindfulness, therapists can recharge their emotional batteries, ensuring they remain effective and empathetic in their work. Movement practices, such as yoga or tai chi, combine physical activity with mindfulness, offering a holistic approach to maintaining physical and mental health. Incorporating mindfulness techniques into daily routines and therapeutic practice not only benefits the therapist's well-being but also significantly enhances their ability to connect with and support their clients.

## Mindfulness Enhances Therapeutic Outcomes

When therapists are attuned and present, they can more accurately assess the needs of the child and respond appropriately. This attunement leads to more tailored and effective therapeutic interventions, as therapists can adjust their techniques based on the real-time feedback they observe in the child's play (Kestly, 2016; Ryan et al., 2012). Furthermore, the trust and safety fostered through mindful presence encourage children to explore deeper issues and emotions, facilitating more profound healing. This mindful approach fosters effective and compassionate therapeutic relationships, ultimately leading to better outcomes for the children and families being served.

Research has shown that mindfulness practices can enhance the therapeutic alliance, a crucial component of successful therapy. When therapists engage in mindfulness, they are better able to remain non-reactive and empathetic, which helps in creating a safe and trusting environment for the child. This environment allows children to express themselves more freely and authentically, which is essential for addressing underlying issues and promoting healing (Hughes & Golding, 2012; Perry, 2013; Siegel, 2010; Siegel & Hartzell, 2013). Mindfulness also enables therapists to manage their own stress and emotional responses, ensuring they remain fully present and focused during sessions (Grepmair et al., 2007).

The integration of mindfulness in therapy has been linked to improved emotional regulation and self-awareness in both therapists and clients. These skills are particularly beneficial in play therapy, where children often communicate complex emotions and experiences through their play. Mindful therapists can observe these expressions with greater clarity and insight, leading to more effective interventions that resonate with the child's needs and experiences (Saunders & Kober, 2020; Semple, 2010; Siegel, 2010).

The benefits of mindfulness in therapeutic settings extend beyond individual sessions. Mindful practices can be incorporated into the daily routines of children and their families, promoting a holistic approach to mental health and well-being. This ongoing practice helps reinforce the therapeutic work in sessions and supports long-term positive outcomes (Kabat-Zinn, 2003).

## Supporting Reflective Practice

Reflective practice in psychotherapy is a continuous process where therapists critically examine their own experiences, thoughts, and actions to enhance their professional effectiveness (Schön, 1983). It involves self-awareness, critical analysis, and reflective thinking to understand how personal experiences and interactions with clients impact therapeutic relationships and outcomes. This practice allows therapists to adapt and improve their techniques, ensuring they provide the most effective care (Mansfield, 2010).

Reflective practice is a cornerstone of effective therapy, enabling therapists to continually evaluate and improve their therapeutic interventions (Fook & Gardner, 2007). Mindfulness significantly enhances a therapist's capacity for reflection by fostering a non-judgmental awareness of their thoughts, feelings, and reactions. This enhanced self-awareness is crucial for identifying countertransference and other unconscious processes that may arise during therapy (Germer et al., 2016). Reflective practice helps in identifying biases, enhancing empathy, and fostering a deeper connection with clients (Finlay, 2008). It encourages ongoing professional development and learning, ensuring that therapists remain responsive to the evolving needs of their clients.

### *Enhancing Self-Awareness and Emotional Regulation for the Therapist*

Mindfulness practice involves paying attention to the present moment with curiosity and openness, which helps therapists become more attuned to their internal states (Germer et al., 2016; Kabat-Zinn, 2003; Kabat-Zinn, 2024). By cultivating a mindful stance, therapists can observe their emotional responses and thoughts without immediately reacting to them. This non-reactive awareness allows therapists to recognize when they are experiencing countertransference – when their own emotional responses to a client are influenced by the therapist's personal history rather than the client's issues (Zuo et al., 2022). Such recognition is essential for maintaining professional boundaries and providing unbiased support to clients.

### *Identifying and Understanding Unconscious Processes for the Therapist*

Unconscious processes, including countertransference, biases, and assumptions, can significantly impact the therapeutic relationship, interventions, and outcomes (Grady, 2015; Lomas et al., 2017; Maharaj et al., 2021; Redlinger-Gross, 2020). Mindfulness practices enhance therapists' ability to bring these unconscious processes into conscious awareness. Techniques such as mindfulness meditation and mindful journaling allow therapists to explore their internal landscapes, uncovering hidden thoughts and feelings that may impact their work (Fabbro et al., 2017; Guendelman et al., 2017). By acknowledging and examining these processes, therapists can prevent them from interfering with the therapeutic alliance and the effectiveness of their interventions (Shapiro & Carlson, 2017). This ongoing reflective practice helps therapists to continually adjust their approaches and maintain a client-centered focus. Countertransference, the therapist's emotional response to the client, is a common phenomenon in therapy. It can provide valuable information about the client-therapist relationship but can also hinder therapeutic progress if left unaddressed (Hayes et al., 2011; Hayes, Gelso et al., 2018). Mindfulness helps therapists recognize and understand their counter-transference reactions by fostering a heightened awareness of their own emotions and bodily sensations (Johnson & Walsh, 2021; Price & Weng, 2021). This awareness enables therapists to differentiate between their own issues and the client's, ensuring that their responses are guided by the client's needs rather than their own unresolved conflicts (Hayes, Hofmann et al., 2018b).

### Developing Empathy and Compassion for Clients

Mindfulness also enhances a therapist's capacity for empathy and compassion (Martin-Allan et al., 2021; Nagaoka et al., 2021). Through mindfulness, therapists learn to be more present and attentive, which can deepen their understanding of clients' experiences. This empathetic attunement fosters a stronger therapeutic alliance and enhances the therapist's ability to respond to clients with genuine compassion. Studies have shown that therapists who practice mindfulness report higher levels of empathy and are better able to manage the emotional demands of their work (Germer et al., 2016).

### Promoting Professional Growth for Therapists

Engaging in reflective practice supported by mindfulness not only benefits the therapeutic process but also promotes professional growth. Therapists who regularly reflect on their practice are more likely to engage in continuous learning and development. Mindfulness encourages a growth mindset, where therapists view challenges as opportunities for learning rather than threats. This mindset supports resilience and adaptability in complex clinical situations (Davis & Hayes, 2011).

### Promoting Non-Judgmental Awareness in the Therapeutic Process

Mindfulness encourages therapists to observe their internal experiences without immediate judgment or reaction. This non-judgmental stance is essential for reflective practice, as it allows therapists to explore their thoughts and emotions with curiosity and openness rather than criticism or avoidance. By acknowledging and accepting their internal experiences, therapists can gain deeper insights into their own motivations, biases, and emotional responses, which is critical for effective self-reflection (Germer et al., 2016).

### Enhancing Sensitivity and Insight

Mindfulness not only increases self-awareness but also enhances a therapist's sensitivity and insight (Baker, 2016). By regularly engaging in mindfulness, therapists can develop a deeper understanding of their own inner workings, which in turn enables them to respond to their clients with greater empathy and attunement. This enhanced sensitivity allows therapists to pick up on subtle cues and dynamics within the therapy session, facilitating more nuanced and effective interventions.

### Developing Effective Interventions

The reflective capacity supported by mindfulness is crucial for developing and implementing effective therapeutic interventions. When therapists have a clear understanding of their own reactions and the dynamics at play in the therapy session, they are better equipped to design interventions that are tailored to the client's needs. This reflective practice ensures that therapeutic techniques are not applied in a one-size-fits-all manner but are thoughtfully adapted to fit the unique context of each client (Mansfield, 2010; Schön, 1983).

Mindfulness fosters a therapist's ability to remain present and attentive, allowing for real-time adjustments based on the client's verbal and non-verbal cues. This adaptability is essential in creating a therapeutic environment where the client feels understood and supported, which can significantly enhance the therapeutic alliance (Siegel, 2010). Furthermore, reflective practice through mindfulness helps therapists identify and mitigate their biases, leading to more culturally sensitive and individualized care (Germer et al., 2016).

Reflective practice also encourages therapists to continually evaluate the effectiveness of their interventions, promoting a cycle of ongoing improvement and professional development. This iterative process is key to maintaining high standards of care and ensuring that therapeutic approaches evolve in response to new insights and client feedback (Fook & Gardner, 2007).

*Maintaining a Positive Outlook*

Therapeutic work, particularly with children and families, can sometimes be challenging and emotionally demanding. With a reflective
practice, mindfulness helps therapists avoid labeling behavior and situations negatively, which is essential for sustaining motivation and passion for their work (Germer et al., 2016). By encouraging an attitude
of gratitude and acceptance, mindfulness practices help therapists focus
on the present moment and appreciate small, positive aspects of their
day-to-day experiences. This can cultivate a more optimistic perspective
(Kabat-Zinn, 2003).

Practices such as keeping a gratitude journal, where therapists write
down things they are thankful for each day, can significantly enhance
their overall sense of well-being (Emmons & McCullough, 2003). This
shift toward gratitude and acceptance helps therapists to view challenges
as opportunities for growth rather than as insurmountable obstacles.
Additionally, mindfulness-based stress reduction (MBSR) programs
have been shown to reduce burnout and improve emotional resilience
among therapists, further contributing to a positive outlook (Shapiro
et al., 2007).

Mindfulness also enables therapists to maintain a balanced perspective,
which is crucial when working with complex and emotionally charged
situations. By practicing mindfulness, therapists can develop a more compassionate and patient approach, which not only benefits their clients but
also enhances their own professional satisfaction and longevity in the
field (Siegel, 2010).

*Enhancing Fulfillment in Reflective Psychotherapy*

Mindfulness helps therapists find greater fulfillment in their professional lives by encouraging them to be fully present and engaged in their
reflective practice. When therapists are mindful, they can connect more
deeply with their clients, experiencing the rewarding moments of breakthroughs and progress more vividly. This presence and engagement can
lead to a greater sense of accomplishment and satisfaction (Siegel, 2010).
Additionally, mindfulness practices such as loving-kindness meditation,
which involves sending positive intentions to oneself and others, can

enhance feelings of compassion and joy, further contributing to professional fulfillment (Germer et al., 2016).

Reflective mindfulness practice allows therapists to continually assess and refine their therapeutic approaches, making the work more dynamic and responsive to client needs. This ongoing self-examination and adaptation not only improve therapeutic outcomes but also keep the practice of therapy intellectually stimulating and personally rewarding (Schön, 1983). By integrating mindfulness into reflective practice, therapists can maintain a balanced perspective, mitigate burnout, and sustain a passion for their work (Shapiro et al., 2007).

## The Ripple Effect on the Therapeutic Environment

The reflective practice cultivated through mindfulness extends beyond the therapist to influence the therapeutic environment. When therapists maintain a centered and resilient attitude, it sets a tone of hope and possibility within the therapy sessions. Clients, especially children and families, often mirror the emotions and attitudes of their therapists. A therapist who exudes hope, delight, positivity, centeredness, and groundedness can help clients feel more secure and motivated to engage in the therapeutic process. This atmosphere enhances the overall experience for clients, making therapy a more effective and enjoyable journey.

This ripple effect begins with the therapist's own practice of mindfulness, which fosters a non-judgmental awareness of their own thoughts and emotions (Germer et al., 2016). By engaging in reflective practice, therapists can continually refine their approaches and maintain a balanced perspective, even when faced with challenging situations (Mansfield, 2010; Schön, 1983). This reflective capacity allows for the development of tailored interventions that address the unique needs of each client, thereby increasing the effectiveness of therapy (Fook & Gardner, 2007).

The integration of mindfulness into reflective practice helps therapists maintain a sense of fulfillment and professional satisfaction. Practices like loving-kindness meditation enhance feelings of compassion and joy, contributing to a positive therapeutic presence (Siegel, 2010). This presence is crucial for building a strong therapeutic alliance, which is foundational for successful therapy (Shapiro et al., 2007).

By promoting an environment of acceptance, gratitude, and resilience, therapists create a therapeutic space where clients feel valued and understood. This environment encourages clients to open and engage deeply in the therapeutic process, leading to more meaningful and lasting outcomes. The cumulative effect of these practices not only benefits individual therapy sessions but also contributes to a more compassionate and effective therapeutic community.

## Practical Ways for Therapists to Incorporate Mindfulness into Daily Life

Practicing mindfulness need not be an overwhelming set of tasks. It can easily be practiced in daily life in the most practical and simple ways.

### Starting the Day with Mindful Quiet Time

Beginning the day with a few moments of quiet sets a positive tone for the rest of the day. This practice can be as short as five to ten minutes and involves sitting quietly, focusing on the breath, and bringing attention to the present moment. This helps you center yourself, ground your presence in the day, and prepare emotionally and mentally for the day ahead. Starting the day with mindfulness can increase focus, reduce stress, and enhance overall well-being.

### Mindful Breathing Exercises between Therapy Sessions

Setting aside a few minutes between therapy sessions for conscious breathing exercises can be highly beneficial for therapists. Conscious breathing activates the parasympathetic nervous system, which promotes relaxation and reduces stress. The 4–7–8 breathing technique, popularized by Dr. Andrew Weil (2011), is a simple yet powerful method for promoting relaxation and reducing stress. This technique involves inhaling for 4 seconds, holding the breath for 7 seconds, and exhaling for 8 seconds. It has roots in ancient yogic practices and has been adapted for modern use to help manage anxiety, improve sleep, and lower blood pressure by calming the mind and body (Cleveland Clinic, 2024; Weil, 2011).

Practicing the 4–7–8 breath regularly can enhance the body's stress response, making it easier to handle upsetting situations or internal tension. It is recommended to perform this technique twice a day for the best results. Although some people might experience lightheadedness when first starting, this usually diminishes with practice as the body adjusts to the slower breathing pace (Cleveland Clinic, 2024). This technique has been found to reduce anxiety and improve sleep, contributing to overall mental health (Tsai et al., 2015).

Deep breathing exercises have been shown to reduce stress and anxiety by stimulating the parasympathetic nervous system, which counteracts the body's stress response. The physiological benefits of deep breathing include a reduction in heart rate and blood pressure, and an increase in feelings of calm and well-being (Jerath et al., 2006). Diaphragmatic breathing, specifically, involves breathing deeply into the diaphragm rather than shallowly into the chest, which enhances oxygen exchange and further promotes relaxation (Ma et al., 2017).

### Mindful Eating

Mindful eating during meals and snacks involves paying full attention to the experience of eating and drinking, both inside and outside the body. This practice encourages savoring each bite, noticing flavors, textures, and smells, and being aware of the body's hunger and fullness cues, leading to a healthier relationship with food and better digestion (Kristeller & Wolever, 2010). For therapists, incorporating mindful eating into both personal life and professional practice can offer significant benefits. Personally, therapists can set aside time for meals without distractions, engage all senses in the eating process, listen to their body's signals, and reflect on food choices. This not only promotes better physical health but also serves as a grounding exercise to reduce stress. By integrating mindful eating into their routine, therapists can enhance their well-being and effectiveness, promoting a holistic approach to health (Kristeller & Wolever, 2011).

### Mindful Walking

Mindful walking means being fully present with the experience of walking, rather than just walking to get from one place to another.

This practice involves paying attention to the sensation of your feet touching the ground, the rhythm of your steps, the movement of your body, and noticing the sights, sounds, and smells around you (Hanh, 2015). For therapists, incorporating mindful walking into both personal life and professional practice can be highly beneficial. Personally, therapists can use mindful walking as a form of meditation to reduce stress and enhance their sense of presence. This can involve setting aside time for short walks during the day, focusing on the physical sensations and surroundings, and using these moments to clear the mind and rejuvenate. Integrating mindful walking into daily routines can enhance the well-being of therapists and their clients, promoting a more mindful and balanced approach to life (Davis et al., 2022; Hanh, 2015; Hanson & Jones, 2015).

### Mindful Listening

Mindful listening, an essential aspect of effective communication, involves fully focusing on the speaker without planning your response. By paying close attention to the words, tone, inflections of voice, and body language, you can enhance your ability to connect with others and improve your communication skills (Weger et al., 2014). This practice fosters deeper understanding and empathy, enabling more meaningful interactions. Research supports the benefits of mindful listening in therapeutic settings, indicating that it can strengthen the therapeutic alliance and improve client outcomes (Watson et al., 2022). Additionally, studies have shown that mindful listening can reduce communication anxiety and increase conversational satisfaction (Jones et al., 2019). For therapists, practicing mindful listening can lead to better client rapport and more effective interventions, as it allows for a deeper comprehension of the client's issues and concerns. Overall, integrating mindful listening into both personal and professional interactions can significantly enhance relational dynamics and contribute to more effective and empathetic communication (Jones et al., 2019; Watson et al., 2022; Weger et al., 2014).

### Mindful Cleaning

Transform routine chores into mindfulness practices by paying full attention to the task at hand. Whether you are washing dishes, sweeping the floor, or folding laundry, focus on the sensory experience – the feel of the water, the sound of the broom, the texture of the fabric. This can make mundane tasks more enjoyable and meditative (Hanh, 2011). For therapists, incorporating mindful cleaning into both personal life and professional practice can offer significant benefits.

Therapists can use mindful cleaning as a way to reduce stress and promote a sense of calm and presence. By engaging fully in the task, they can transform a routine chore into a meditative exercise that enhances their overall well-being. Research supports the benefits of mindful cleaning, indicating that it can reduce stress and improve mental well-being (Irving et al., 2009). Engaging in mindful cleaning can also foster a sense of gratitude and appreciation for one's surroundings, further enhancing emotional and mental health (Grider et al., 2021, 2023). Overall, incorporating mindful cleaning into daily routines can provide a simple yet powerful way to enhance mindfulness and improve quality of life (Champagne Clean, 2023).

### Mindful Technology Use

Mindful technology use involves setting specific times for checking emails, social media, or browsing the internet, and being fully present during these activities. For therapists, practicing mindful technology use can significantly enhance their professional and personal well-being. By avoiding multitasking and noticing their feelings and reactions to what they see and read, therapists can develop a healthier relationship with technology and reduce stress associated with constant connectivity (Duke & Montag, 2017).

Therapists can start by scheduling dedicated times for digital activities, ensuring that these periods do not overlap with therapy sessions or personal relaxation time. This approach helps in maintaining boundaries and prevents the digital overload that can lead to burnout. During these scheduled times, therapists should engage with their devices mindfully, paying attention to their posture, the content they are consuming, and their emotional responses. This practice can enhance their awareness of how technology affects their mood and productivity, allowing them to make more intentional choices about their digital consumption (Duke & Montag, 2017).

Therapists can use digital tools to support their mindfulness practice, such as apps designed for meditation and relaxation. These tools can provide structured guidance for mindfulness exercises, helping therapists to incorporate regular mindfulness practices into their daily routines. By leveraging technology in a mindful way, therapists can enhance their self-care practices and ensure they are mentally and emotionally prepared to support their clients (Goyal et al., 2014).

### Mindful Driving

Mindful driving involves paying close attention to the various sensations and experiences associated with driving, such as the feel of the steering wheel, the sound of the engine, and the scenery passing by. This practice encourages drivers to avoid distractions and stay present in the moment, which not only enhances the driving experience but also improves safety on the road (McKenna, 2014). For therapists, incorporating mindful driving into their routine can offer significant personal and professional benefits.

By practicing mindful driving, therapists can reduce the stress often associated with commuting and use the time as an opportunity for mindfulness practice. Paying attention to the sensations of driving can transform a potentially stressful activity into a calming and centering experience. This can involve noticing the texture of the steering wheel, the sensation of the seat, the sounds of the tires on the road, and the visual landscape outside the car. This heightened awareness can help therapists arrive at their destinations feeling more relaxed and prepared for their sessions.

Mindful driving can lead to improved emotional regulation. When therapists or clients encounter challenging driving situations, such as heavy traffic or aggressive drivers, mindfulness can help them remain calm and composed. This practice fosters a non-reactive mindset, allowing individuals to respond to stressors with greater equanimity (Shapiro et al., 2007). This can reduce the likelihood of road rage and improve overall driving experiences.

### Mindful Gardening

Mindful gardening involves focusing on the physical sensations of digging, planting, and watering, while also paying attention to the colors, shapes, and growth of the plants. This connection with nature can be deeply calming and grounding (Gonzalez et al., 2010). For therapists, incorporating mindful gardening into their routine can offer significant personal and professional benefits.

Therapists can use gardening to decompress and reconnect with nature after a busy day. Tending to plants requires attention and care that can help therapists shift their focus from the stresses of work to the nurturing of life. This practice can be particularly grounding, as it involves direct contact with the earth and a tangible connection to the natural world. Studies have shown that gardening can reduce stress, improve mood, and enhance overall well-being (Soga et al., 2017).

Additionally, mindful gardening can enhance therapists' observational skills. Paying close attention to the details of plant growth and health can sharpen their ability to notice subtle changes, a skill that is equally valuable in therapeutic settings. This enhanced attention to detail can improve their ability to observe and respond to clients' needs during sessions (Kaplan, 1995).

By engaging with nature mindfully, therapists can find relaxation, enhance their observational skills, and introduce clients to a therapeutic activity that promotes healing and well-being.

### Mindful Journaling

Mindful journaling involves spending a few minutes each day writing about your thoughts and feelings without judgment. This practice, often referred to as free-flow writing, allows for the exploration of experiences, emotions, and reactions in a non-critical way. Reflecting on one's inner life through writing can significantly increase self-awareness and emotional intelligence (Pennebaker & Chung, 2011). For therapists, mindful journaling can serve as a powerful tool for personal and professional development.

Therapists can use mindful journaling to process their own experiences and emotions, which is crucial for maintaining emotional balance and preventing burnout. By writing regularly, therapists can gain deeper insights into their own mental and emotional states, helping them to better manage stress and enhance their overall well-being. This practice can improve their ability to empathize with others, as it fosters a greater understanding of their own emotional responses and how these might influence their relationships with others (Baikie & Wilhelm, 2005).

Mindful journaling can be integrated with other mindfulness practices to create a comprehensive approach to mental health. For instance, clients can combine journaling with meditation or mindfulness exercises to deepen their self-awareness and promote a more profound sense of inner peace and clarity. This holistic approach can lead to more effective and lasting therapeutic outcomes (Kabat-Zinn, 2003).

### Mindful Creative Expression

Engaging in mindful creative expression involves immersing oneself in activities such as drawing, painting, pottery, coloring, crocheting, knitting, dancing, singing, or crafting with a focus on the process rather than the outcome. This practice encourages noticing the colors, shapes, and textures, and allowing oneself to express freely without self-criticism. By focusing on the present moment and the act of creation, individuals can experience a significant reduction in stress and an increase in mindfulness (Drake & Winner, 2011). For therapists, integrating mindful creative expression into both personal and professional life can provide numerous benefits.

Therapists can use mindful creative expression to enhance their well-being. This creative process can serve as a form of meditation, helping to quiet the mind and reduce stress. Creating without judgment fosters a sense of freedom and self-expression, which can be particularly therapeutic. Research has shown that engaging in creative activities can improve mood and lower cortisol levels, a biomarker of stress (Kaimal et al., 2016). By incorporating mindful creative expression into their routine, therapists can maintain a balanced and grounded state, which is essential for their demanding profession.

Mindful creative expression also promotes a state of flow, where individuals become fully absorbed in their activities, leading to enhanced concentration and enjoyment (Csikszentmihalyi, 1990). This state of flow can be deeply fulfilling and can help clients build resilience and coping skills. Furthermore, the non-judgmental aspect of mindful creative expression helps therapists cultivate self-compassion and reduce negative self-talk, which are critical components of emotional healing (Neff, 2003a, Neff, 2003b).

Mindful creative expression is a versatile and powerful practice that can benefit therapists. By engaging in creative activities with mindfulness, individuals can experience reduced stress, increased self-awareness, and improved emotional well-being.

### Mindful Listening to Music

Mindful listening to music involves selecting a piece of music and listening to it with full attention, focusing on the different instruments, rhythms, melodies, and emotions conveyed in the music. This practice can significantly enhance one's appreciation of music and bring a sense of calm and presence (Diaz, 2011). For therapists, incorporating mindful listening to music into their routine can offer numerous personal and professional benefits.

Mindful listening to music can serve as a powerful tool for stress reduction and emotional regulation. By dedicating time to listen attentively to music, therapists can create a space for relaxation and mental rejuvenation. This practice encourages a deep engagement with the music, allowing therapists to experience its emotional nuances and calming effects fully. Research has shown that music can influence physiological processes such as heart rate and blood pressure, contributing to overall well-being (Koelsch, 2015; Thaut & Hoemberg, 2014). By integrating mindful music listening into their self-care routine, therapists can enhance their resilience and maintain a balanced emotional state.

Mindful listening to music can enhance the therapeutic relationship. Sharing and discussing music can create a meaningful connection between therapist and client, providing a shared experience that can deepen rapport and trust. This practice can also serve as a grounding exercise during therapy sessions, helping therapists to center themselves and become more present in the moment (Hernandez-Ruiz et al., 2021). By engaging with music mindfully, individuals can experience reduced stress, increased emotional awareness, and improved mental well-being.

### Seated Meditation

While there are many traditions and styles of meditation, seated meditation involves sitting quietly and focusing on the breath, a mental image, or a specific repeated mantra, helping therapists settle the cascade of racing thoughts and reduce stress in the mind and body. Research has shown that regular meditation practice can significantly reduce stress, anxiety, and depression while enhancing emotional well-being and cognitive function (Goyal et al., 2014; Khoury et al., 2015; Sharma & Sharma, 2024). In the beginning stages of learning to meditate, it can be helpful to follow along with a guided meditation. Prominent meditation teachers such as Tara Brach (2003, 2019) and Sharon Salzberg (1995) offer excellent options available online.

Guided meditations provide structure and support, making it easier for beginners to develop a consistent practice. These sessions often include instructions on posture, breathing, and mindfulness techniques, which can help new meditators stay focused and engaged. Tara Brach's meditations often incorporate elements of compassion and self-acceptance, making them particularly beneficial for therapists who may be dealing with the emotional burdens of their clients (Brach, 2019). Sharon Salzberg's teachings emphasize loving-kindness (metta) meditation, which can help therapists cultivate a sense of empathy and compassion, both for themselves and others (Salzberg, 1995).

Research supports the benefits of seated meditation for mental health professionals. A study by Shapiro, Brown, and Biegel (2007) found that therapists who participated in an eight-week MBSR program reported significant reductions in stress and anxiety, as well as improvements in self-compassion and overall well-being. Another study by Fortney and Taylor (2010) highlighted the positive impact of meditation on reducing burnout and increasing resilience among healthcare providers.

Seated meditation also has physiological benefits. It can lower blood pressure, improve heart rate variability, and reduce cortisol levels, which are biomarkers of stress (Black & Slavich, 2016; Pascoe et al., 2017). These physical health benefits complement the psychological advantages, making meditation a comprehensive tool for enhancing overall health.

Seated meditation is a powerful practice for therapists, offering numerous psychological and physiological benefits. Following guided meditations by renowned teachers like Tara Brach and Sharon Salzberg can help beginners develop a robust meditation practice, leading to reduced stress, increased self-compassion, and improved mental and physical well-being.

## Mindful Gazing

Mindful gazing involves being fully present while watching a sunrise, sunset, starry sky, clouds, flowing river, or candle flame. This practice can be highly effective in cultivating mindfulness because it encourages deep, focused engagement with the present moment. By fully immersing themselves in the visual experience and observing colors, movements, and patterns without distraction or judgment, individuals can train their minds to maintain concentration and resist distractions, which is a fundamental aspect of mindfulness (Kabat-Zinn, 2003). The repetitive and rhythmic nature of natural phenomena, such as the flow of a river or the flicker of a candle flame, can have a soothing effect on the mind, helping to reduce stress and anxiety by shifting focus away from worries and into a state of calm observation (Hanh, 2011). Engaging the visual sense fully through mindful gazing also enhances present-moment awareness and can lead to a greater appreciation of the beauty and intricacy of the natural world (De Smet & De Cruz, 2013). Furthermore, observing natural phenomena can evoke feelings of awe, peace, and connectedness, counteracting negative emotions and promoting overall well-being (Stellar et al., 2017). This holistic sensory immersion helps individuals connect more deeply with their environment, regulate their emotional state, and cultivate a greater sense of inner peace and clarity.

## Creating a Foundation of Self-Care

Observing mindfulness with daily practice does not require significant time investment but can yield substantial benefits. Therapists can begin their day with a brief mindfulness meditation, set aside a few minutes between sessions for deep breathing exercises, or practice mindful walking during breaks. These small, intentional practices can accumulate to create a robust foundation of self-care. Regularly engaging in mindfulness exercises helps therapists maintain a consistent practice, making it easier to stay grounded and resilient amid the demands of their profession. Over time, these practices become ingrained habits that support ongoing emotional and mental well-being.

Incorporating mindfulness into daily practice offers therapists a practical and effective way to enhance their emotional and mental well-being. These practices do not require significant time investment but can lead to substantial benefits, creating a foundation of self-care that supports both therapists and their clients. By integrating mindfulness into their routines and therapeutic approaches, therapists can foster a more balanced, present, and resilient professional life.

## Evidence-Based Benefits of Mindfulness-Based Practice for Therapists

Numerous studies (Mettler et al., 2022) have highlighted the benefits of mindfulness for mental health professionals. Research indicates that therapists who engage in mindfulness practices report lower levels of stress and higher levels of job satisfaction (Ruiz-Fernandez et al., 2020). These practices enhance therapists' reflective capacities, allowing them to respond to clients' needs with greater sensitivity and insight (Guendelman et al., 2017). Moreover, mindfulness can improve therapists' emotional regulation, helping them maintain a calm and composed demeanor, even in challenging therapeutic situations (Dobkin et al., 2016).

### Science Supports Mindfulness for Therapists' Stress

One of the most significant benefits of mindfulness for therapists is the reduction of stress levels (Askey-Jones, 2018; Mohammed et al., 2018; Price & Weng, 2021; Ruíz-Fernández et al., 2020; Suyi et al., 2017). Chronic stress can impair a therapist's ability to provide effective care and can lead to burnout. Studies have shown that mindfulness practices, such as meditation and mindful breathing, activate the body's relaxation response, reducing the production of stress hormones like cortisol.

### Clinical Studies

Research has demonstrated that therapists who participated in an eight-week MBSR program reported significant reductions in perceived stress and anxiety levels (Irving et al., 2009; Michalak et al., 2020; Shapiro et al., 2007).

### Neuroscientific Evidence

Neuroimaging studies (Bauer et al., 2019; Doll et al., 2016; Gotink et al., 2016; Hatchard et al., 2017; Lutz et al., 2014; Marchand, 2014) have shown that mindfulness practices can alter brain structures involved in stress regulation, such as the amygdala and prefrontal cortex, enhancing the brain's ability to manage stress effectively.

## Mindfulness Supports Therapists' Vocational Satisfaction

Mindfulness practices contribute to higher levels of job satisfaction among mental health professionals (Hülsheger et al., 2013). Job satisfaction is crucial for retaining skilled therapists and ensuring the quality of care provided to clients. Mindfulness helps therapists find greater fulfillment in their work by fostering a positive and engaged mindset.

### Improved Work Engagement

Mindfulness enhances therapists' ability to be present and engaged during sessions, leading to more meaningful interactions with clients. This presence and engagement can increase job satisfaction by making the work more rewarding and impactful (Baggs et al., 2024; Zerpa et al., 2024; Ziede & Norcross, 2024).

### Enhanced Professional Relationships

Mindfulness can strengthen professional relationships with colleagues and supervisors by improving empathy and communication skills, contributing to a more supportive and satisfying work environment (Mesmer-Magnus et al., 2017).

### Client-Centered Interventions

By enhancing their sensitivity and insight, therapists can develop more client-centered interventions that address everyone's unique needs and concerns (Baker, 2016; Lee, 2013)

### Mindful Supervision and Peer Support

Engaging in mindful supervision and peer support groups can enhance reflective practice and provide additional support for integrating mindfulness into clinical work (Glassburn et al., 2019; Johnson et al., 2020; Schat et al., 2016).

The evidence-based benefits of mindfulness for therapists are well-documented, highlighting its positive impact on stress reduction, job satisfaction, reflective capacities, sensitivity, insight, and emotional regulation

(Ablett, 2023; Mohammed et al., 2018). By incorporating mindfulness practices into their daily routines and professional development, therapists can enhance their well-being and effectiveness, ultimately providing better care for their clients.

## Resources for Developing a Mindfulness Practice

Here is a detailed list of resources to help you integrate mindfulness into your daily life and therapeutic practice.

### Books

*Wherever You Go, There You Are* by Jon Kabat-Zinn (2024)

Offering a classic introduction to mindfulness, this book provides practical advice and insights into integrating mindfulness into everyday life. Kabat-Zinn's accessible writing style makes this a perfect read for both beginners and experienced practitioners.

*The Miracle of Mindfulness* by Thich Nhat Hanh (1975)

Thich Nhat Hanh, a renowned Vietnamese Zen Buddhist monk, provides a gentle and profound guide to mindfulness in this book. He offers simple techniques and reflections to help readers cultivate mindfulness in their daily activities.

*Radical Acceptance* by Tara Brach (2003)

Tara Brach combines mindfulness and compassion in this insightful book, exploring how accepting ourselves and our experiences can lead to profound healing and transformation. This book is particularly useful for therapists looking to deepen their understanding of self-compassion.

*The Mindful Therapist* by Daniel J. Siegel (2010)

This book explores the application of mindfulness in therapeutic practice, offering therapists insights into how mindfulness can enhance their work. Siegel provides practical exercises and reflections to help therapists integrate mindfulness into their personal and professional lives.

*Mindfulness in Psychotherapy* by Frank W. Bond and Paul Gilbert (2006)

This book provides a comprehensive overview of how mindfulness can be integrated into psychotherapy. It covers theoretical foundations, practical applications, and case studies, offering valuable insights for therapists looking to incorporate mindfulness into their practice.

### Online Courses

Online courses offer structured and comprehensive training in mindfulness practices. Here are some highly regarded options.

#### Mindfulness-Based Stress Reduction (MBSR) Online Courses

These courses provide an in-depth exploration of MBSR techniques, designed to help participants reduce stress and improve overall well-being. Kabat-Zinn's courses are based on decades of research and clinical practice.

#### The Science of Well-Being

This course, taught by Professor Laurie Santos from Yale University, explores the science behind what makes us happy and how we can apply these insights to our own lives. It includes mindfulness practices as part of the curriculum and is available for free on Coursera.

#### Oxford Mindfulness Center

The center offers a range of mindfulness courses, including mindfulness-based cognitive therapy (MBCT) and Mindfulness for Life, both of which are available online. These courses are designed to integrate mindfulness into daily life and improve mental health.

#### Insight Timer Guided Meditations and Courses

Insight Timer is a popular app that provides a vast library of guided meditations, mindfulness courses, and community support. It's a great resource for therapists looking to integrate mindfulness into their daily routines.

### Workshops and Retreats

Attending workshops and retreats can deepen your mindfulness practice through immersive experiences and expert guidance. Here are some notable options.

#### The Art of Living Retreat Center

Nestled in the Blue Ridge Mountains of North Carolina, this retreat center offers programs focused on mindfulness, meditation, and yoga.

The Art of Living Retreat Center provides various retreats that cater to different needs, from stress reduction to personal growth, all within a tranquil and supportive environment.

### Blue Cliff Monastery

Founded by Zen Master Thich Nhat Hanh, Blue Cliff Monastery in Pine Bush, New York, offers mindfulness retreats in the Plum Village tradition. These retreats emphasize mindful living, meditation, and the practice of mindfulness in daily activities. The serene environment and teachings from monastic and lay practitioners provide a supportive space for deepening mindfulness practice.

### The Dancing Spirit Ranch

Situated in the Flathead Valley, in Montana this retreat center offers mindfulness retreats that focus on nature immersion, meditation, and personal growth. The beautiful landscape, including views of Glacier National Park, enhances the mindfulness experience.

### Elohee Center

Located in the Blue Ridge Mountains of North Georgia, the Elohee Center offers various mindfulness retreats focused on rest, relaxation, and holistic wellness. The center features miles of trails, a 100-foot waterfall, and a tranquil spa, providing an ideal setting for mindfulness practice and self-discovery.

### The Esalen Institute

Esalen, in Big Sur, California, offers immersive mindfulness retreats that combine meditation, mindful movement, and contemplative practices in a serene coastal setting. These retreats are led by experienced instructors and aim to help participants cultivate greater awareness and presence, integrating mindfulness into daily life through practical tools and techniques. The natural beauty of Esalen's environment enhances the experience, providing a perfect backdrop for personal reflection and growth.

### Feathered Pipe Ranch

Located near Helena, Montana, Feathered Pipe Ranch offers a variety of mindfulness and wellness retreats. These programs include yoga, meditation, and holistic healing practices in a serene natural setting, promoting deep relaxation and self-discovery. The ranch's secluded environment amid forests and meadows provides an ideal backdrop for mindfulness practice.

### Florida Community of Mindfulness

The Florida Community of Mindfulness (FCM) offers numerous retreats throughout the year in Tampa and other locations. These retreats typically include meditation sessions, mindful movements, and Dharma talks. FCM provides a nurturing environment for deepening mindfulness practice and integrating mindfulness into daily life.

### Insight Meditation Society (IMS)

Based in Barre, Massachusetts, Insight Meditation Society (IMS) provides a range of meditation retreats, including mindfulness retreats, led by esteemed teachers in the Vipassana tradition. The center offers silent retreats that vary in length, providing an immersive environment for developing mindfulness and insight.

### The Insight Center

Located in downtown Chicago, The Insight Center provides MBSR programs and integrative psychotherapy. Their retreats and workshops focus on enhancing mindfulness, reducing stress, and promoting overall well-being.

### Kripalu Center for Yoga & Health

Located in Stockbridge, Massachusetts, the Kripalu Center offers mindfulness retreats that combine meditation, yoga, and contemplative practices. The retreats are designed to help participants cultivate mindfulness and integrate it into their daily lives. Kripalu's holistic approach and beautiful natural surroundings enhance the retreat experience.

### Mountain Cloud Zen Center

Located in Santa Fe, New Mexico, Mountain Cloud Zen Center provides Zen meditation retreats. These retreats offer an immersive experience in mindfulness and Zen practices, suitable for both beginners and experienced meditators.

*Omega Institute (Rhinebeck, NY)*

The Omega Institute offers a variety of mindfulness workshops and retreats led by renowned teachers. These programs provide an opportunity to disconnect from daily stresses and immerse oneself in mindfulness practice.

*Retreat in the Pines*

Situated in Mineola, Texas, this center offers women's mindfulness retreats that include yoga, meditation, and nature walks. The retreats are designed to help participants relax, rejuvenate, and connect with themselves in a peaceful forest setting.

*Rocky Mountain Ecodharma Retreat Center*

Located near Boulder, Colorado, RMERC offers eco-dharma retreats that integrate meditation with nature. The center focuses on silent meditation retreats, nature-based mindfulness practices, and retreats for underserved communities. The 180-acre site includes meadows, forests, and wildlife, providing a tranquil setting for deepening mindfulness and connecting with nature.

*Sedona Mago Center for Well-Being and Retreat*

Situated in the picturesque landscapes of Sedona, Arizona, this center offers numerous mindfulness and wellness retreats. Programs include meditation, tai chi, qigong, and spiritual healing practices designed to enhance physical, emotional, and spiritual well-being.

*Serenbe*

Serenbe, situated in Chattahoochee Hills near Atlanta, is a wellness community offering a variety of mindfulness and wellness retreats. Activities include yoga classes, nature walks, and farm-to-table dining experiences. The community is designed to connect visitors with nature, providing a peaceful environment for mindfulness practice.

*Shambhala Mountain Center*

Located in the Colorado Rockies, the Shambhala Mountain Center offers a wide range of mindfulness and meditation retreats. These retreats are based on Buddhist teachings and Shambhala principles, aiming to create a peaceful and mindful community. Programs vary in length and focus, providing options for beginners and advanced practitioners.

### Spirit Rock Meditation Center

Spirit Rock in Woodacre, California is a leading meditation center that offers both online and in-person retreats focused on mindfulness and insight meditation. Their programs are designed to support personal growth and professional development for therapists.

### Zen Den Yoga School and Retreat Center

Located in Boca Raton, Florida, Zen Den offers a combination of yoga, meditation, and wellness retreats. These retreats focus on holistic health and mindfulness, providing various yoga styles, meditation practices, and relaxation techniques to enhance overall well-being.

## Apps

Mobile apps can provide convenient access to mindfulness practices and resources. Here are some recommended apps.

### Insight Timer

This app offers a wide range of guided meditations, courses, and a supportive community. It's suitable for both beginners and experienced practitioners.

### Headspace

Headspace provides structured mindfulness programs, including meditation courses and mindfulness exercises designed to reduce stress, improve focus, and enhance overall well-being.

### Calm

Calm offers guided meditations, sleep stories, and relaxation exercises. It's designed to help users manage stress, improve sleep, and develop a regular mindfulness practice.

*10% Happier*

This app features practical mindfulness and meditation courses, guided by expert teachers. It focuses on making mindfulness accessible and useful in everyday life.

### Professional Organizations

Joining professional organizations can provide ongoing support, resources, and a community of like-minded professionals. Here are two prominent organizations.

*American Mindfulness Research Association (AMRA)*

American Mindfulness Research Association (AMRA) is dedicated to supporting scientific research on mindfulness and its applications. Membership offers access to the latest research, resources, and networking opportunities with other professionals in the field.

*Association for Contextual Behavioral Science (ACBS)*

Association for Contextual Behavioral Science (ACBS) is an international organization focused on advancing cognitive and behavioral sciences, including mindfulness-based approaches. Membership includes access to conferences, workshops, and a community of practitioners and researchers.

*Center for Mindfulness in Medicine, Health Care, and Society (CFM)*

This organization was founded at the University of Massachusetts Medical School and is a pioneer in the field of MBSR. They offer training programs for professionals, conduct research, and provide resources for integrating mindfulness into various sectors.

*International Mindfulness Teachers Association (IMTA)*

This organization sets standards for mindfulness teachers and provides certification. They aim to ensure the quality and integrity of mindfulness teaching worldwide by supporting teachers with resources, training, and professional development.

*Mindfulness in Education Network (MiEN)*

This organization is dedicated to supporting mindfulness in educational settings. The network connects educators and professionals interested in integrating mindfulness into schools and educational programs. They provide resources, training, and a community for sharing best practices.

*Mindfulness-Based Professional Training Institute (MBPTI)*

This organization is located at the University of California, San Diego, and offers professional training in mindfulness-based interventions. They provide certification programs, workshops, and resources for practitioners and researchers.

Developing a mindfulness practice is a valuable investment of time and energy for therapists. These resources provide a comprehensive foundation for integrating mindfulness into your personal and professional life, enhancing your well-being and effectiveness as a therapist. Whether through reading, online courses, workshops, apps, or professional organizations, there are numerous ways to deepen your mindfulness practice and enrich your therapeutic skills.

## Shifting the Therapist's Way of Being with Clients

Integrating mindfulness into psychotherapy involves a fundamental shift in the therapist's approach and presence. Mindfulness encourages therapists to embody qualities such as openness, acceptance, and nonjudgment, which are crucial for effective therapeutic relationships. This shift goes beyond applying techniques and requires therapists to cultivate a mindful way of being that permeates all aspects of their professional practice.

### Therapeutic Presence

By practicing mindfulness, therapists develop a heightened state of awareness and presence. This presence allows them to be fully attuned to their clients' needs, fostering a deeper connection and understanding. The quality of being present is not just about physical proximity but involves a genuine engagement and attentiveness that clients can feel and trust.

## Conclusion

As the rest of this book provides theoretical and practical ways to utilize Mindfulness-based Play Therapy®, it is imperative to emphasize the importance of consistent mindfulness practice for therapists. This practice not only supports the therapist's well-being but also enhances the quality of the therapeutic alliance with clients. By bridging mindfulness and psychotherapy, therapists can enhance their therapeutic effectiveness and contribute to more positive outcomes for their clients. In the following chapters, we will explore how mindfulness-based practices can be integrated into play therapy to support children and families. Next, there will be exploration of the neurobiology of mindfulness, then examination of how Mindfulness-based Play Therapy® can be applied to all of the historically significant and seminal play therapy theories. Specific techniques and exercises that can be used in play therapy sessions will be presented, offering practical guidance for incorporating mindfulness into therapeutic practice. Through this integration, therapists can create a more holistic and effective approach to therapy, fostering resilience, emotional regulation, and overall well-being in their clients.

## References

Ablett, M. (2023). *Mindfulness practice uses in countertransference: A phenomenological study.* Institute for Clinical Social Work (Chicago).

American Psychological Association. (2021). The ethical imperative of self-care. *Monitor on Psychology*, *52*(4). Retrieved from https://www.apa.org/monitor/2021/04/feature-imperative-self-care

Ash, M., Harrison, T., Pinto, M., DiClemente, R., & Negi, L. T. (2021). A model for cognitively-based compassion training: theoretical underpinnings and proposed mechanisms. Social Theory & Health, 19, 43–67. https://doi.org/10.1057/s41285-019-00124-x

Askey-Jones, R. (2018). Mindfulness-based cognitive therapy: An efficacy study for mental health care staff. *Journal of Psychiatric and Mental Health Nursing*, *25*, 380–389. https://doi.org/10.1111/jpm.12472

Baggs, A., Duhel, O., Justice, E., & Henderson, F. (2024). Mindfulness practice and expressions of wellness: Experiences of doctoral counselor education and supervision students. *Journal of Creativity in Mental Health*, 1–14. https://doi.org/10.1080/15401383.2024.2345366

Baikie, K. A., & Wilhelm, K. (2005). Emotional and physical health benefits of expressive writing. *Advances in Psychiatric Treatment*, *11*(5), 338–346. https://doi.org/10.1192/apt.11.5.338

Baker, S. (2016). Working in the present moment: The impact of mindfulness on trainee psychotherapists' experience of relational depth. *Cancer Prevention Research*, *16*, 5–14. https://doi.org/10.1002/CAPR.12038

Bays, J. C. (2017). *Mindful eating: A guide to rediscovering a healthy and joyful relationship with food* (Revised ed.). Shambhala Publications.

Black, D. S., & Slavich, G. M. (2016). Mindfulness meditation and the immune system: A systematic review of randomized controlled trials. *Annals of the New York Academy of Sciences*, *1373*(1), 13–24. https://doi.org/10.1111/nyas.12998.

Bond, F. W., & Gilbert, P. (2006). Historical aspects of mindfulness and self-acceptance in psychotherapy. *Journal of Rational-Emotive & Cognitive-Behavior Therapy*, *24*(1), 3–28.

Bostock, S., Crosswell, A. D., Prather, A. A., & Steptoe, A. (2019). Mindfulness on-the-go: Effects of a mindfulness meditation app on work stress and well-being. *Journal of Occupational Health Psychology*, *24*(1), 127–138. https://doi.org/10.1037/ocp0000118

Brach, T. (2003). *Radical acceptance: Embracing your life with the heart of a Buddha.* Bantam Books.

Brach, T. (2019). *Radical compassion: Learning to love yourself and your world with the practice of RAIN.* Viking.

Bronfenbrenner, U. (1979). *The ecology of human development: Experiments by nature and design.* Harvard University Press.

Burton, A., Burgess, C., Dean, S., Koutsopoulou, G. Z., & Hugh-Jones, S. (2017). How effective are mindfulness-based interventions for reducing stress among healthcare professionals? A systematic review and meta-analysis. *Stress and Health, 33*(1), 3–12. https://doi.org/10.1002/smi.2673

Caballero, C., Scherer, E., West, M. R., Mrazek, M. D., Gabrieli, C. F., & Gabrieli, J. D. (2019). Greater mindfulness is associated with better academic achievement in middle school. Mind, Brain, and Education, *13*(3), 157–166. https://doi.org/10.1111/mbe.12200

Champagne Clean. (2023). The Zen of mindful cleaning: Finding inner peace through tidying. *Champagne Clean.* Retrieved from Champagne Clean.

Cleveland Clinic. (2024). 4-7-8 Breathing method for sleep and relaxation. Retrieved from Cleveland Clinic. Available at: https://health.clevelandclinic.org/4-7-8-breathing

Crenshaw, D. A., & Stewart, A. L. (2014). Healing the wounds of childhood trauma: Mindfulness, compassion, and play therapy. *Journal of Clinical Psychology, 70*(11), 1033–1043. https://doi.org/10.1002/jclp.22116

Csikszentmihalyi, M. (1990). *Flow: The psychology of optimal experience.* Harper & Row.

Davis, L., & Hayes, J. (2011). What are the benefits of mindfulness? A practice review of psychotherapy-related research. *Psychotherapy, 48*(2), 198–208. https://doi.org/10.1037/a0022062

Davis, P., Scott, T., & Engle, D. (2022). The impact of mindfulness-based practices on employee well-being: A meta-analysis. *Journal of Occupational Health Psychology, 27*(3), 315–333. https://doi.org/10.1037/ocp0000317

De Smet, J., & De Cruz, H. (2013). Delighting in natural beauty: Joint attention and the phenomenology of nature aesthetics. *European Journal for Philosophy of Religion, 5*(4), 167–186.

Diaz, F. M. (2011). Mindfulness, music, and emotion: Integrating mindfulness meditation with music listening to reduce stress and anxiety. *Psychomusicology: Music, Mind, and Brain, 21*(1-2), 67–75. https://doi.org/10.1037/h0094004

Doll, M., Jandhyala, R., & Von Scheve, C. (2016). Emotions in conflict: Understanding emotional processes in violent political conflict. *Sociology Compass, 10*(8), 674–687. https://doi.org/10.1111/soc4.12385

Drake, J. E., & Winner, E. (2011). Confronting assumptions about art and mental illness. *Journal of Psychiatric Research, 45*(2), 260–263. https://doi.org/10.1016/j.jpsychires.2010.06.001

Duke, E., & Montag, C. (2017). Mindfulness, personality, and internet addiction: A review of the literature. *Journal of Behavioral Addictions, 6*(1), 27–35. https://doi.org/10.1556/2006.6.2017.007

Dye, L., Burke, M. G., & Wolf, C. (2020). Teaching mindfulness for the self-care and well-being of counselors-in-training. *Journal of Creativity in Mental Health*, 15(2), 140–153.

Emmons, R. A., & McCullough, M. E. (2003). Counting blessings versus burdens: An experimental investigation of gratitude and subjective well-being in daily life. *Journal of Personality and Social Psychology, 84*(2), 377–389. https://doi.org/10.1037/0022-3514.84.2.377

Fabbro, F., Crescentini, C., Matiz, A., Clarici, A., & Fabbro, F. (2017). Effects of mindfulness meditation on conscious and non-conscious components of the mind. *Applied Sciences, 7*(4), 349. https://doi.org/10.3390/app7040349

Finlay, L. (2008). *Reflecting on 'reflective practice'. Practice-based professional learning paper 52*, The Open University.

Fook, J., & Gardner, F. (2007). *Practising critical reflection: A resource handbook.* McGraw-Hill Education.

Fortney, L., & Taylor, M. (2010). Mindfulness in addiction treatment: State of the field and implications for clinical practice. *Journal of Addictive Behaviors, 35*(9), 1082–1089. https://doi.org/10.1016/j.addbeh.2010.07.008

Gamaiunova, A., Lucas, M., & Den Hartigh, L. (2022). The influence of mindfulness on student-athlete performance: A meta-analysis. *Psychology of Sport and Exercise, 61,* 102199. https://doi.org/10.1016/j.psychsport.2022.102199

Gardi, C., Fazia, T., Stringa, B., & Giommi, F. (2022). A short mindfulness retreat can improve biological markers of stress and inflammation. *Psychoneuroendocrinology, 135,* 105579.

Germer, C. K., Siegel, R. D., & Fulton, P. R. (Eds.). (2016). *Mindfulness and psychotherapy* (2nd ed.). Guilford Press.

Glassburn, S. L., McGuire, L. E., & Lay, K. (2019). Reflection as self-care: Models for facilitative supervision. *Reflective Practice, 20,* 692–704. https://doi.org/10.1080/14623943.2019.1674271

Gonzalez, M. T., Hartig, T., Patil, G. G., Martinsen, E. W., & Kirkevold, M. (2010). Therapeutic horticulture in clinical depression: A prospective study of active components. *Journal of Advanced Nursing, 66*(9), 2002–2013.

Good, D. J., Lyddy, C. J., Glomb, T. M., Bono, J. E., Brown, K. W., Duffy, M. K., Baer, R. A., Brewer, J. A., & Lazar, S. W. (2016). Contemplating mindfulness at work: An integrative review. *Journal of Management, 42*(1), 114–142. https://doi.org/10.1177/0149206315617003

Gotink, R. A., Meijboom, R., Vernooij, M. W., Smits, M., & Hunink, M. G. M. (2016). 8-week mindfulness-based stress reduction induces brain changes similar to traditional long-term meditation practice – A systematic review. *Brain and Cognition, 108,* 32–41. https://doi.org/10.1016/j.bandc.2016.07.001

Goyal, M., Singh, S., Sibinga, E. M. S., Gould, N. F., Rowland-Seymour, A., Sharma, R., Berger, Z., Sleicher, D., Maron, D. D., Shihab, H. M., Ranasinghe, P. D., Linn, S., Saha, S., Bass, E. B., & Haythornthwaite, J. A. (2014). Meditation programs for psychological stress and well-being: A systematic review and meta-analysis. *JAMA Internal Medicine, 174*(3), 357–368. https://doi.org/10.1001/jamainternmed.2013.13018

Grider, H. S., Douglas, S. M., & Raynor, H. A. (2021). The influence of mindful eating and/or intuitive eating approaches on dietary intake: A systematic review. *Journal of the Academy of Nutrition and Dietetics, 121*(4), 709–727.

Grensman, A., Acharya, B. D., & Wändell, P. (2021). Effects of mindfulness-based interventions on stress and well-being in healthcare professionals: A systematic review. *Journal of Clinical Medicine, 10*(3), 493. https://doi.org/10.3390/jcm10030493

Grepmair, L., Mitterlehner, F., Loew, T., Bachler, E., Rother, W., & Nickel, M. (2007). Promoting mindfulness in psychotherapists in training influences the treatment results of their patients: A randomized, double-blind, controlled study. *Psychotherapy and Psychosomatics, 76*(6), 332–338.

Guendelman, S., Medeiros, S., & Rampes, H. (2017). Mindfulness and emotion regulation: Insights from neurobiological, psychological, and clinical studies. *Frontiers in Psychology, 8,* 220.

Hanh, T. N. (2011). *The miracle of mindfulness: An introduction to the practice of meditation.* Beacon Press.

Hanh, T. N. (2015). *The art of living: Peace and freedom in the here and now.* HarperOne.

Hanson, T., & Jones, J. (2015). Is there evidence that walking groups have health benefits? A systematic review and meta-analysis. *British Journal of Sports Medicine, 49*(11), 710–715.

Hatchard, T., Mioduszewski, O., Zambrana, A., O'Farrell, E., Caluyong, M. B., Poulin, P. A., & Smith, A. (2017). Neural changes associated with mindfulness-based stress reduction (MBSR): Current knowledge, limitations, and future directions. *Psychology & Neuroscience, 10*, 41–56. https://doi.org/10.1037/pne0000073

Hayes, J. A., Gelso, C. J., & Goldberg, S. (2018a). Countertransference management and effective psychotherapy: Meta-analytic findings. *Psychotherapy, 55*(4), 496–507. https://doi.org/10.1037/pst0000193

Hayes, J. A., Gelso, C. J., & Hummel, A. M. (2011). Managing countertransference. *Psychotherapy, 48*(1), 88–97. https://doi.org/10.1037/a0022182

Hayes, S. C., Hofmann, S. G., & Stanton, C. E. (2018b). Open, aware, and active: Contextual approaches as an emerging trend in the behavioral and cognitive therapies. *Annual Review of Clinical Psychology, 14*(1), 259–289. https://doi.org/10.1146/annurev-clinpsy-050817-084917

Hernandez-Ruiz, E., Sebren, A., Alderete, C., Bradshaw, L., & Fowler, R. (2021). Effect of music on a mindfulness experience: An online study. *The Arts in Psychotherapy, 75*, 101827.

Hölzel, B. K., Lazar, S. W., Gard, T., Schuman-Olivier, Z., Vago, D. R., & Ott, U. (2011). How does mindfulness meditation work? Proposing mechanisms of action from a conceptual and neural perspective. *Perspectives on Psychological Science, 6*(6), 537–559. https://doi.org/10.1177/1745691611419671

Hughes, D., & Golding, K. S. (2012). *Creating loving attachments: Parenting with PACE to nurture confidence and security in the troubled child.* Jessica Kingsley Publishers.

Hülsheger, U. R., Alberts, H. J., Feinholdt, A., & Lang, J. W. (2013). Benefits of mindfulness at work: The role of mindfulness in emotion regulation, emotional exhaustion, and job satisfaction. *Journal of Applied Psychology, 98*(2), 310–325. https://doi.org/10.1037/a0031313

Hyland, P. K., Lee, R. A., & Mills, M. J. (2015). Mindfulness at work: A new approach to improving individual and organizational performance. Industrial and organizational Psychology, *8*(4), 576–602. https://doi.org/10.1017/iop.2015.41

Irving, J. A., Dobkin, P. L., & Park, J. (2009). Cultivating mindfulness in health care professionals: A review of empirical studies of mindfulness-based stress reduction (MBSR). *Complementary Therapies in Clinical Practice, 15*(2), 61–66.

Jerath, R., Edry, J. W., Barnes, V. A., & Jerath, V. (2006). Physiology of long pranayamic breathing: Neural respiratory elements may provide a mechanism that explains how slow deep breathing shifts the autonomic nervous system. *Medical Hypotheses, 67*(3), 566–571. https://doi.org/10.1016/j.mehy.2006.02.042

Johnson, D. A., Ivers, N. N., Avera, J., & Frazee, M. (2020). Supervision guidelines for fostering state-mindfulness among supervisees. *The Clinical Supervisor, 39*, 128–145.

Johnson, M. H., & Walsh, M. J. (2021). Associations between specific mindfulness practices and in-session relational factors. *Journal of Counseling & Development.* https://doi.org/10.1002/jcad.12390

Jones, S. M., Bodie, G. D., & Hughes, S. D. (2019). The impact of mindfulness on empathy, active listening, and perceived provisions of emotional support. *Communication Research, 46*(6), 838–865.

Kabat-Zinn, J. (1990). *Full catastrophe living: Using the wisdom of your body and mind to face stress, pain, and illness.* Delacorte Press.

Kabat-Zinn, J. (1992). Mindfulness meditation: Health benefits of an ancient Buddhist practice. In Y. Ishii (Ed.), *Comparative and psychological study on meditation* (pp. 105–117). Eburon.

Kabat-Zinn, J. (1994). *Wherever you go, there you are: Mindfulness meditation in everyday life.* Hachette Books.

Kabat-Zinn, J. (2003). Mindfulness-based interventions in context: Past, present, and future. *Clinical Psychology: Science and Practice, 10*(2), 144–156. https://doi.org/10.1093/clipsy.bpg016

Kabat-Zinn, J. (2023). *Wherever you go, there you are: Mindfulness meditation in everyday life.* Hachette Books.

Kaimal, G., Ray, K., & Muniz, J. (2016). Reduction of cortisol levels and participants' responses following art making. *Art Therapy: Journal of the American Art Therapy Association, 33*(2), 74–80. https://doi.org/10.1080/07421656.2016.1166832

Kaplan, R. (1995). The restorative benefits of nature: Toward an integrative framework. *Journal of Environmental Psychology, 15*(3), 169–182. https://doi.org/10.1016/0272-4944(95)90001-2

Kestly, T. A. (2016). Presence and play: Why mindfulness matters. *International Journal of Play Therapy, 25*(1), 14.

Khoury, B., Sharma, M. K., Rush, S. E., & Fournier, C. (2015). Mindfulness-based stress reduction for healthy individuals: A meta-analysis. *Journal of Psychosomatic Research, 78*(6), 519–528. https://doi.org/10.1016/j.jpsychores.2015.03.009

Koelsch, S. (2015). Music-evoked emotions: Principles, brain correlates, and implications for therapy. *Annals of the New York Academy of Sciences, 1337*(1), 193–201. https://doi.org/10.1111/nyas.12684

Kristeller, J. L., & Wolever, R. Q. (2010, 2011). Mindfulness-based eating awareness training for treating binge eating disorder: The conceptual foundation. *Eating Disorders, 19*(1), 49–61. https://doi.org/10.1080/10640266.2011.533605

Lomas, T., Medina, J. C., Ivtzan, I., Rupprecht, S., & Eiroa-Orosa, F. J. (2017). The impact of mindfulness on the wellbeing and performance of educators: A systematic review of the empirical literature. *Teaching and Teacher Education, 61*, 132–141. https://doi.org/10.1016/j.tate.2016.10.008

Lutz, J., Herwig, U., Opialla, S., Hittmeyer, A., Jäncke, L., Rufer, M., Grosse Holtforth, M., & Brühl, A. B. (2014). Mindfulness and emotion regulation – An fMRI study. *Social Cognitive and Affective Neuroscience, 9*(6), 776–785. https://doi.org/10.1093/scan/nst043

Ma, X., Yue, Z. Q., Gong, Z. Q., Zhang, H., Duan, N. Y., Shi, Y. T., Wei, G. X., & Li, Y. F. (2017). The effect of diaphragmatic breathing on attention, negative affect and stress in healthy adults. *Frontiers in Psychology, 8*, 874.

Maharaj, A. S., Bhatt, N. V., & Gentile, J. P. (2021). Bringing it in the room: Addressing the impact of racism on the therapeutic alliance. *Innovations in Clinical Neuroscience, 18*(7–9), 39.

Mansfield, S. (2010). *Reflective practice: Writing and professional development* (279 pp.). Education in the North. Sage. ISBN 978848602120.

Marchand, W. R. (2014). Mindfulness meditation practices as adjunctive treatments for psychiatric disorders. *Psychiatric Clinics of North America, 35*(1), 141–152. https://doi.org/10.1016/j.psc.2013.01.002

Martin-Allan, J., Leeson, P., & Lovegrove, W. (2021). The effect of mindfulness and compassion meditation on state empathy and emotion. *Mindfulness, 12*(7), 1768–1778.

McKenna, F. P. (2014). Exploring mindfulness interventions in driver safety training. *Transportation Research Part F: Traffic Psychology and Behaviour, 27*(2), 21–28. https://doi.org/10.1016/j.trf.2014.01.001

Mesmer-Magnus, J., Manapragada, A., Viswesvaran, C., & Allen, J. W. (2017). Trait mindfulness at work: A meta-analysis of the personal and professional correlates of trait mindfulness. *Human Performance*, *30*, 79–98. https://doi.org/10.1080/08959285.2017.1307842

Mettler, J., Khoury, B., Zito, S., Sadowski, I., & Heath, N. L. (2023). Mindfulness-based programs and school adjustment: A systematic review and meta-analysis. *Journal of School Psychology*, 97, 43–62.

Michalak, J., Steinhaus, K., & Heidenreich, T. (2020). (How) do therapists use mindfulness in their clinical work? A study on the implementation of mindfulness interventions. *Mindfulness*, *11*(2), 401–410.

Mohammed, W. A., Pappous, A., Muthumayandi, K., & Sharma, D. (2018). The effect of mindfulness meditation on therapists' body-awareness and burnout in different forms of practice. *European Journal of Physiotherapy*, *20*, 213–224. https://doi.org/10.1080/21679169.2018.1452980

Nagaoka, M., Hashimoto, Z., Takeuchi, H., & Sado, M. (2021). Effectiveness of mindfulness-based interventions for people with dementia and mild cognitive impairment: A meta-analysis and implications for future research. *PLoS One*, *16*(8), e0255128.

Neff, K. (2003a). Self-compassion: An alternative conceptualization of a healthy attitude toward oneself. *Self and Identity*, *2*(2), 85–101.

Neff, K. D. (2003b). The development and validation of a scale to measure self-compassion. *Self and Identity*, *2*(3), 223–250. https://doi.org/10.1080/15298860309027

Pascoe, M. C., Thompson, D. R., Jenkins, Z. M., & Ski, C. F. (2017). Mindfulness mediates the physiological markers of stress: Systematic review and meta-analysis. *Journal of Psychiatric Research*, *95*, 156–178. https://doi.org/10.1016/j.jpsychires.2017.08.004

Pennebaker, J. W., & Chung, C. K. (2011). Expressive writing: Connections to physical and mental health. *Handbook of health psychology* (pp. 263–284). Guilford Press.

Perry, B. D. (2014). *Creative interventions with traumatized children*. Guilford Publications.

Phan, M. L., Renshaw, T. L., Caramanico, J., Greeson, J. M., MacKenzie, E., Atkinson-Diaz, Z., Doppelt, N., Tai, H., Mandell, D. S., & Nuske, H. J. (2022). Mindfulness-based school interventions: A systematic review of outcome evidence quality by study design. *Mindfulness*, *13*(7), 1591–1613. https://doi.org/10.1007/s12671-022-01885-9

Price, C. J., & Weng, H. Y. (2021). Facilitating adaptive emotion processing and somatic reappraisal via sustained mindful interoceptive attention. *Frontiers in Psychology*, *12*, 578827. https://doi.org/10.3389/fpsyg.2021.578827

Redlinger-Gross, S. (2020). Mindful parenting: Integrating mindfulness into family therapy. *Family Process*, *59*(4), 1741–1758. https://doi.org/10.1111/famp.12547

Rudaz, M., Twohig, M. P., Ong, C. W., & Levin, M. E. (2017). Mindfulness and acceptance-based trainings for fostering self-care and reducing stress in mental health professionals: A systematic review. *Journal of Contextual Behavioral Science*, *6*(4), 380–390.

Ruíz-Fernández, M. D., Pérez-García, E., Ortega-Galán, Á. M., & Cabrera-Troya, J. (2020). The benefits of self-compassion in mental health professionals: A systematic review. *International Journal of Environmental Research and Public Health*, *17*(18), 6601. https://doi.org/10.3390/ijerph17186601

Ryan, A., Safran, J. D., Doran, J. M., & Muran, J. C. (2012). Therapist mindfulness, alliance and treatment outcome. *Psychotherapy Research*, *22*(3), 289–297.

Salzberg, S. (1995). *Facets of Metta*. https://doi.org/10.1080/14639947.2013.832494

Salzberg, S. (1995). *Lovingkindness: The revolutionary art of happiness*. Shambhala Publications.

Saunders, D., & Kober, H. (2020). Mindfulness-based intervention development for children and adolescents. *Mindfulness, 11*(8), 1868–1883.

Schat, A., van Noorden, M. S., Noom, M. J., Giltay, E. J., van der Wee, N. J., de Graaf, R., Ten Have, M., Vermeiren, R. R., & Zitman, F. G. (2016). A cluster analysis of early onset in common anxiety disorders. *Journal of Anxiety Disorders, 44*, 1–8. https://doi.org/10.1016/j.janxdis.2016.09.001

Schön, D. A. (1983). *The reflective practitioner: How professionals think in action.* Basic Books.

Shapiro, S. L., Brown, K. W., & Biegel, G. M. (2007). Teaching self-care to caregivers: Effects of mindfulness-based stress reduction on the mental health of therapists in training. *Training and Education in Professional Psychology, 1*(2), 105–115. https://doi.org/10.1037/1931-3918.1.2.105

Shapiro, S. L., & Carlson, L. E. (2017). *The art and science of mindfulness: Integrating mindfulness into psychology and the helping professions* (2nd ed.). American Psychological Association.

Shapiro, S. L., Carlson, L. E., Astin, J. A., & Freedman, B. (2006). Mechanisms of mindfulness. *Journal of Clinical Psychology, 62*(3), 373–386. https://doi.org/10.1002/jclp.20237

Sharma, D., & Sharma, B. R. (2024). The impact of yoga and meditation on mental and physical well-being. *Journal of Ayurveda and Integrated Medical Sciences, 9*(5), 144–153.

Siegel, D. J. (2010). *The mindful therapist: A clinician's guide to mindsight and neural integration.* Norton.

Siegel, D. J., & Hartzell, M. (2013). *Parenting from the inside out: How a deeper self-understanding can help you raise children who thrive.* Penguin.

Soga, M., Gaston, K. J., & Yamaura, Y. (2017). Gardening is beneficial for health: A meta-analysis. *Preventive Medicine Reports, 5*, 92–99. https://doi.org/10.1016/j.pmedr.2016.11.007

Stellar, J. E., Gordon, A., Anderson, C. L., Piff, P. K., McNeil, G. D., & Keltner, D. (2018). Awe and humility. *Journal of Personality and Social Psychology, 114*(2), 258–269. https://doi.org/10.1037/pspi0000109

Sternisko, A., Cichocka, A., & Van Bavel, J. J. (2020). The dark side of social movements: social identity, non-conformity, and the lure of conspiracy theories. *Current Opinion in Psychology, 35*, 1–6. https://doi.org/10.1016/j.copsyc.2020.02.007

Suyi, Y., Meredith, P. J., & Khan, A. (2017). Effectiveness of mindfulness intervention in reducing stress and burnout for mental health professionals in Singapore. *The Journal of Science and Healing, 13*, 319–326. https://doi.org/10.1016/j.explore.2017.06.001

Teper, R., Segal, Z. V., & Inzlicht, M. (2013). Inside the mindful mind: How mindfulness enhances emotion regulation through improvements in executive control. *Current Directions in Psychological Science, 22*(6), 449–454.

Thaut, M. H., & Hoemberg, V. (2014). *Handbook of neurologic music therapy.* Oxford University Press.

Tsai, H. J., Kuo, T. B., Lee, G. S., & Yang, C. C. (2015). Efficacy of paced breathing for insomnia: Enhances vagal activity and improves sleep quality. *Psychological Reports, 116*(2), 519–532. https;//doi.org.10.1111/psyp.12333

Watson, T., Walker, O., Cann, R., & Varghese, A. K. (2022). The benefits of mindfulness in mental healthcare professionals. *F1000Research, 10.* https://doi.org/10.12688/f1000research.73729.2

Weger, H., Castle Bell, G., Minei, E. M., & Robinson, M. C. (2014). The relative effectiveness of active listening in initial interactions. *International Journal of Listening, 28*(1), 13–31. https://doi.org10.1080/10904018.2013.813234

Weil, A. (2011). *Spontaneous happiness: A new path to emotional well-being*. Little, Brown and Company.

Wheeler, M. S., Arnkoff, D. B., & Glass, C. R. (2017). The neuroscience of mindfulness: How mindfulness alters the brain and facilitates emotion regulation. *Mindfulness, 8*(6), 1471–1487.

Wonders, L. L. (2021). Theoretical roots and branches of the evolving field of play therapy. In *Play therapy and telemental health* (pp. 3–24). Routledge.

Wonders, L. L., & Affee, M. L. (Eds.). (2024). *Play therapy treatment planning with children and families: A Guide for mental health professionals*. Taylor & Francis.

Zhao, X. (2019). Mindfulness and creativity: The mediating role of psychological safety. *Frontiers in Psychology, 10*, 2424. https://doi.org/10.3389/fpsyg.2019.02424

Zuo, B., Wang, C., & Hu, W. (2022). Enhancing therapists' reflective capacities through mindfulness: A longitudinal study. *Journal of Clinical Psychology, 78*(6), 1024–1039. https://doi.org/10.1002/jclp.23234

Zerpa, A. E., Miró, M. T., Díez, E., & Alonso, M. A. (2024). Promoting mindfulness in training psychotherapists in a university setting: A pilot study. *Revista de Psicodidáctica (English ed.), 29*(1), 86–95. https://doi.org/10.1016/j.psicoe.2023.12.002

Ziede, J. S., & Norcross, J. C. (2024). Personal therapy and self-care in the making of psychologists. In *Psychologists in making* (pp. 53–86). Routledge.

# 3

# THE NEUROBIOLOGY OF MINDFULNESS AND PLAY IN CHILD DEVELOPMENT

## Introduction

Understanding nervous system science is important to support the integration of mindfulness and play into therapeutic settings for children and families. Both mindfulness and play contribute significantly to healthy brain development, supporting emotional regulation, cognitive flexibility, and social skills (Wonders, 2022). This chapter delves into the neurobiology of mindfulness and children's brain development, the neurobiological benefits of play, and the critical role of mirror neurons in attachment and therapeutic relationships, all supported by current research literature.

## The Role of Play in Child Development

Play is a fundamental activity for children's development, offering a natural context for learning and growth. Recent research underscores the multifaceted benefits of play, particularly in promoting neurobiological development and supporting healthy brain function and structure. Play is universally recognized as a crucial element in children's development (Dankiw et al., 2020; Fleer, 2021; Souto-Manning, 2017). Play facilitates cognitive, emotional, social, and physical growth, and it provides children with opportunities to explore, experiment, and understand the world around them, leading to enhanced learning and development (Fisher, 2019).

 DOI: 10.4324/9781003468585-3

## Cognitive Development

Research indicates that play significantly contributes to cognitive development. Through play, children engage in problem-solving, decision-making, and creative thinking, which stimulate neural pathways and enhance brain plasticity, critical for learning and memory (Lillard et al., 2013). Vygotsky's theory of cognitive development emphasizes the importance of social interaction in play, which helps children develop higher-order thinking skills (Vygotsky, 1978). Play allows children to explore and experiment with different scenarios, promoting cognitive flexibility and executive function (Diamond & Lee, 2011). Additionally, play has been shown to improve language skills, as children often use more complex vocabulary and sentence structures during imaginative play (Weisberg et al., 2013). Studies have also demonstrated that play-based learning environments foster better academic outcomes compared to more traditional, structured educational approaches (Hirsh-Pasek et al., 2009). These findings underscore the critical role of play in cognitive development, supporting its inclusion in early childhood education and beyond.

## Emotional and Social Development

Play also has a pivotal role in emotional and social development. It allows children to express their emotions, develop empathy, and build social skills. Pretend play, for instance, enables children to explore different roles and perspectives, fostering emotional regulation and social understanding (Hoffmann & Russ, 2016). Through play, children learn to navigate complex social dynamics, negotiate roles, and resolve conflicts, which are essential skills for healthy social interactions (Goncu & Gauvain, 2012). Play therapy has been shown to be effective in helping children process emotions and develop coping strategies (Landreth, 2012). It provides a safe space for children to express their feelings and work through trauma or anxiety in a supportive environment (Bratton et al., 2005).

Engaging in play helps children build resilience by allowing them to experience and overcome challenges in a controlled setting. This process not only supports emotional growth but also enhances problem-solving abilities and adaptive functioning (Milteer et al., 2012). Social play promotes the development of interpersonal skills such as cooperation, sharing, and empathy. Children learn to understand others' feelings and viewpoints, which is crucial for developing compassion and building meaningful relationships (Nielsen, 2012).

Additionally, the shared joy and mutual engagement in play activities strengthen bonds between children, fostering a sense of belonging and community. These social interactions are foundational for developing a sense of identity and self-worth (Frost et al., 2012). The emotional and social skills acquired through play are not only beneficial during childhood but also serve as a foundation for healthy, adaptive functioning in adulthood.

### Neurobiological Development
#### Brain Structure and Function

Cotman et al. (2007) emphasizes that physical activity, often encompassing play, increases the production of brain-derived neurotrophic factor (BDNF), which is crucial for neuronal growth, synaptic plasticity, and cognitive function. Higher BDNF levels correlate with improved memory and learning capabilities (Cohen-Corey et al., 2010). This is crucial for the development of the prefrontal cortex (PFC), which governs executive functions such as planning, decision-making, and self-control (Diamond & Lee, 2011). Research by Vaynman et al. (2004) shows that engaging in physical activities, including play, enhances synaptic plasticity through the action of BDNF. This synaptic enhancement supports learning and memory formation.

#### Stress Reduction and Emotional Regulation

Play also influences the neuroendocrine system by reducing stress hormones like cortisol and promoting the release of endorphins and oxytocin, which enhance feelings of well-being and social bonding (Panksepp, 2007). These biochemical changes support emotional regulation and resilience, essential for healthy psychological development (Pellis & Pellis, 2013). Engaging in playful activities triggers the brain's reward systems, fostering positive emotions and reducing the impact of stressors. This neurobiological response not only alleviates immediate stress but also builds a foundation for better stress management in the future.

Research has shown that children who engage in regular play exhibit lower levels of cortisol, a stress hormone, compared to those who do not engage in such activities (Slopen et al., 2014). Lower cortisol levels are associated with reduced anxiety and improved emotional stability. Moreover, the release of endorphins during play acts as a natural painkiller and mood booster, creating a sense of euphoria and relaxation (Burgdorf & Panksepp, 2006).

Oxytocin, often referred to as the "love hormone," plays a crucial role in social bonding and emotional regulation. Playful interactions, especially those involving physical touch and social engagement, increase oxytocin levels, thereby enhancing trust and emotional closeness among peers and caregivers (Carter, 2014). This hormone is vital for forming secure attachments and fostering a supportive social environment, which are key factors in emotional resilience.

The dynamic nature of play allows children to practice coping mechanisms and adaptive behaviors in a low risk setting. This experiential learning process helps them develop strategies for managing stress and regulating emotions effectively (Gray, 2013). Through imaginative play and role-playing, children experiment with different responses to challenging situations, which can translate to better emotional control and problem-solving skills in real-life scenarios.

*Motor Skills and Physical Health*

Physical play, such as running, jumping, and climbing, is vital for developing motor skills and overall physical health. Engaging in these activities enhances coordination, balance, and strength, contributing to the development of the cerebellum and motor cortex (Pellegrini, 2013). The cerebellum is responsible for motor control and coordination, while the motor cortex is involved in the planning, controlling, and executing voluntary movements. By participating in physical play, children not only improve their gross motor skills but also fine-tune their neuromuscular connections, which are crucial for precise and coordinated movements (Stodden et al., 2008).

These activities also promote cardiovascular health and overall physical well-being. Regular physical play increases heart rate and improves circulation, strengthening the cardiovascular system and reducing the risk of heart disease (Janssen & LeBlanc, 2010). Additionally, physical activity helps regulate body weight by burning calories and increasing metabolism, which is essential in combating childhood obesity (Tremblay et al., 2011).

Physical play supports the development of bone density and muscle mass. Weight-bearing activities, such as jumping and climbing, stimulate bone growth and help maintain bone strength, reducing the risk of osteoporosis later in life (Gunter et al., 2012). The repetitive movements involved in physical play also enhance muscle endurance and flexibility, contributing to overall physical fitness.

Engaging in diverse physical activities from an early age fosters lifelong healthy habits. Children who participate in regular physical play are more likely to continue being active as adults, promoting sustained physical health and well-being (Telama et al., 2005). Additionally, physical play has psychological benefits, such as reducing symptoms of anxiety and depression, and improving mood and cognitive function, thus supporting holistic development (Biddle & Asare, 2011).

*Educational Implications*

Given the extensive benefits of play, it is imperative to integrate play-based learning approaches in educational settings. Research indicates that play-based curricula significantly improve academic outcomes, enhance student engagement, and foster a love for learning (Miller & Almon, 2009). Such curricula emphasize active, hands-on learning experiences where children can explore, experiment, and discover at their own pace, which supports cognitive and socio-emotional development (Bodrova & Leong, 2007).

Integrating play into the curriculum helps children develop essential skills such as critical thinking, creativity, and problem-solving. These skills are crucial for success in the 21st century, where adaptability and innovation are highly valued (Rushton et al., 2010). Additionally, play-based learning promotes intrinsic motivation and self-regulation, as children engage in activities they are genuinely interested in, which fosters a deeper, more meaningful learning experience (Stipek et al., 1998).

Schools and educators ideally will include play to support holistic development and prepare children for future challenges. By creating an environment that values and incorporates play, educators can help students develop a well-rounded skill set that includes not only academic knowledge but also social, emotional, and physical competencies (Zigler & Bishop-Josef, 2006a). This holistic approach to education recognizes that children learn best when they are active participants in their learning process, and when their educational experiences are enjoyable and relevant to their lives.

Play-based learning can help bridge educational inequalities. It provides all children, regardless of their background, with opportunities to engage in enriching and stimulating activities that promote development across multiple domains (Golinkoff et al., 2006). By ensuring that play is an integral part of the curriculum, schools can support the diverse needs of all learners, fostering an inclusive and supportive educational environment.

The benefits of play-based learning are well-documented, and the evidence supports its implementation in educational settings to enhance student outcomes and well-being. Elevating play as a priority in schools not only prepares children for academic success but also equips them with the skills and dispositions necessary to navigate and thrive in an ever-changing world.

## The Neurobiology of Mindfulness and Children's Brain Development

During childhood, the brain exhibits heightened neuroplasticity, making it an optimal period for interventions that promote cognitive and emotional development (Goldberg, 2022; Kadosh, 2013). Mindfulness practices have been shown to improve cognitive control, reduce anxiety, and enhance social-emotional learning in children (Zenner et al., 2014). These changes are supported by findings that mindfulness can increase functional connectivity in the brain, leading to better integration of cognitive and emotional processes (Roeser et al., 2013). Research has shown that mindfulness practices can lead to structural and functional changes in the brain, enhancing areas associated with attention, emotion regulation, and executive function (Davidson & McEwen, 2012; Hölzel et al., 2011). Neuroimaging research indicates that mindfulness can increase gray matter density in brain regions involved in learning, memory, and emotional regulation, such as the hippocampus and PFC (Hölzel et al., 2011). These findings suggest that incorporating mindfulness practices into childhood education and therapy could support the development of essential skills that promote lifelong mental health and well-being.

### Brain Structures Involved with Mindfulness Practice

#### Mindfulness and the Prefrontal Cortex (PFC)

The PFC is crucial for complex cognitive behavior, decision-making, and social behavior. Mindfulness practices have been shown to increase the thickness and activity of the PFC, which can improve executive functions in children, such as self-control, planning, and problem-solving (Tang et al., 2012).

#### Mindfulness and the Amygdala

This brain region is central to processing emotions, particularly fear and anxiety. The amygdala plays a pivotal role in the developing brain of a child, as it is highly active during childhood and adolescence when emotional processing and regulation are still maturing. It acts as an alarm system, detecting potential threats and triggering fight-or-flight responses. However, in the absence of proper emotional regulation, an overactive amygdala can lead to heightened anxiety and fear-based reactions. Studies have shown that mindfulness practices can reduce the reactivity of the amygdala by promoting a calmer state of mind and fostering the use of the prefrontal cortex to moderate emotional responses (Hölzel et al., 2011). This shift not only decreases anxiety but also enhances emotional regulation, allowing children to respond more thoughtfully rather than impulsively to stressors. Additionally, by calming the amygdala, mindfulness supports the developing brain's ability to build resilience and a sense of safety, which are essential for healthy emotional and psychological growth (Davidson & McKewen, 2012; Siegal, 2012).

#### Mindfulness and the Hippocampus

The hippocampus encodes, consolidates, and retrieves memories and regulates emotions. The hippocampus helps children integrate new experiences and build emotional regulating skills. The hippocampus grows and develops during childhood and adolescence, making it sensitive to stress, trauma, and nurturing. Chronic stress can lower hippocampus volume and function, affecting memory and emotional equilibrium (McEwen

& Morrison, 2013). However, consistent mindfulness practice increases hippocampus volume, improving memory and stress resilience (Bauer et al., 2019).

Mindfulness activities like focused breathing and body awareness strengthen hippocampus–prefrontal cortex brain connections, helping children manage emotions and respond carefully to stressors. Neuroplasticity improves coping and lowers amygdala overactivation-induced anxiety (Hölzel et al., 2011). Mindfulness helps children integrate emotional experiences with cognitive knowledge, which improves academic performance and emotional intelligence (Davidson et al., 2012). The hippocampus plays a role in learning and remembering. These findings show that mindfulness can help youngsters establish a healthy hippocampus, which enhances emotional regulation and cognitive performance throughout life.

*Mindfulness and Functional Connectivity between Brain Structures*

Mindfulness enhances the functional connectivity between the PFC, amygdala, and hippocampus. The PFC, responsible for executive functions such as decision-making, attention, and regulating emotions, works closely with the amygdala, which processes emotions, and the hippocampus, which is critical for memory formation and emotional regulation. Improved connectivity between these regions facilitates better top-down regulation of emotions, enabling children to manage stress and emotional responses more effectively (Tang et al., 2015).

In children, the development of functional connectivity between these brain regions is crucial for emotional and cognitive development. The PFC-amygdala pathway is particularly important for emotional regulation. Stronger connectivity in this pathway means that the PFC can more effectively modulate the emotional responses generated by the amygdala, leading to better emotional control and reduced anxiety and reactivity (Creswell et al., 2007). This top-down regulation is essential for managing stress and maintaining emotional balance.

Mindfulness practices have been shown to strengthen these neural connections. For instance, mindfulness meditation increases the functional connectivity between the PFC and the amygdala, thereby enhancing the ability to regulate emotions (Zeidan et al., 2011). This is particularly beneficial for children, as their brains are highly plastic and responsive to interventions that promote healthy development. Enhanced connectivity not only aids in emotional regulation but also supports improved attention and cognitive flexibility, which are crucial for academic and social success (Roeser et al., 2013).

Additionally, the hippocampus, which plays a key role in memory and learning, also benefits from mindfulness practices. Studies have shown that mindfulness can increase hippocampal volume and improve its functional connectivity with both the PFC and the amygdala (Hölzel et al., 2011). This triadic connectivity supports better memory processing, emotional regulation, and stress resilience, contributing to overall mental health and cognitive development in children.

By enhancing the functional connectivity between these critical brain regions, mindfulness practices help children develop better emotional regulation, improved cognitive function, and greater resilience to stress. This neural development supports not only immediate emotional and cognitive benefits but also long-term psychological well-being (Tang et al., 2015).

### Mindfulness and Neurotransmitter Changes

Mindfulness practices can significantly alter levels of critical neurotransmitters such as serotonin and dopamine, which are involved in mood regulation and reward processing. These biochemical changes contribute to a more balanced emotional state and increased resilience to stress in children.

Serotonin, often referred to as the "feel-good" neurotransmitter, plays a crucial role in regulating mood, anxiety, and happiness. Mindfulness practices, including meditation and deep breathing exercises, have been shown to increase serotonin levels, thereby improving mood, and reducing symptoms of anxiety and depression (Young, 2007). By enhancing serotonin production, mindfulness helps stabilize emotional responses, leading to a more consistent and positive mood.

Dopamine, another key neurotransmitter, is associated with the brain's reward system and is crucial for motivation, pleasure, and learning. Mindfulness practices can increase dopamine levels, which enhances feelings of enjoyment and motivation (Kjaer et al., 2002). This increase in dopamine not only improves mood but also encourages engagement in positive activities, further reinforcing the benefits of mindfulness practices.

Research supports these effects, showing that mindfulness interventions can lead to significant changes in brain chemistry. For example, studies have demonstrated that mindfulness meditation can alter the function and structure of the brain areas responsible for mood regulation and emotional processing, such as the PFC and the amygdala (Hölzel et al., 2011). These changes are associated with increased production of serotonin and dopamine, which contribute to improved emotional stability and resilience.

Additionally, mindfulness practices have been shown to reduce levels of cortisol, the stress hormone, further supporting emotional regulation and stress resilience (Tang et al., 2007). Lower cortisol levels indicate a reduced stress response, which is crucial for maintaining mental health and preventing the negative effects of chronic stress.

Overall, the neurotransmitter changes induced by mindfulness practices help children develop a more balanced emotional state and increase resilience to stress. These biochemical benefits support children's holistic development, contributing to their overall well-being and mental health.

## The Neurobiology of Play and Its Benefits for Brain Development

A recent study highlights the diverse advantages of play, specifically in enhancing neurobiological development and maintaining healthy brain function and structure (Achterberg & Vanderschuren, 2023). Play is widely acknowledged as a fundamental component in the development of children (Dankiw et al., 2020; Fleer, 2021; Souto-Manning, 2017). Play promotes cognitive, emotional, social, and physical development, allowing children to investigate, test, and comprehend their surroundings, resulting in improved learning and growth (Fisher, 2019).

### Brain Structures Involved with Play

*Play and the Prefrontal Cortex (PFC)*

Engaging in play activities stimulates the PFC, which is essential for planning, decision-making, and social interactions. Play encourages the development of executive functions and problem-solving skills, which are critical for navigating complex social environments (Diamond & Lee, 2011).

*Play and the Amygdala*

Play significantly affects the amygdala in children, enhancing emotional regulation and stress resilience. Social and pretend play engage the amygdala, helping children practice managing their emotions and navigating complex social interactions, which fosters better emotional control (Panksepp, 2007; Lillard et al., 2013). Physical play reduces cortisol levels, decreases stress and anxiety, and promotes neuroplasticity in the amygdala, which supports improved emotional regulation (Ginsburg, 2007; Pellis & Pellis, 2013). These activities help develop the functional connectivity between the amygdala and the PFC, essential for top-down emotional regulation and overall psychological well-being (Ginsburg, 2007; Lillard et al., 2013).

*Play and the Cerebellum*

The cerebellum, responsible for motor control and coordination, is activated during physical play. Activities such as running, jumping, and balancing enhance cerebellar function, which is crucial for both motor and cognitive development (Diamond, 2000).

*Play and the Basal Ganglia*

The basal ganglia are involved in habit formation and reward processing. Play activates this area, reinforcing learning and memory consolidation through repetitive and rewarding experiences, making play an essential part of healthy development (Gray, 2013).

*Play and Neurotransmitter and Hormonal Effects*

Play increases the release of dopamine, a neurotransmitter associated with pleasure and reward, promoting motivation and learning (Trezza et al., 2010; Vanderschuren et al., 2016). Additionally, play reduces levels of cortisol, the stress hormone, creating a more conducive environment for healthy brain development (Panksepp, 2007).

*Play and Social and Emotional Development*

Play provides a platform for children to explore social roles, practice empathy, and develop emotional intelligence. These experiences enhance neural networks related to social cognition and emotional regulation, which are crucial for forming healthy interpersonal relationships (Pellis & Pellis, 2007).

*Play and Cognitive Flexibility and Creativity*

Engaging in imaginative and pretend play fosters cognitive flexibility and creativity. These activities require children to think divergently, solve problems, and adapt to new situations, promoting robust neural connections and cognitive agility (Russ & Wallace, 2013).

## Mirror Neurons, Attachment Theory, and Brain Development

Mirror neurons are specialized brain cells that respond both when an individual performs an action and when they observe the same action performed by another (Rizzolatti & Craighero, 2004). These neurons were first discovered in the premotor cortex of macaque monkeys and have since been identified in humans. They play a critical role in understanding the actions, intentions, and emotions of others, which is foundational to empathy and social learning (Rizzolatti & Craighero, 2004). During early childhood, the brain undergoes significant development, and mirror neurons contribute substantially to this process. Mirror neurons are integral to imitation, a primary mechanism through which children learn new skills and behaviors (Mizrachi & Maor, 2024). Through imitation, children develop motor skills, language, and social behaviors by observing and mimicking adults and peers (Meltzoff & Decety, 2003).

### Mirror Neurons and Brain Development

Mirror neurons are in various brain regions, including the premotor cortex and the inferior parietal lobule (Bonnini et al., 2022). These neurons are essential for imitation learning, a fundamental mechanism for developing social and cognitive skills in children (Iacoboni, 2009). Activating mirror neurons allows children to mimic and internalize behaviors observed in others, which is crucial for learning new skills and understanding social cues.

Research has shown that mirror neurons play a vital role in developing empathy, language acquisition, and motor skills. For example, a study by Rizzolatti and Craighero (2004) highlights that mirror neurons facilitate the understanding of others' actions by mapping observed actions onto the observer's motor system, creating a shared neural representation. This shared representation is crucial for imitation, as it enables children to replicate actions accurately, thereby acquiring new motor skills. Imitation is not limited to motor actions but extends to more complex behaviors, including emotional expressions and social interactions (Gallese, 2003). The role of mirror neurons in language development is also significant, with Iacoboni (2009) suggesting that these neurons contribute to the ability to understand and produce speech by linking the auditory perception of speech sounds with the corresponding motor actions of speech production. This neural mechanism supports the hypothesis that language evolution may have been grounded in the mirror neuron system, facilitating the development of communication skills in humans (Arbib, 2010).

In terms of social cognition, mirror neurons are implicated in the ability to understand and respond to the emotions and intentions of others. A study by Decety and Jackson (2004) indicates that the activation of mirror neurons when observing others' emotional expressions can lead to a similar emotional experience in the observer, fostering empathy. This empathic response is essential for social bonding and effective interpersonal interactions, as it allows individuals to resonate with the emotional states of others.

Mirror neurons are a critical component of the neural architecture underlying imitation learning and social cognition. Their activation enables children to learn new skills, acquire language, and develop empathy, all of which are fundamental for their social and cognitive development. The extensive research on mirror neurons underscores their importance in various aspects of human behavior and highlights their potential implications for understanding developmental disorders and enhancing educational practices.

### Attachment Theory and Mirror Neurons

Attachment theory, developed by John Bowlby, asserts that early interactions with caregivers are crucial for future emotional and social development (Bowlby, 1969, 1988). Mirror neurons play a key role in these interactions by allowing infants to resonate with their caregivers' emotional states (Gallese, 2003). For instance, when a caregiver smiles or shows affection, the infant's mirror neurons activate similar neural circuits, promoting emotional bonding and secure attachment. This mirroring process helps infants internalize and understand their caregivers' emotions and intentions, which is essential for developing empathy and social competence (Siegel, 2012). Secure attachment, formed through sensitive and responsive caregiving, lays the foundation for healthy interpersonal relationships throughout life. When caregivers respond sensitively to their child's needs, the child's mirror neurons help them understand and replicate these nurturing behaviors, reinforcing the attachment bond (Schore, 2012). This early emotional attunement and bonding is critical for the child's overall psychological development and their ability to form healthy relationships in adulthood.

### Play Therapy and Mirror Neurons

Play therapy leverages the natural way children express themselves through play to help them process emotions and experiences. This therapeutic approach takes advantage of the activation of mirror neurons during play, which are crucial for understanding and empathizing with the actions and emotions of others (Gallese et al., 2004). Mirror neurons fire both when an individual performs an action and when they observe the same action performed by another, facilitating empathy and emotional resonance.

During play therapy, children often engage in activities that mirror real-life scenarios, allowing them to reenact and process their internal conflicts in a safe and controlled environment. The activation of mirror neurons enables children to connect with the emotions and actions of their therapists and peers, fostering a deeper understanding of their own experiences and those of others (Gallo-Lopez & Schaefer, 2005). This mirroring effect is essential in helping children externalize their feelings and work through their emotional and psychological challenges.

For instance, when a child sees a therapist demonstrating a coping strategy through play, their mirror neurons are activated, enabling the child to empathize and understand the action on a deeper level. This neural mirroring helps children internalize therapeutic interventions, making them more effective. Additionally, observing peers during group play therapy sessions can also activate mirror neurons, promoting social learning and emotional development (Rizzolatti & Craighero, 2004).

Play therapy provides a non-threatening context for children to explore their feelings and behaviors. The use of toys and imaginative scenarios allows children to project their inner thoughts and emotions onto external objects, making it easier for them to communicate and process complex emotions (Landreth, 2012). The empathetic response generated by mirror neurons during these interactions enhances the therapeutic alliance, helping children feel understood and supported.

Overall, the activation of mirror neurons during play therapy significantly contributes to its effectiveness, allowing children to empathize with others, understand their own emotions, and develop healthier coping mechanisms in a nurturing and supportive environment.

### Mindfulness and Mirror Neurons

Mindfulness practices can significantly enhance children's awareness of their thoughts and emotions and improve their ability to regulate these experiences. Mindfulness involves observing one's own mental states, which parallels the function of mirror neurons in observing and understanding the states of others (Siegel, 2007). Engaging in mindfulness can strengthen neural pathways associated with empathy and self-regulation, contributing to overall emotional and social well-being (Britton et al., 2014). Mindfulness encourages children to pay attention to their inner experiences in a non-judgmental manner, leading to better emotional regulation and stability (Zelazo & Lyons, 2012). The activation of mirror neurons during mindfulness practices allows children to connect with their emotions and those of others, enhancing their capacity for empathy.

Furthermore, mindfulness practices can recalibrate the mirror neuron system, especially in children who have experienced trauma or attachment disruptions, thereby improving their capacity for social connection and empathy (Cozolino, 2014). This recalibration fosters a safer environment for children to process their emotions, leading to improved social and emotional outcomes. By strengthening these neural pathways, mindfulness helps children develop skills necessary for empathy, emotional resilience, and social competence, contributing to their overall psychological well-being (Greenberg & Harris, 2012). Overall, integrating mindfulness practices into children's routines supports the development of empathy, emotional regulation, and resilience, promoting their holistic development and mental health.

## Relational Connections in the Therapeutic Alliance

Mirror neurons facilitate the development of the essential therapeutic alliance between client and therapist by allowing the child to feel understood and mirrored by the therapist, which is essential for building trust and emotional safety (Siegel, 2012). When therapists attune to the child's emotional states and reflect them back through empathetic engagement, the child's mirror neurons activate, strengthening the relational bond. This connection is crucial for effective therapy, as it creates a safe space for the child to explore emotions and behaviors.

Play therapy utilizes children's natural inclination to play and the therapist's ability to engage empathetically. This relational connection can enhance therapy's effectiveness by promoting emotional regulation, social skills, and cognitive development. The presence of a supportive and attuned therapist can help children process and express emotions, leading to therapeutic breakthroughs and long-term benefits (Gaskill & Perry, 2014; Grayson, 2024).

The interplay between mirror neurons, attachment, and therapeutic relationships further highlights the importance of empathy and attunement in child therapy. Mirror neurons play a critical role in observing and understanding the states of others, which is fundamental for empathy and emotional resonance (Gallese et al., 2004). Mindfulness practices, by enhancing self-awareness and emotional regulation, can recalibrate the mirror neuron system, especially in children who have experienced trauma or attachment disruptions, improving their capacity for social connection and empathy (Cozolino, 2014; Siegel, 2007). Integrating these insights into therapeutic practices ensures a holistic approach that leverages the interconnected benefits of mindfulness and play, ultimately supporting the comprehensive development and well-being of children.

## Conclusion

The neurobiological benefits of mindfulness and play support various aspects of children's brain development. By integrating these practices into therapeutic settings, practitioners can offer a comprehensive approach to fostering healthy development and resilience in children, feeling confident in the science literature that explains the why and the how. Mindfulness enhances the functional connectivity between key brain regions like the PFC, amygdala, and hippocampus, promoting better emotional regulation and stress resilience (Tang et al., 2015). Similarly, play stimulates neural pathways and enhances brain plasticity, which is critical for learning, memory, and emotional processing (Ginsburg, 2007; Pellegrini, 2013). Understanding and utilizing the neurobiological mechanisms underlying mindfulness, play, and relational connections can enhance therapeutic outcomes and support children's overall well-being.

# References

Achterberg, E. J. M., & Vanderschuren, L. J. M. J. (2023). The neurobiology of social play behaviour: Past, present and future. *Neuroscience and Biobehavioral Reviews, 152*, 105319. https://doi.org/10.1016/j.neubiorev.2023.105319

Arbib, M. A. (2010). Mirror system activity for action and language is embedded in the integration of dorsal and ventral pathways. *Brain and Language, 112*(1), 12–24. https://doi.org/10.1016/j.bandl.2009.10.001

Bauer, C. C. C., Caballero, C., Scherer, E., West, M. R., Mrazek, M. D., Phillips, D. T., Whitfield-Gabrieli, S., & Gabrieli, J. D. E. (2019). Mindfulness training reduces stress and amygdala reactivity to fearful faces in middle-school children. *Behavioral Neuroscience, 133*(6), 569–585. https://doi.org/10.1037/bne0000337

Burgdorf, J., & Panksepp, J. (2006). The neurobiology of positive emotions. *Neuroscience and Biobehavioral Reviews, 30*(2), 173–187. https://doi.org/10.1016/j.neubiorev.2005.06.001

Biddle, S. J., & Asare, M. (2011). Physical activity and mental health in children and adolescents: A review of reviews. *British Journal of Sports Medicine, 45*(11), 886–895.

Bodrova, E., & Leong, D. J. (2007). *Tools of the mind: The Vygotskian approach to early childhood education* (2nd ed.). Merrill/Prentice Hall.

Bonnini, S., & Borghesi, M. (2022). Relationship between mental health and socio-economic, demographic and environmental factors in the COVID-19 lockdown period—A multivariate regression analysis. *Mathematics, 10*(18), 3237. https://doi.org/10.3390/math10183237

Bowlby, J. (1969). *Attachment and loss: Vol. 1. Attachment*. Basic Books.

Bowlby, J. (1988). *A secure base: Parent–child attachment and healthy human development*. Basic Books.

Bratton, S. C., Ray, D., Rhine, T., & Jones, L. (2005). The efficacy of play therapy with children: A meta-analytic review of treatment outcomes. *Professional Psychology: Research and Practice, 36*(4), 376–390.

Britton, W. B., Lepp, N. E., Niles, H. F., Rocha, T., Fisher, N. E., & Gold, J. S. (2014). A randomized controlled pilot trial of classroom-based mindfulness meditation compared to an active control condition in sixth-grade children. *Journal of School Psychology, 52*(3), 263–278.

Carter, C. S. (2014). Oxytocin pathways and the evolution of human behavior. *Annual Review of Psychology, 65*, 17–39.

Cohen-Cory, S., Kidane, A. H., Shirkey, N. J., & Marshak, S. (2010). Brain-derived neurotrophic factor and the development of structural neuronal connectivity. *Developmental Neurobiology*, *70*(5), 271–288. https://doi.org/10.1002/dneu.20774

Cotman, C. W., Berchtold, N. C., & Christie, L. A. (2007). Exercise builds brain health: Key roles of growth factor cascades and inflammation. *Trends in Neurosciences*, *30*(9), 464–472. https://doi.org/10.1016/j.tins.2007.06.011

Cozolino, L. (2014). *The neuroscience of human relationships: Attachment and the developing social brain* (2nd ed.). Norton.

Creswell, J. D., Way, B. M., Eisenberger, N. I., & Lieberman, M. D. (2007). Neural correlates of dispositional mindfulness during affect labeling. *Psychosomatic Medicine*, *69*(6), 560–565.

Dankiw, K. A., Tsiros, M. D., Baldock, K. L., & Kumar, S. (2020). The impacts of unstructured nature play on health in early childhood development: A systematic review. *PLoS One*, *15*(2), e0229006. https://doi.org/10.1371/journal.pone.0229006

Davidson, R. J., & McEwen, B. S. (2012). Social influences on neuroplasticity: Stress and interventions to promote well-being. *Nature Neuroscience*, *15*(5), 689–695.

Decety, J., & Jackson, P. L. (2004). The functional architecture of human empathy. *Behavioral and Cognitive Neuroscience Reviews*, *3*(2), 71–100.

Diamond, A. (2000). Close interrelation of motor development and cognitive development and of the cerebellum and prefrontal cortex. *Child Development*, *71*(1), 44–56. https://doi.org/10.1111/1467-8624.00117

Diamond, A., & Lee, K. (2011). Interventions shown to aid executive function development in children 4 to 12 years old. *Science*, *333*(6045), 959–964.

Fisher, K. R. (2019). The impact of play on development. In S. A. Kessler (Ed.), *Contemporary perspectives on play in early childhood education* (pp. 43–61). Peter Lang Publishing.

Fleer, M. (2021). Play in the early years. *Early Childhood Research Quarterly*, *55*, 1–10.

Frost, J. L. (2012). The changing culture of play. *International Journal of Play*, *1*(2), 117–130. https://doi.org/10.1080/21594937.2012.698461

Gallese, V. (2003). The roots of empathy: The shared manifold hypothesis and the neural basis of intersubjectivity. *Psychopathology*, *36*(4), 171–180.

Gallese, V., Keysers, C., & Rizzolatti, G. (2004). A unifying view of the basis of social cognition. *Trends in Cognitive Sciences*, *8*(9), 396–403. https://doi.org/10.1016/j.tics.2004.07.002

Gallo-Lopez, L., & Schaefer, C. E. (2005). *Play therapy with children in crisis* (3rd ed.). Guilford Press.

Gaskill, R., & Perry, B. (2014). The neurobiological power of play: Using the neurosequential model of therapeutics to guide play in the healing process. In C. A. Malchiodi & D. A. Crenshaw (Eds.), *Creative arts and play therapy for attachment problems* (pp. 178–194). The Guilford Press.

Ginsburg, K. R. (2007). The importance of play in promoting healthy child development and maintaining strong parent-child bonds. *Pediatrics*, *119*(1), 182–191.

Goldberg, S. (2022). The role of neuroplasticity in mindfulness practices: A review. *Mindfulness and Neuroplasticity Journal*, *10*(2), 110–126.

Golinkoff, R. M., & Hirsh-Pasek, K. (2006). Baby wordsmith: From associationist to social sophisticate. *Current Directions in Psychological Science*, *15*(1), 30–33.

Göncü, A., & Gauvain, M. (2012). Sociocultural approaches to educational psychology: Theory, research, and application. In K. R. Harris, S. Graham, T. Urdan, C. B. McCormick, G. M. Sinatra, & J. Sweller (Eds.), *APA educational psychology handbook, Vol. 1. Theories, constructs, and critical issues* (pp. 125–154). American Psychological Association. https://doi.org/10.1037/13273-006

Gray, P. (2013). *Free to learn: Why unleashing the instinct to play will make our children happier, more self-reliant, and better students for life.* Basic Books.

Grayson, D. (2024). Therapeutic play and the development of neural pathways. *Journal of Child Psychology and Psychiatry, 65*(4), 459–475.

Greenberg, M. T., & Harris, A. R. (2012). Nurturing mindfulness in children and youth: Current state of research. *Child Development Perspectives, 6*(2), 161–166.

Gunter, K. B., Almstedt, H. C., & Janz, K. F. (2012). Physical activity in childhood may be the key to optimizing lifespan skeletal health. *Exercise and Sport Sciences Reviews, 40*(1), 13–21.

Hoffmann, J., & Russ, S. W. (2016). Pretend play, creativity, and emotion regulation in children. *Psychology of Aesthetics, Creativity, and the Arts, 10*(3), 296–308.

Hirsh-Pasek, K., Golinkoff, R. M., Berk, L. E., & Singer, D. G. (2009). *A mandate for playful learning in preschool: Presenting the evidence.* Oxford University Press.

Hölzel, B. K., Carmody, J., Vangel, M., Congleton, C., Yerramsetti, S. M., Gard, T., & Lazar, S. W. (2011). Mindfulness practice leads to increases in regional brain gray matter density. *Psychiatry Research: Neuroimaging, 191*(1), 36–43.

Iacoboni, M. (2009). Imitation, empathy, and mirror neurons. *Annual Review of Psychology, 60*, 653–670.

Janssen, I., & LeBlanc, A. G. (2010). Systematic review of the health benefits of physical activity and fitness in school-aged children and youth. *International Journal of Behavioral Nutrition and Physical Activity, 7*(1), 40.

Kadosh, K. C. (2013). Neuroplasticity in child development: The role of the prefrontal cortex. *Developmental Neuroscience, 35*(5), 449–462.

Kjaer, T. W., Bertelsen, C., Piccini, P., Brooks, D., Alving, J., & Lou, H. C. (2002). Increased dopamine tone during meditation-induced change of consciousness. *Brain Research. Cognitive Brain Research, 13*(2), 255–259. https://doi.org/10.1016/s0926-6410(01)00106-9

Landreth, G. L. (2012). *Play therapy: The art of the relationship.* Routledge.

Lillard, A. S., Lerner, M. D., Hopkins, E. J., Dore, R. A., Smith, E. D., & Palmquist, C. M. (2013). The impact of pretend play on children's development: A review of the evidence. *Psychological Bulletin, 139*(1), 1–34. https://doi.org/10.1037/a0029321

McEwen, B. S., & Morrison, J. H. (2013). The brain on stress: Vulnerability and plasticity of the prefrontal cortex over the life course. *Neuron, 79*(1), 16–29. https://doi.org/10.1016/j.neuron.2013.06.028

Meltzoff, A. N., & Decety, J. (2003). What imitation tells us about social cognition: A rapprochement between developmental psychology and cognitive neuroscience. *Philosophical Transactions of the Royal Society of London. Series B: Biological Sciences, 358*(1431), 491–500.

Miller, E., & Almon, J. (2009). *Crisis in the kindergarten: Why children need to play in school.* Alliance for Childhood.

Milteer, R. M., Ginsburg, K. R., & Mulligan, D. A. (2012). The importance of play in promoting healthy child development and maintaining strong parent-child bonds. *Pediatrics, 129*(1), e204–e213.

Mizrachi, H., & Maor, G. (2024). Shadow theater for children with ASD: The integrative role of mirror neurons, empathy, and social learning to facilitate self-regulation. *Education & Training in Autism & Developmental Disabilities, 59*(2), 179.

Nielsen, T. (2012). Social play and development in children. *Child Development Perspectives, 6*(4), 244–251.

Panksepp, J. (2007). Neuroevolutionary sources of laughter and social joy: Modeling primal human laughter in laboratory rats. *Behavioral Brain Research, 182*(2), 231–244.

Pellegrini, A. D. (2013). *The role of play in human development.* Oxford University Press.

Pellis, S., & Pellis, V. (2013). *The playful brain: Venturing to the limits of neuroscience*. Simon and Schuster.

Pellis, S. M., & Pellis, V. C. (2007). Rough-and-tumble play and the development of the social brain. Current Directions in Psychological Science, *Sage Journal, 16*(2), 95–98. https://doi.org/10.1111/j.1467-8721.2007.00483.x

Rizzolatti, G., & Craighero, L. (2004). The mirror-neuron system. *Annual Review of Neuroscience, 27*, 169–192.

Roeser, R. W., Schonert-Reichl, K. A., Jha, A., Cullen, M., Wallace, L., Wilensky, R., Oberle, E., Thomson, K., Taylor, C., & Harrison, J. (2013). Mindfulness training and reductions in teacher stress and burnout: Results from two randomized, wait-list-control field trials. *Journal of Educational Psychology, 105*(3), 787–804.

Rushton, S., Eitelgeorge, J., & Zickafoose, R. (2010). Connecting neuroscience, cognitive, and educational theories and applying them to the classroom. *Educational Psychology Review, 22*(1), 49–70.

Russ, S. W., & Wallace, C. E. (2013). Pretend play and creative processes. *American Journal of Play, 6*(1), 136–148.

Schore, A. N. (2012). *The science of the art of psychotherapy*. W. W. Norton & Company.

Siegel, D. J. (2007). *The mindful brain: Reflection and attunement in the cultivation of well-being*. Norton.

Siegel, D. J. (2012). *The developing mind: How relationships and the brain interact to shape who we are* (2nd ed.). Guilford Press.

Slopen, N., McLaughlin, K. A., & Shonkoff, J. P. (2014). Interventions to improve cortisol regulation in children: A systematic review. *Pediatrics, 133*(2), 312–326. https://doi.org/10.1542/peds.2013-1632

Souto-Manning, M. (2017). Is play a privilege or a right? And what's our responsibility? On the role of play for equity in early childhood education. *Early Child Development and Care, 187*(5–6), 785–787.

Stipek, D. J., Feiler, R., Byler, P., Ryan, R., Milburn, S., & Salmon, J. M. (1998). Good beginnings: What difference does the program make in preparing young children for school? *Journal of Applied Developmental Psychology, 19*(1), 41–66.

Stodden, D. F., Goodway, J. D., Langendorfer, S. J., Roberton, M. A., Rudisill, M. E., Garcia, C., & Garcia, L. E. (2008). A developmental perspective on the role of motor skill competence in physical activity: An emergent relationship. *Quest, 60*(2), 290–306.

Tang, Y. Y., Hölzel, B. K., & Posner, M. I. (2015). The neuroscience of mindfulness meditation. *Nature Reviews Neuroscience, 16*(4), 213–225.

Tang, Y. Y., Ma, Y., Wang, J., Fan, Y., Feng, S., Lu, Q., Yu, Q., Sui, D., Rothbart, M. K., Fan, M. & Posner, M. I. (2007). Short-term meditation training improves attention and self-regulation. *Proceedings of the national Academy of Sciences, 104*(43), 17152–17156.

Tang, Y. Y., Rothbart, M. K., & Posner, M. I. (2012). Neural correlates of establishing, maintaining, and switching brain states. *Trends in Cognitive Sciences, 16*(6), 330–337.

Telama, R., Yang, X., Viikari, J., Välimäki, I., Wanne, O., & Raitakari, O. (2005). Physical activity from childhood to adulthood: A 21-year tracking study. *American Journal of Preventive Medicine, 28*(3), 267–273.

Tremblay, M. S., LeBlanc, A. G., Kho, M. E., Saunders, T. J., Larouche, R., Colley, R. C., Goldfield, G., & Gorber, S. C. (2011). Systematic review of sedentary behaviour and health indicators in school-aged children and youth. *International Journal of Behavioral Nutrition and Physical Activity, 8*(1), 98. https://doi.org/10.1186/1479-5868-8-98

Trezza, V., Baarendse, P. J., & Vanderschuren, L. J. (2010). The pleasures of play: Pharmacological insights into social reward mechanisms. *Trends in Pharmacological Sciences, 31*(10), 463–469.

Vanderschuren, L. J., Achterberg, E. J., & Trezza, V. (2016). The neurobiology of social play and its rewarding value in rats. *Neuroscience and Biobehavioral Reviews, 70,* 86–105. https://doi.org/10.1016/j.neubiorev.2016.07.025

Vaynman, S., Ying, Z., & Gomez-Pinilla, F. (2004). Hippocampal BDNF mediates the efficacy of exercise on synaptic plasticity and cognition. *The European Journal of Neuroscience, 20*(10), 2580–2590. https://doi.org/10.1111/j.1460-9568.2004.03720.x

Vygotsky, L. S. (1978). *Mind in society: The development of higher psychological processes.* Harvard University Press.

Weisberg, D. S., Hirsh-Pasek, K., & Golinkoff, R. M. (2013). Embracing complexity: Rethinking the relation between play and learning: Comment on Lillard et al. (2013). *Psychological Bulletin, 139*(1), 35–39. https://doi.org/10.1037/a0030077

Wonders, L. L. (2022). Cultivating mindfulness through use of nature in play therapy. In *Nature-based play and expressive therapies* (pp. 113–126). Routledge.

Young, S. N. (2007). How to increase serotonin in the human brain without drugs. *Journal of Psychiatry & Neuroscience, 32*(6), 394–399. https://www.ncbi.nlm.nih.gov/pmc/articles/PMC2077351/

Zeidan, F., Johnson, S. K., Diamond, B. J., David, Z., & Goolkasian, P. (2010). Mindfulness meditation improves cognition: Evidence of brief mental training. *Consciousness and Cognition, 19*(2), 597–605. https://doi.org/10.1016/j.concog.2010.03.014

Zelazo, P. D., & Lyons, K. E. (2012). The potential benefits of mindfulness training in early childhood: A developmental social cognitive neuroscience perspective. *Child Development Perspectives, 6*(2), 154–160. https://doi.org/10.1111/j.1750-8606.2012.00241.x

Zenner, C., Herrnleben-Kurz, S., & Walach, H. (2014). Mindfulness-based interventions in schools-a systematic review and meta-analysis. *Frontiers in Psychology, 5,* 603. https://doi.org/10.3389/fpsyg.2014.00603

Zigler, E., Singer, D. G., & Bishop-Josef, S. J. (2004). *Children's play: The roots of reading* (1st ed.). Zero to Three Press. http://catalog.hathitrust.org/api/volumes/oclc/53967066.html

# 4

# THE ROLE OF MINDFULNESS IN ENHANCING THERAPEUTIC ALLIANCE

## Introduction

A strong therapeutic alliance is recognized as a cornerstone of effective psychotherapy (Anderson & Perlman, 2020; Aponte, 2022; Eubanks & Babl, 2024; Macneil et al., 2009; Krupnik, 2023). Before we dive more deeply into the therapeutic alliance's specific interest in play therapy and why mindfulness is such a vital component, it's important to understand the therapeutic alliance as a concept in the context of the history of psychotherapy. In this chapter, we will explore the importance of therapeutic alliance as commonly agreed to be an essential factor, if not the most essential factor, in the effectiveness of all psychotherapy regardless of the theoretical orientation.

## Common Factors Theory

The common factors theory says that certain elements, such as the therapeutic alliance, empathy, and the therapist's positive regard, are more predictive of successful therapy outcomes than the specific techniques used (Eubanks & Babl, 2024). This theory suggests that these common factors are present across various therapeutic approaches and are essential for effective treatment. Although randomized controlled trials have yet to prove that the therapeutic relationship is the sole basis for effective

DOI: 10.4324/9781003468585-4

therapy, research indicates a strong correlation between this alliance and positive outcomes (Koole & Tschacher, 2016).

Key elements of the common factors theory include the following.

### Therapeutic Alliance

As previously mentioned, the collaborative and affective bond between therapist and client is central.

### Empathy

The therapist's ability to understand and share the feelings of the client.

### Positive Regard

The therapist's acceptance and support of the client, regardless of what the client says or does.

### Therapeutic Presence

The therapist's ability to be fully present and engaged with the client during sessions. This perspective emphasizes that the therapist-client relationship is a primary driver of therapeutic success, highlighting the importance of fostering a strong alliance in all therapeutic contexts. By focusing on these common factors, therapists can enhance the effectiveness of their interventions, regardless of their theoretical orientation.

## The Importance of Therapeutic Alliance in Psychotherapy

The theory of therapeutic alliance as a common factor in psychotherapy suggests that the relationship quality between therapist and client is the primary determinant of therapeutic success, transcending the specific theoretical orientation or techniques employed (Eubanks & Babl, 2024). This perspective, supported by extensive research and meta-analyses (Ahn & Wamphold, 1997; Bailey & Ogles, 2023; Benish et al., 2007; Laska et al., 2014; Wamphold, 2010), supposes that elements such as empathy, trust, mutual respect, and collaboration are universal drivers of positive outcomes in therapy. Prominent researchers like Carl Rogers (1942), along with John Norcross and Bruce Wampold (2010), have demonstrated that the therapist's ability to form a strong, supportive bond with the client significantly impacts the effectiveness of treatment. The common factors theory underscores that regardless of whether a therapist practices cognitive-behavioral therapy, psychodynamic therapy, humanistic therapy, or any other modality, the therapeutic alliance remains the key element in facilitating meaningful change and healing for clients (Castonguay et al., 2010; Flückiger et al., 2018). In cognitive-behavioral therapy, for example, the quality of the therapeutic alliance significantly predicts treatment success, as it does in psychodynamic and humanistic therapies. This suggests that while the specific techniques of each modality are important, the relational factors shared across therapies play a crucial role in the healing process (Castonguay et al., 2006). The robust empirical support for the common factors theory highlights the importance of focusing on the therapeutic alliance to enhance therapy effectiveness, regardless of the specific therapeutic approach used (Flückiger et al., 2012; Horvath et al., 2011). This alliance, characterized by trust, mutual respect, and collaboration between therapist and client, significantly influences treatment outcomes across various modalities, including play therapy. A positive therapeutic alliance enhances client engagement, fosters trust, and provides a secure base for exploring difficult emotions and experiences.

### The Therapeutic Alliance: Definition and Key Components

The therapeutic alliance refers to the collaborative and affective bond between therapist and client, a fundamental aspect of effective psychotherapy (Rodgers et al., 2010). This alliance is crucial for facilitating client engagement and promoting positive therapeutic outcomes (Horvath et al., 2011). It involves three primary components.

### Agreement on Goals

Both therapist and client share a mutual understanding and agreement on the goals of therapy. This agreement ensures that both parties are working toward the same objectives, essential for maintaining focus and direction in the therapeutic process. Research highlights that goal agreement positively correlates with therapy outcomes, aligning the therapist's interventions with the client's needs and expectations (Bordin, 1979; Tryon & Winograd, 2011).

*Agreement on Tasks*

They also agree on the tasks or interventions that will be used to achieve these goals. This component involves collaborative discussions about the therapeutic techniques and strategies that will be employed, ensuring that the client is actively involved in their treatment plan. Studies have shown that when clients understand and agree with the therapeutic tasks, their motivation and commitment to the process increase, leading to better outcomes (Kazantzis et al., 2010).

*Bond*

There is an emotional bond characterized by mutual trust, respect, and confidence in each other. This bond is built through empathic listening, validation, and genuine positive regard from the therapist. The strength of the therapeutic bond is a significant predictor of therapy success, as it creates a safe and supportive environment where clients feel understood and validated (Norcross & Lambert, 2018). A strong emotional bond helps clients to open and engage deeply in the therapeutic process, facilitating personal growth and healing (Flückiger et al., 2012).

These components work together to create a supportive environment where clients feel understood and validated, which is crucial for the therapeutic process. The therapeutic alliance is considered one of the most robust predictors of treatment success across different therapeutic modalities (Wampold & Imel, 2015). It underscores the importance of a collaborative, goal-oriented, and emotionally supportive relationship in fostering effective therapy.

### Research Evidence Supporting the Therapeutic Alliance

Meta-analyses have consistently shown that the quality of the therapist-client relationship accounts for a substantial portion of the variance in therapy outcomes, regardless of the specific therapeutic modality employed (Ahn & Wamphold, 1997; Bailey & Ogles, 2023; Benish et al., 2007; Elliott et al., 2018; Gelso et al., 2018; Laska et al., 2014; Martin et al., 2000; Stubbe, 2007; Wamphold, 2010). This indicates that the strength of the therapeutic alliance is a critical predictor of treatment success.

Studies by prominent researchers such as Carl Rogers (1942) and John Norcross with Bruce Wampold (2010) highlight the critical components of this relationship, including empathy, warmth, and genuineness.

*Carl Rogers* (1942) emphasized the importance of unconditional positive regard, empathy, and congruence (genuineness) as fundamental therapist qualities. He believed that these elements create a growth-promoting climate that facilitates change.

*John Norcross* (2011) has extensively researched the impact of the therapeutic relationship on treatment outcomes, finding that the alliance is a robust predictor of success across different therapeutic approaches.

*Bruce Wampold* (2010) has contributed significantly to understanding the common factors that contribute to effective psychotherapy. His research shows that the therapist-client relationship is one of the most important elements influencing outcomes, often outweighing the specific techniques used.

Crenshaw and Kenney-Noziska (2014) discuss how the topic of therapeutic presence has not been given as much consideration in the sub-field of play therapy as it has in the larger field of psychotherapy with adults noting the exceptions of Virginia Axline, Clark Moustakas, and Garry Landreth, all influenced by Carl Rogers' person-centered psychotherapy theoretical orientation. Rogers' publications not only highlighted the significance of the therapeutic relationship but also conducted pioneering research that established the therapist's warmth, empathy, and genuineness as fundamental elements of the therapeutic relationship (Crenshaw & Kenney-Noziska, 2014). The quality of a therapist's therapeutic presence in session with a client is a determining factor of the quality of the therapeutic relationship. Mindfulness practiced by the therapist with the client lends to the quality of therapeutic presence.

## Application across Therapeutic Modalities

According to common factors theory, the importance of the therapeutic alliance transcends specific therapeutic modalities, making it a universal element of effective therapy (Eubanks & Babl, 2024). Regardless of a therapist's chosen theoretical orientation, the quality of the therapist-client relationship remains a key determinant of successful outcomes. For example, in CBT, the therapeutic alliance helps clients feel safe and supported as they challenge and change maladaptive thoughts and behaviors. In psychodynamic therapy, a strong alliance allows clients to explore unconscious processes and past experiences within a secure and trusting relationship. In humanistic therapy, the emphasis on empathy, unconditional positive regard, and congruence directly aligns with the principles of a strong therapeutic alliance. In all of play therapy, the therapist's ability to create a warm, accepting, and attuned relationship with the child in the playroom is essential for facilitating emotional expression and healing (Crenshaw & Kenney-Noziska, 2014).

## Enhancing the Therapeutic Alliance through Mindfulness

Mindfulness practices can significantly enhance the therapeutic alliance by improving the therapist's capacity for presence, empathy, and attunement. By cultivating mindfulness, therapists can develop greater self-awareness and emotional regulation, which in turn allows them to be more fully present and engaged with their clients. This presence is crucial for building a strong therapeutic alliance, as it conveys to clients that they are seen, heard, and valued. Mindfulness itself has been regarded as a common factor and a core psychotherapy process that is achieved through a collaborative process between therapist and client within all psychotherapy orientations (Martin, 1997).

Mindfulness practices, as explained in Chapter 2, help therapists stay grounded and focused during sessions with clients. This increased presence enhances the therapist's ability to attune to the client's emotional state and respond with greater empathy and sensitivity. By being more attuned, therapists can better understand and address the client's needs, fostering a deeper and more meaningful therapeutic relationship.

The therapeutic alliance is a universally recognized common factor in effective psychotherapy, crucial for achieving positive treatment outcomes. Research (Bratton et al., 2005; Jensen et al., 2017; McBride & Greeson, 2023) consistently demonstrates that the quality of the therapist-client relationship significantly influences therapeutic success, regardless of the specific modality employed. The common factors theory highlights the importance of elements such as empathy, warmth, and positive regard, which are central to building a strong alliance. By focusing on these common factors and incorporating mindfulness practices, therapists can enhance their capacity to create a supportive and collaborative therapeutic environment, ultimately facilitating more effective and meaningful therapeutic interventions.

## The Therapeutic Relationship in Play Therapy

The significance of the therapeutic relationship in play therapy was first articulated by Virginia Axline (1947) in her pioneering work. Axline (1947) emphasized that a genuine, accepting, and empathic relationship is the foundation for effective therapeutic intervention with children. Her principles of play therapy underscore the importance of the therapist's ability to create a non-judgmental and supportive environment where children can freely express themselves and explore their emotions.

Axline's (1947) Eight Principles of non-directive play therapy highlight the importance of therapist qualities such as warmth, acceptance, and permissiveness. These principles lay the groundwork for creating a therapeutic space where children feel safe and understood, allowing them to engage in the therapeutic process fully. According to Axline (1947), the therapeutic relationship must be built on the following principles:

1. Developing a warm and friendly relationship with the child.
2. Accepting the child unconditionally, without judgment.
3. Creating a permissive environment where the child feels free to express thoughts and feelings.
4. Recognizing and reflecting the child's feelings to promote self-understanding.
5. Maintaining respect for the child's ability to solve their own problems.
6. Refraining from directing the child's actions or conversation.
7. Allowing the child to lead the way in the play process.
8. Establishing therapeutic limits to anchor the therapy to the real world.

Garry Landreth (2012) further emphasized the centrality of the therapeutic relationship in play therapy. In his seminal text, *Play Therapy:*

*The Art of the Relationship*, Landreth (2012) asserts that the quality of the therapist-client relationship is the most critical factor in facilitating therapeutic change. He introduces the concept of "therapeutic presence," which involves the therapist being fully attuned to the child in the moment, providing a consistent and supportive presence that fosters trust and security. Landreth (2012) describes therapeutic presence as the therapist's ability to be fully engaged, emotionally available, and responsive to the child's needs and expressions during sessions. This presence helps create a safe space where the child feels valued and understood, which is essential for effective therapy.

Landreth (2012) also highlights the importance of creating a permissive and accepting environment, where children can explore their feelings and experiences without fear of judgment. He emphasizes that the therapeutic relationship itself is a powerful agent of change, asserting that the genuine, empathetic connection between therapist and child facilitates the child's emotional healing and growth. According to Landreth (2012), the therapist's role is to provide unconditional positive regard, empathy, and congruence, mirroring the child's emotions and experiences to foster self-awareness and self-acceptance.

Dee Ray (2011), in her book *Advanced Play Therapy*, builds upon Landreth's (1991) foundation by exploring the nuances and complexities of the therapeutic relationship in greater depth. Ray (2011) emphasizes that the therapeutic relationship in play therapy is not just a backdrop for interventions but is an active, dynamic process that requires continuous attention and nurturing. She discusses the concept of "relational safety," which involves creating an environment where the child feels emotionally secure enough to explore difficult and painful experiences. Ray (2011) argues that this sense of safety is fundamental to the therapeutic process and is cultivated through the therapist's attunement, responsiveness, and authenticity.

Ray (2011) also delves into the importance of cultural competence and sensitivity in building and maintaining the therapeutic relationship. She highlights that therapists must be aware of and respect the cultural backgrounds and unique experiences of each child, adapting their approach to meet the diverse needs of their clients. By doing so, therapists can foster a more inclusive and supportive therapeutic environment.

Ray (2011) explores the role of countertransference in the therapeutic relationship, emphasizing the need for therapists to be aware of their own emotional responses and biases. She provides strategies for managing countertransference, such as self-reflection, supervision, and ongoing professional development, to ensure that the therapist's reactions do not interfere with the therapeutic process.

VanFleet et al. (2010), in *Child-Centered Play Therapy*, add another layer of depth to the understanding of the therapeutic relationship. VanFleet et al. (2010) emphasize the importance of a strong, supportive relationship as the foundation for all therapeutic work with children. She discusses the principles of child-centered play therapy, which prioritize the child's autonomy and capacity for self-directed healing within the context of a nurturing relationship. VanFleet et al. (2010) highlight that the therapist's role is to provide a safe, accepting, and empathetic environment where children can freely express themselves and work through their issues at their own pace.

VanFleet et al. (2010) also explore the practical aspects of building and maintaining a therapeutic relationship, offering detailed guidance on how therapists can communicate acceptance and understanding to the child. She stresses the importance of consistent, non-judgmental engagement and the therapist's ability to genuinely connect with the child. This connection helps the child feel respected and valued, which is crucial for fostering trust and facilitating therapeutic progress.

Axline (1947), Landreth (2012), Ray (2011), and VanFleet et al. (2010) highlight the transformative power of the therapeutic relationship in play therapy. Their works emphasize the importance of empathy, presence, and attunement in creating a therapeutic alliance that supports the child's emotional and psychological growth. By focusing on these relational qualities, therapists can facilitate more effective and meaningful therapeutic interventions, helping children navigate their emotional landscapes and achieve greater well-being.

Lisa Dion (2018), the founder and teacher of Synergetic Play Therapy® (SPT), places significant emphasis on the quality of the therapist-client relationship and the critical role of attunement to self and other in the moment together in therapy. In her work, Dion (2018) posits that therapeutic attunement is the foundation of effective therapy, asserting that genuine, attuned connections between therapist and child are essential for facilitating healing and growth. Attunement, in the context of SPT, involves the therapist's ability to be fully present with the child, accurately sensing and responding to the therapist's own internal responses and sensations as well as the child's emotional and physiological states. This deep level of attunement helps co-regulate the child's nervous system, creating a sense of safety and trust.

Dion (2018) explains that through attunement, therapists can reflect the child's internal experiences more accurately, thereby validating and supporting the child's emotional world. This process not only strengthens the therapeutic alliance but also empowers children to process and integrate their experiences more effectively. Dion (2018) emphasizes that the therapist's ability to attune is greatly enhanced by the practice of mindfulness. Mindfulness helps therapists maintain a state of regulation and presence, allowing them to be more attuned, receptive, and responsive to the child's needs as presented in session.

In her teachings, Dion (2018) advocates for therapists to use mindfulness techniques to improve their emotional regulation and presence during sessions. Practices such as mindful breathing, body awareness, self-regulation, mindful movement, and meditation enable therapists to remain grounded and centered, which is crucial for maintaining attunement with the child. By cultivating mindfulness, therapists can better manage their own emotional responses and stay fully engaged with the child, even in the face of challenging behaviors or intense emotional expressions.

Dion (2018) also highlights the importance of self-awareness in the therapeutic process. She encourages therapists to use mindfulness to become more aware of their own internal states and potential triggers, which can affect their ability to attune to the child. By staying mindful, therapists can ensure that their own emotional reactions do not interfere with the therapeutic process, allowing them to provide a more supportive and empathetic presence.

Dion and Norton (2024) discuss how the therapeutic relationship in SPT is not just about using specific techniques but about the therapist's authentic engagement and emotional presence. They stress that the therapist must be attuned to their own internal experiences to effectively attune to the child, facilitating a collaborative and healing environment. This approach underscores the importance of the therapist's self-regulation and authenticity in modeling healthy emotional responses for the child (Dion & Norton, 2024).

These insights align with broader research on the therapeutic alliance, which consistently finds that the quality of the therapeutic relationship, characterized by trust, empathy, and attunement, is a key determinant of successful therapy outcomes across various modalities (Flückiger et al., 2012; Horvath et al., 2011).

## Mindfulness and Therapeutic Presence

Axline (1947), Landreth (2012), Ray (2011), VanFleet et al. (2010), and Dion (2018, 2024) all emphasize the idea that the therapeutic relationship itself is a powerful agent of change. They all point to the therapist's ability to be fully present, accepting, and empathetic creating a space where children can explore their feelings and experiences without fear of judgment. This quality of therapeutic presence is at the heart of effective play therapy and is enhanced through the practice of mindfulness.

Mindfulness practice helps therapists develop that deeper level of presence. Mindfulness practice increases the therapist's capacity to stay grounded and focused, allowing them to be fully present with the child during sessions. This presence is crucial for building a strong therapeutic alliance, as it conveys to the child that they are seen, heard, and valued.

By practicing mindfulness, therapists can cultivate a state of non-judgmental awareness, which enhances their ability to empathize with and attune to the child's emotional state. This empathetic attunement is essential for creating a therapeutic environment where the child feels safe to express themselves. Mindfulness allows therapists to be more attuned to the subtle cues of the child's behavior, helping them respond with greater sensitivity and understanding.

Mindfulness also plays a critical role in helping therapists manage their own emotional responses. Therapists often encounter emotional expressions and externalizing behaviors in child clients, or challenging dynamics with caregivers which can create high levels of stress for therapists. Mindfulness practices can help therapists maintain emotional balance, reducing the risk of burnout and enhancing their capacity to provide consistent support. By staying calm and composed, therapists can model emotional regulation for the child, further reinforcing the therapeutic alliance.

### Enhancing Empathy and Attunement

Empathy and attunement are key components of the therapeutic alliance, particularly in play therapy. Mindfulness enhances these qualities by fostering a state of open, non-judgmental awareness. When therapists practice mindfulness, they become more attuned to their own internal experiences, which in turn helps them attune to the experiences of their clients. This heightened attunement allows therapists to respond to the child's needs in a more empathic and understanding manner.

Mindfulness also enhances the therapist's ability to stay present and fully engaged during sessions. This presence is crucial in play therapy, where the child relies on the therapist to provide a safe and consistent environment. By being fully present, therapists can better understand the child's play and the underlying emotions and experiences being expressed. This deeper understanding helps build trust and rapport, strengthening the therapeutic alliance.

### Building a Safe and Supportive Environment

A strong therapeutic alliance in play therapy is built on creating a safe and supportive environment where children feel free to express themselves. Mindfulness helps therapists cultivate the qualities necessary to create such an environment. By practicing mindfulness, therapists can develop greater patience, acceptance, and compassion, which are essential for building a trusting relationship with the child.

In a mindful state, therapists are better able to create a non-judgmental space where children can explore their feelings and experiences without fear of criticism or rejection. This non-judgmental approach helps children feel understood and accepted, which is crucial for their emotional and psychological well-being. By fostering a safe and supportive environment, therapists can facilitate deeper emotional exploration and healing for the child.

## Conclusion

The quality of the therapist-client relationship significantly influences therapeutic outcomes, with empathy, presence, and attunement being key components. Mindfulness practices enhance these qualities, enabling therapists to create a safe, supportive, and non-judgmental therapeutic environment. By fostering a strong therapeutic alliance through mindfulness, therapists can facilitate more effective and meaningful therapeutic interventions for children and families.

Mindfulness enhances the therapist's capacity for presence, empathy, and attunement, all of which are essential for creating a strong therapeutic alliance. By practicing mindfulness, therapists can create a safe and supportive environment where children feel seen, heard, and valued. This strong therapeutic alliance is the foundation for effective play therapy, allowing for deeper emotional exploration and healing. On this foundation, we can now examine the transtheoretical nature of Mindfulness-based Play Therapy® by demonstrating how mindfulness easily interfaces with all of the seminal and historically significant play therapy theories as established by the Association for Play Therapy (Association for Play Therapy, n.d.).

## References

Ahn, H., & Wamphold, B. (1997). Where oh where are the specific ingredients? A meta-analysis of component studies in counseling and psychotherapy. *Journal of Counseling Psychology, 48*(3), 251–257.

Anderson, T., & Perlman, M. R. (2020). Therapeutic interpersonal skills for facilitating the working alliance. In J. N. Fuertes (Ed.), *Working alliance skills for mental health professionals* (pp. 43–68). Oxford University Press. https://doi.org/10.1093/med-psych/9780190868529.003.0003

Aponte, H. J. (2022). The soul of therapy: The therapist's use of self in the therapeutic relationship. *Contemporary Family Therapy, 44*(2), 136–143.

Association for Play therapy. (n.d.). https://www.a4pt.org/general/custom.asp?page=Publications

Axline, V. M. (1947). *Play therapy: The inner dynamics of childhood.* Houghton Mifflin.

Bailey, R. J., & Ogles, B. M. (2023). *Common factors therapy: A principle-based treatment framework.* American Psychological Association.

Benish, S. G., Imel, Z. E., & Wampold, B. E. (2007). The relative efficacy of bona fide psychotherapies for treating post-traumatic stress disorder: A meta-analysis of direct comparisons. *Clinical Psychology Review, 28*(6), 746–759.

Bordin, E. S. (1979). The generalizability of the psychoanalytic concept of the working alliance. *Psychotherapy: Theory, Research, & Practice, 16*(3), 252–260.

Bratton, S. C., Ray, D., Rhine, T., & Jones, L. (2005). The efficacy of play therapy with children: A meta-analytic review of treatment outcomes. *Professional Psychology: Research and Practice, 36*(4), 376–390.

Castonguay, L. G., Constantino, M. J., & Grosse Holtforth, M. (2006). The therapeutic alliance: Research and theory. In J. C. Norcross, L. E. Beutler, & R. F. Levant (Eds.), *Psychotherapy research: A handbook for practitioners.* Oxford University Press.

Castonguay, L. G., Constantino, M. J., McAleavey, A. A., & Goldfried, M. R. (2010). The therapeutic alliance in cognitive-behavioral therapy. In J. C. Muran & J. P. Barber (Eds.), *The therapeutic alliance: An evidence-based guide to practice* (pp. 150–171). The Guilford Press.

Crenshaw, D. A., & Kenney-Noziska, S. (2014). Therapeutic presence in play therapy. *International Journal of Play Therapy, 23*(1), 31–43.

Dion, L. (2018). *Synergetic play therapy: How to guide the child to success.* Norton.

Dion, L., & Norton, R. (2024). A synergetic play therapy® approach to treatment planning. In L. L. Wonders & M. L. Affee (Eds.), *Play therapy treatment planning with children and families.* Routledge.

Elliott, R., Watson, J., Greenberg, L. S., & Timulak, L. (2018). Therapist empathy and client outcome: An updated meta-analysis. *Psychotherapy, 55*(4), 399–410.

Eubanks, C. F., & Babl, A. (2024). Are common factors responsible for therapeutic change? In F. T. L. Leong, J. L. Callahan, M. J. Constantino, & C. F. Eubanks (Eds.), *APA handbook of psychotherapy: Evidence-based practice, practice-based evidence, and contextual participant-driven practice* (pp. 43–61). American Psychological Association.

Flückiger, C., Del Re, A. C., Wampold, B. E., & Horvath, A. O. (2018). The alliance in adult psychotherapy: A meta-analytic synthesis. *Psychotherapy, 55*(4), 316–340.

Flückiger, C., Del Re, A. C., Wampold, B., Symmonds, D., & O Horath, A. (2012). The alliance in adult psychotherapy: A meta-analytic synthesis. *Psychotherapy, 55*(4), 316–340.

Gelso, C. J., Kivlighan, D. M., & Markin, R. D. (2018). The real relationship and its role in psychotherapy outcome: A meta-analysis. *Psychotherapy, 55*, 434–444. https://doi.org/10.1037/pst0000183

Horvath, A. O., Del Re, A. C., Flückiger, C., & Symonds, D. (2011). Alliance in individual psychotherapy. *Psychotherapy (Chicago, Ill.), 48*(1), 9–16. https://doi.org/10.1037/a0022186

Jensen, S. A., Biesen, J. N., & Graham, E. R. (2017). A meta-analytic review of play therapy with emphasis on outcome measures. *Professional Psychology: Research and Practice, 48*, 390–400. https://doi.org/10.1037/pro0000148

Kazantzis, N., Fairburn, C. G., Padesky, C. A., Reinecke, M., & Teesson, M. (2014). Unresolved issues regarding the research and practice of cognitive behavior therapy: The case of guided discovery using socratic questioning. *Behaviour Change, 31*(1), 1–17. https://doi.org/10.1017/bec.2013.29

Koole, S. L., & Tschacher, W. (2016). Synchrony in psychotherapy: A review and an integrative framework for the therapeutic alliance. *Frontiers in Psychology, 7*, 862. https://doi.org/10.3389/fpsyg.2016.00862

Krupnik, V. (2023). The therapeutic alliance as active inference: The role of trust and self-efficacy. *Journal of Contemporary Psychotherapy, 53*(3), 207–215.

Landreth, G. L. (2012). *Play therapy: The art of the relationship.* Routledge.

Laska, K. M., Gurman, A. S., & Wampold, B. E. (2014). Expanding the lens of evidence-based practice in psychotherapy: A common factors perspective. *Psychotherapy: Theory, Research, Practice, Training, 51*, 467–481.

Macneil, C. A., Hasty, M. K., Evans, M., Redlich, C., & Berk, M. (2009). The therapeutic alliance: Is it necessary or sufficient to engender positive outcomes? *Acta Neuropsychiatrica, 21*(2), 95–98. https://doi.org/10.1111/j.1601-5215.2009.00372.x

Martin, D. J., Garske, J. P., & Davis, M. K. (2000). Relation of the therapeutic alliance with outcome and other variables: A meta-analytic review. *Journal of Consulting and Clinical Psychology, 68*(3), 438–450. https://doi.org/10.1037/0022-006X.68.3.438

Martin, J. R. (1997). Mindfulness: A proposed common factor. *Journal of Psychotherapy Integration, 7*(4), 291–312. https://doi.org/10.1023/B:JOPI.0000010885.18025.BC

McBride, E. E., & Greeson, J. M. (2023). Mindfulness, cognitive functioning, and academic achievement in college students: The mediating role of stress. *Current Psychology (New Brunswick, N.J.), 42*(13), 10924–10934. https://doi.org/10.1007/s12144-021-02340-z

Norcross, J. C., & Lambert, M. J. (2018). *Psychotherapy relationships that work: Evidence-based responsiveness* (3rd ed.). Oxford University Press.

Norcross, J. C., & Wampold, B. E. (2011). Evidence-based therapy relationships: Research conclusions and clinical practices. *Psychotherapy, 48*(1), 98–102.

Ray, D. C., Armstrong, S. A., Balkin, R. S., & Jayne, K. M. (2015). Child-centered play therapy in the schools: Review and meta-analysis. *Psychology in Schools, 52*(2), 107–123. https://doi.org/10.1002/pits.21798

Rodgers, R. F., Cailhol, L., Bui, E., Klein, R., Schmitt, L., & Chabrol, H. (2010). L'alliance thérapeutique en psychothérapie: apports de la recherche empirique [Therapeutic alliance in psychotherapy: The contribution of empirical research]. *L'Encephale, 36*(5), 433–438. https://doi.org/10.1016/j.encep.2010.02.005

Rogers, C. (1942). *Counseling and psychotherapy: Newer concepts in practice.* Houghton Mifflin.

Stubbe, D. (2007). *Child and adolescent psychiatry: A practical guide.* Lippincott Williams & Wilkins.

Tryon, G. S., & Winograd, G. (2011). Goal consensus and collaboration. *Psychotherapy (Chicago, Ill.), 48*(1), 50–57. https://doi.org/10.1037/a0022061

VanFleet, R., Sywulak, A. E., & Sniscak, C. C. (2010). *Child-centered play therapy.* Guilford Press.

Wampold, B. E. (2010). *The great psychotherapy debate: Models, methods, and findings.* Routledge.

Wampold, B., & Imel, Z. E. (2015). *The great psychotherapy debate: The evidence for what makes psychotherapy work* (2nd ed.). Routledge.

# 5

# MINDFULNESS IN ADLERIAN PLAY THERAPY

## Introduction

Adlerian Play Therapy (AdPT), a historically significant and seminal play therapy approach pioneered by Terri Kottman, builds on Alfred Adler's Individual Psychology. AdPT emphasizes the importance of social connections and the individual's pursuit of significance and belonging within their social context (Kerley & Wassenaar, 2024; Kottman, 1995, 2020a; Kottman & Warlick, 1990). Grounded in Adler's concepts of inferiority and compensation, social interest, and early childhood experiences, AdPT has evolved into a comprehensive framework for understanding and addressing children's emotional and behavioral issues through play. Integrating Mindfulness-based Play Therapy® (MBPT) with AdPT can enhance therapeutic outcomes by promoting self-awareness, emotional regulation, and present-moment focus. This fusion leverages the strengths of both approaches, creating a powerful, holistic method that aligns with Adlerian goals of fostering a child's sense of belonging, social interest, and overall psychological well-being.

## History and Foundation of Adlerian Play Therapy

AdPT, pioneered by Terri Kottman, is grounded in Alfred Adler's Individual Psychology (Kerley & Wassenaar, 2024; Kottman, 1995, 2020b; Kottman & Warlick, 1990). This approach highlights the

96                    DOI: 10.4324/9781003468585-5

significance of social connections and the individual's quest for significance and belonging. Adler's theory suggests that human behavior is intentional and goal oriented. He proposed that people are driven by their need to overcome inferiority and find significance within their social contexts (Kerley & Wassenaar, 2024; Kottman, 1995, 2020a; Kottman & Warlick, 1990).

AdPT evolved from the broader principles of Adler's Individual Psychology, which emphasized the holistic understanding of individuals within their social context. Adler, an Austrian psychiatrist and a contemporary of Freud, broke away from Freudian theories to develop his own approach, focusing on the social nature of human beings and their drive for success and belonging. His concepts of inferiority and compensation, social interest, and the importance of early childhood experiences laid the groundwork for later therapeutic approaches, including AdPT (Ansbacher & Ansbacher, 1956).

In the 1990s, Terri Kottman, the founder of AdPT, began integrating Adler's theories with play therapy techniques. Kottman recognized that play is a natural medium for children to express themselves, work through their issues, and develop problem-solving skills. By combining Adlerian principles with play therapy, Kottman created a therapeutic approach that is both child-friendly and deeply rooted in a well-established psychological framework (Kottman, 1995; Kottman & Warlick, 1990).

Kottman's work emphasized the importance of understanding the child's lifestyle, which includes their beliefs, feelings, and behaviors as they interact within their social world. This perspective aligns with Adler's belief in the uniqueness of the individual and the importance of social interest and community feeling. Over the years, AdPT has continued to evolve, incorporating new insights and techniques to better address the needs of children in therapy (Kerley & Wassenaar, 2024; Kottman, 2020a).

Integrating mindfulness into AdPT can enhance the therapeutic process by fostering self-awareness, emotional regulation, and present-moment focus for both the therapist and the child. Mindfulness practices help children become more aware of their thoughts and feelings, enabling them to manage their emotions more effectively and develop a stronger sense of self and belonging.

## AdPT's Key Principles

### Social Embeddedness

AdPT recognizes that humans are inherently social beings who thrive on connections and relationships with others. This principle emphasizes the fundamental human need to belong and be a part of a community. It acknowledges that a child's behavior and feelings are deeply influenced by their social interactions and the environments they are part of. Understanding the child's social context, including their family dynamics, friendships, and school environment, is crucial in AdPT. This perspective helps therapists address issues of isolation, rejection, or social conflicts, fostering a sense of belonging and community in the child (Kottman, 2001).

### Goal-Directed Behavior

AdPT posits that all behavior is purposeful and directed toward achieving specific goals, whether they are conscious or unconscious. This principle stems from the idea that humans are motivated by their desires to fulfill their needs and aspirations. In the context of therapy, understanding the underlying goals behind a child's behavior can provide insights into their motivations and needs. For example, a child displaying aggressive behavior might be seeking attention or attempting to assert control in situations where they feel powerless. Recognizing these goal-directed behaviors allows therapists to guide children toward more constructive ways to achieve their goals, thereby promoting healthier behavior patterns (Sweeney, 2009).

### Subjective Perception

This principle highlights that each individual's perception of reality is subjective and shaped by personal experiences, beliefs, and emotions. In AdPT, therapists strive to understand the child's unique perspective and how it influences their feelings and behaviors. By acknowledging that each child has a subjective view of the world, therapists can validate their experiences and help them develop a more balanced and positive perception of themselves and their surroundings. This understanding also aids in addressing any distorted perceptions or misconceptions the child may have, fostering a more accurate and empowering self-view (Watts & Garza, 2008).

## Holistic Nature

AdPT views individuals as whole, unique beings who cannot be understood in isolation from their various parts. This holistic approach considers the physical, emotional, cognitive, and social aspects of a child's life as interconnected and interdependent. Rather than focusing solely on symptoms or specific issues, AdPT aims to understand the child as a complete person. This perspective encourages therapists to consider the broader context of the child's life, including their strengths, interests, and challenges, and to integrate various therapeutic interventions that address the child's overall well-being. By embracing the holistic nature of the child, therapists can create more comprehensive and effective treatment plans that support the child's growth and development in all areas of their life (Carlson & Kjos, 2002).

## Phases of Adlerian Play Therapy

1. **Building the Egalitarian Relationship**
2. **Exploring the Child's Lifestyle and Functioning at Life Tasks**
3. **Helping the Child Gain Insight**
4. **Reorienting/Reeducating the Child**

Adlerian play therapists advocate for an egalitarian relationship with clients, promoting a sense of agency and choice. Adlerian play therapists believe that every child can find healthy coping mechanisms, improve their sense of belonging, and contribute meaningfully to society. A unique aspect of AdPT is its emphasis on shared power and decision-making, involving the child in cleaning up and taking turns in choosing activities. AdPT is a strengths-based approach founded on encouragement and mutual respect (Kerley & Wassenaar, 2024; Kottman, 1995, 2020a; Meany-Walen, 2020).

## Integrating Mindfulness into Adlerian Play Therapy

### Phase 1: Building the Relationship

Establishing a strong therapeutic alliance that is egalitarian is crucial in AdPT. Mindfulness can enhance this phase by helping therapists remain present and attuned to the child, creating a safe and trusting environment. Phase 1 calls for a child-led, non-directive approach (Kottman, 1995).

*Mindful Presence*

In AdPT, mindful presence is essential for establishing a strong therapeutic alliance that is egalitarian, which is the foundation of effective therapy. The palpable sense of presence that the therapist exemplifies is particularly crucial during Phase 1, as it involves creating an environment where the child feels genuinely respected, seen, heard, and understood as an equal to the therapist. In AdPT, the therapist wants the child to feel like they are partners in the experience of play therapy together. Mindful presence helps in building that quality of rapport with the child by demonstrating genuine interest and attention. When therapists are fully present, children feel valued and respected, which is fundamental to Adlerian principles of social interest and encouragement. This deep connection can significantly enhance the child's willingness to engage in therapy. Trust is a key component of the therapeutic relationship. By maintaining mindful presence, therapists convey a sense of safety and reliability. This consistent attunement reassures the child that the therapist is a stable and attentive figure in their lives, fostering a sense of security that is crucial for exploring deeper emotional issues. Mindfulness helps therapists remain calm and centered, which in turn helps regulate the child's emotional state. This regulation is important in the initial phase of therapy, where the child is learning to trust the therapeutic process and the therapist.

*Examples of Mindful Presence in Phase 1*

**Mindful Breathing before Sessions**: Before a session begins, the therapist can engage with their own breath in a mindful way. Imagine a therapist who uses mindful breathing to envision connecting with the Adlerian concept of social interest, community connection, and a sense of belonging (Gemeinschaftsgefühl). Before each session, the therapist might spend five minutes practicing mindful breathing while visualizing a moment of connection with the child. The therapist might focus on the breath while recalling a recent instance where the child expressed joy or made a significant breakthrough in their play. This visualization reinforces the therapist's commitment to fostering the child's sense of belonging and significance within the therapeutic relationship.

**Modeling Mindful Breathing during Sessions:** During the session, therapists can model mindful breathing in a way that the child can observe. For example, if a child appears anxious or agitated, the therapist might demonstrate taking a few deep breaths, inviting the child to do the same. This non-directive, child-led approach aligns with Adlerian principles by allowing the child to choose whether or not to participate, thereby respecting their autonomy.

**Attunement to Play:** While the child engages in non-directed play, the therapist remains fully present, observing and reflecting on the child's actions and expressions. For example, if a child is building a structure with blocks, the therapist might notice aloud, "I see you're putting a lot of effort into building that tower. It looks very important to you." This kind of attuned observation helps the child feel understood and validates their efforts, reinforcing the Adlerian concept of encouragement.

**Responding to Non-Verbal Cues:** Children often communicate their feelings and thoughts through non-verbal cues in their play. A therapist practicing mindful presence will notice these cues and respond appropriately. For instance, if a child's play becomes more aggressive or chaotic, the therapist might gently say, "I notice that the play has become very fast and intense. I wonder how your body feels right now." This reflective statement shows the child that the therapist is attuned and curious about their inner world, encouraging deeper exploration and connection.

*Reflective Observations*

In AdPT, reflective observations are a critical aspect of the therapeutic process, especially during Phase 1. Mindfulness enhances the therapist's ability to engage in reflective listening and watching, which involves fully attending to the child's verbal and non-verbal communication. This deep listening and attunement help the child feel seen and heard, fostering a strong therapeutic alliance built on trust and connection. Reflective observations validate the child's experiences by mirroring their feelings and actions. This validation is crucial in Adlerian theory, as it reinforces the child's sense of significance and belonging. This consistent attention builds trust, making the child more likely to open and engage deeply in the therapeutic process. Reflective observations encourage children to explore and express their thoughts and feelings more freely. By feeling understood, children are empowered to communicate more openly, which is essential for their emotional and psychological development.

*Examples of Reflective Observations in Phase 1*

**Tracking Play Behavior:** Mindful therapists track the child's play behavior, noticing and reflecting on what the child is doing. For instance, if a child is repeatedly stacking and knocking down blocks, the therapist might reflect, "I see you're building the tower again and again, and then knocking it down. It seems important to see it fall." This kind of reflection helps the child feel that their actions and underlying feelings are acknowledged and understood.

**Reflecting Verbal Expressions:** When a child verbalizes thoughts or feelings, the therapist uses reflective listening to mirror these expressions. For example, if a child says, "I'm making a fort to keep everyone out," the therapist might respond, "You're building a fort that's very strong to keep others away. It sounds like you want to feel safe and protected." This response shows that the therapist is deeply attuned to the child's verbal communication, reinforcing a sense of safety and validation.

**Noticing Non-Verbal Cues:** Mindfulness enhances the therapist's ability to pick up on non-verbal cues, such as body language, facial expressions, and tone of voice. If a child is playing quietly but with a tense expression, the therapist might observe, "I notice you're playing very quietly, but your face looks tense. I wonder what you're feeling right now." This observation helps the child become aware of their own non-verbal expressions and can lead to a deeper exploration of their emotions.

**Encouraging Reflection:** Reflective observations can also encourage the child to reflect on their own actions and feelings. For instance, if a child switches abruptly from one type of play to another, the therapist might say, "You were building a castle, and now you've quickly moved to the drawing table. I'm curious about what made you decide to change." This kind of reflective questioning encourages the child to think about their motivations and emotions, fostering self-awareness and insight.

**Using Mindful Language:** The therapist uses language that encourages mindfulness, such as wondering aloud if the child can "notice" certain aspects of their play or their feelings. For instance, "I wonder if you notice how your body feels when you play with the clay?" Mindful language helps the child develop a habit of self-awareness and reflection, which are key components of mindfulness.

### Phase 2: Exploring the Child's Lifestyle and Functioning at Life Tasks

Phase 2 involves the therapist and child collaboratively examining the child's experiences, feelings, and behaviors to gain a deeper understanding of their lifestyle patterns and mistaken beliefs (Kerley & Wassenaar, 2024; Kottman, 1995, 2020a; Kottman & Warlick, 1990). Mindfulness helps therapists and children gain deeper insights into these aspects (Germer et al., 2016). The use of directive and non-directive play techniques combined and alternately allows the child to express themselves freely while also providing opportunities for the therapist to guide the exploration.

#### Mindful Observation

Therapists can use mindful observation to attentively watch the child's play, noticing subtle cues and behaviors that reveal insights into their lifestyle and goals. The same strategies outlined previously for Phase 1 can be applied here in Phase 2.

#### Body Awareness

Teaching children mindfulness techniques, such as body check-ins, can significantly enhance their self-awareness and emotional regulation. In Adlerian theory, understanding the child's lifestyle involves recognizing how they perceive and respond to the world around them. Body awareness exercises help children tune into their bodily sensations, which are often closely linked to their emotions and thoughts. For instance, a child who experiences anxiety might notice tightness in their chest or a racing heart. By identifying these physical cues, the child can begin to understand how their body responds to stress and anxiety, which is a critical step in exploring their overall functioning.

Adlerian theory emphasizes a holistic approach to understanding individuals, considering the interconnectedness of their physical, emotional, and social experiences. Body awareness aligns with this holistic view by integrating mindfulness of physical sensations into the therapeutic process. This practice helps children recognize the interplay between their bodies and their emotional and social experiences, leading to a more comprehensive understanding of their lifestyle.

By becoming more aware of their physical sensations, children can better understand how their bodies react in different social situations, such as interacting with peers or family members. This awareness can help them develop greater empathy and social interest, as they learn to recognize and manage their emotional responses in a way that promotes healthier relationships and a sense of belonging.

Teaching body awareness techniques empowers children to take an active role in their own emotional regulation and self-understanding. This empowerment is a core Adlerian principle, as it encourages children to develop a sense of competence and confidence in managing their feelings and behaviors. For example, a therapist might guide a child through a body check-in exercise, asking them to notice any areas of tension or discomfort and to describe these sensations. This practice not only enhances the child's self-awareness but also provides opportunities for the therapist to offer encouragement and support.

### *Examples of Body Awareness Interventions in Phase 2*

**The Body Clues Activity:** During sessions, therapists can incorporate body check-ins as a regular practice. For example, at the beginning of a session, the therapist can invite the child to scan their body from toes to nose and use crayons, markers, or stickers to mark different areas on a cut-out of a gingerbread person to note clues in the form of sensations they notice in various parts of their body. This exercise helps children become more attuned to their bodily states and can be a starting point for discussing how these sensations relate to their emotional experiences.

**Connecting Body Awareness to Life Tasks:** By linking body awareness activity to specific life tasks, therapists can help children understand how their physical sensations impact their functioning in different areas.

For instance, a child might notice that their stomach feels uneasy before school. The therapist can invite the child to explore this sensation further, helping the child realize that this physical response may be linked to feelings of anxiety about school tasks or social interactions. This understanding can lead to strategies for managing these sensations, thereby improving the child's functioning at school.

**Bibliotherapy and Mindfulness:** The therapist can select a children's book that tells a story and has a character to which the child can relate. While reading the story together, the therapist encourages the child to notice their emotions and body sensations. The therapist might wonder aloud if the character or the situation in the story feels familiar to the child. The therapist can guide the child through a body scan or mindful breathing before starting the story to become more attuned and present. This mindfulness practice helps the child stay connected to their feelings and enhances the therapeutic impact of the metaphor.

### Phase 3: Helping the Child Gain Insight

In AdPT, Phase 3 focuses on helping children develop insight into their thoughts, feelings, and behaviors. The aim is to foster a deeper understanding of the child's internal world and how it influences their interactions with others and their functioning in various life tasks. Insight development is a crucial aspect of AdPT, as it aligns with Adlerian principles of promoting self-awareness, understanding, and personal growth. *Mindful Reflective Inquiry* is a technique that involves guiding children to become more aware of their emotional responses and relate them to their own lives through playful activities. This method is grounded in several key Adlerian concepts and therapeutic goals.

### Holistic Understanding

Adlerian theory emphasizes understanding the individual as a whole, considering their physical, emotional, and social experiences. *Mindful Reflective Inquiry* helps children integrate these aspects by connecting their emotional experiences with physical sensations and social interactions. This holistic approach enables children to see the interconnectedness of their feelings, thoughts, and behaviors.

*Encouragement and Empowerment*

Adlerian therapy aims to encourage and empower individuals by helping them understand their agency and ability to effect change in their lives. Through reflective inquiry, children learn to identify and articulate their emotions, which empowers them to manage their feelings more effectively. This process encourages a sense of competence and confidence, reinforcing the Adlerian principle of encouragement.

*Social Interest and Community Feeling*

Developing insight into one's emotions and behaviors helps children understand their role within their social context. *Mindful Reflective Inquiry* fosters social interest and connection to community (Gemeinschaftsgefühl) by encouraging children to consider how their emotions and actions affect their relationships with others. This awareness promotes empathy and a sense of belonging, which are central to Adlerian theory.

*Understanding Lifestyle*

Adlerian theory says that each individual has a unique lifestyle, or way of perceiving and interacting with the world, shaped by early experiences and social context. Reflective inquiry helps uncover aspects of the child's lifestyle by exploring their habitual emotional responses and coping strategies. This understanding is crucial for helping children develop healthier ways of relating to themselves and others.

## Mindful Reflective Inquiry

Mindful Reflective Inquiry in AdPT involves using playful activities to introduce and explore various emotions and scenarios, with the therapist guiding the child to reflect on their experiences.

### Relating Play to Real Life

By using mindful reflective inquiry during play, therapists help children draw connections between the emotions and scenarios they encounter in play and their own lives. This practice aligns with Adlerian principles of fostering insight and understanding the individual's lifestyle. For example, if a child enacts a puppet scenario where the puppet feels jealous of a sibling, the therapist might gently explore if the child has similar feelings, thereby helping the child understand and articulate their emotions.

## *Developing a Coherent Narrative*

Reflective inquiry helps children develop a coherent narrative about their experiences. This process is vital for Adlerian therapy, which emphasizes the importance of understanding and integrating one's life story. Through repeated reflective inquiries, children learn to identify patterns in their emotions and behaviors, gaining insights into how they cope with different situations and how they can make positive changes.

### *Examples of Mindful Inquiry in Phase 3*

**Feelings Charades**: In this activity, the therapist and child act out different emotions while the other guesses the emotion. This game helps children recognize and label emotions in a fun and engaging way. During the game, the therapist can use the whisper technique to ask, "What does it feel like in your body when you feel happy/sad/angry?" This question encourages the child to connect the physical sensations with the emotional experience, fostering deeper insight.

**Feelings Bingo:** This game involves a bingo card with different emotions instead of numbers. As emotions are called out, the child marks them on their card. When a child gets a bingo, the therapist can ask, "Have you ever felt this emotion? Can you tell me about a time when you felt it?" This inquiry helps the child reflect on their personal experiences and understand the context of their emotions.

**Puppet Play:** Using puppets, the therapist can create scenarios that depict various emotional situations. For example, a puppet might feel scared about going to school or excited about a birthday party. The therapist can then ask the child, "What do you think this puppet is feeling right now? Have you ever felt this way?" This technique allows the child to project their own feelings onto the puppet, making it easier to discuss and explore difficult emotions.

### *Phase 4: Reorienting/Reeducating the Child*

In the final phase of AdPT, the focus shifts to helping children integrate the insights gained from earlier phases into practical changes in behavior, thoughts, and emotions. Phase 4 emphasizes reorienting the child's lifestyle toward more adaptive and positive patterns and reeducating them to adopt new, healthier ways of thinking and behaving

(Kerley & Wassenaar, 2024; Kottman, 1995, 2020a; Kottman & Warlick, 1990). Mindfulness plays a crucial role in this phase, supporting the child in developing healthier ways of achieving significance and belonging.

*Mindful Practices*

Introducing regular mindfulness practices in a playful and engaging manner can help children cultivate presence, awareness, and compassion for themselves and others. These practices foster self-awareness and social interest, which are central to Adlerian theory. For example, a therapist might use a **mindful finger maze** on paper, where the child traces a path with their finger while focusing on their breath. This activity promotes concentration, patience, and a sense of calm. Another effective practice is **love-and-kindness meditation**, where the therapist guides the child to send kind thoughts to themselves and others. This practice encourages empathy, social interest, and a positive self-concept.

*Mindful Decision-Making*

Engaging children in mindful decision-making during play teaches them to approach situations with greater awareness and consideration. This process enhances their ability to make positive choices, reflecting the Adlerian goal of fostering self-directed behavior. For instance, during a play session, the therapist might present a scenario where the child must decide how to resolve a conflict between toy figures. The therapist can guide the child to pause, take a few deep breaths, and think about the possible outcomes of different choices. This practice not only improves decision-making skills but also reinforces the importance of considering the impact of one's actions on others.

*Examples for Mindful Practices and Decision Making in Phase 4*

**Mindful Reflection**: At the end of a play session, the therapist can invite the child to reflect mindfully on their experiences. For example, the therapist might say, "Let's take a moment to think about what we did today. How did it feel when you made that choice for your puppet? What did you notice about yourself during our game?" This reflection helps the child internalize the lessons learned and apply them to real-life situations.

**Positive Reinforcement:** Using mindfulness to reinforce positive behaviors is another key aspect of Phase 4. When a child demonstrates a new, healthier behavior, the therapist can acknowledge it mindfully, saying, "I noticed you took a deep breath before deciding how to share the toys. That was a great way to stay calm and think about what's best for everyone." This positive reinforcement encourages the child to continue practicing mindfulness and making positive choices.

**Role-Playing Scenarios:** Role-playing different scenarios allows children to practice new behaviors in a safe and supportive environment. The therapist can set up scenarios that reflect common challenges the child faces, such as dealing with peer pressure or managing frustration. By guiding the child through mindful reflection and decision-making during these role-plays, the therapist helps the child develop practical skills that can be applied outside of therapy.

**Creating a Mindfulness Routine:** Helping children establish a regular mindfulness routine can solidify the gains made in therapy. The therapist might work with the child to create a simple daily routine that includes mindfulness activities, such as a few minutes of breathing exercises in the morning or a gratitude practice before bed. This routine reinforces the child's ability to stay present and make thoughtful choices throughout their day.

## Conclusion

Incorporating mindfulness into AdPT is a process through which therapists learn about the child's lifestyle through the therapeutic alliance, non-directive play with mindful observations, various play-based interventions, and frequent consultation with primary adults in the child's life (Kerley & Wassernaar, 2023). Mindfulness can be woven throughout this process to tailor interventions that best meet the child's needs and their system. Integrating mindfulness into AdPT enhances the therapeutic process by fostering self-awareness, emotional regulation, and present-moment focus for both the therapist and the child. By incorporating mindfulness into the four phases of AdPT – building the relationship, exploring the child's lifestyle, helping the child gain insight, and reorienting/reeducating the child – therapists can create a more effective and compassionate therapeutic environment. This integration supports the Adlerian goals of improving the child's sense of belonging, fostering social interest, and helping the child feel connected to society.

## References

Ansbacher, H. L., & Ansbacher, R. R. (1956). *The individual psychology of Alfred Adler*. Basic Books.

Carlson, J., & Kjos, D. (2002). *Adlerian therapy: Theory and practice*. American Psychological Association.

Germer, C. K., Siegel, R. D., & Fulton, P. R. (2016). *Mindfulness and psychotherapy* (2nd ed.). Guilford Press.

Kerley, S., & Wassenaar, E. (2024). Play therapy treatment planning with children and families. In K. R. O'Connor & L. D. Bratton (Eds.), *An Adlerian play therapy approach to treatment planning* (1st ed., pp. 41–50). Routledge.

Kottman, T. (1995). *Adlerian play therapy*. W. W. Norton & Company.

Kottman, T. (2001). Adlerian play therapy. In G. L. Landreth (Ed.), *Innovations in play therapy: Issues, process, and special populations* (pp. 45–67). Brunner-Routledge.

Kottman, T., & Warlick, C. (1990). Adlerian play therapy. *Journal of Individual Psychology*, *46*(4), 491–502.

Kottman, T. (2020a). Adlerian play therapy: A personal and professional journey. *The Journal of Individual Psychology*, *76*, 162–175. https://doi.org/10.1353/jip.2020.0004

Kottman, T. (2020b). *Play therapy: Basics and beyond*. American Counseling Association.

Meany-Walen, K. (2020). Adlerian play therapy: Building a therapeutic relationship through mindfulness. *International Journal of Play Therapy*, *29*(2), 102–114. https://doi.org/10.1037/pla0000120

Sweeney, T. J. (2009). *Adlerian counseling and psychotherapy* (5th ed.). Routledge.

Watts, R. E., & Garza, Y. (2008). Adlerian therapy as a relational constructivist approach. *Journal of Constructivist Psychology*, *21*(3), 224–242. https://doi.org/10.1080/10720530802071499

# 6

## MINDFULNESS IN CHILD-CENTERED PLAY THERAPY

### Introduction

Child-Centered Play Therapy (CCPT) emphasizes the creation of a safe and accepting environment where children can freely express themselves through play. The therapist's role is to provide a non-directive, empathetic, and supportive presence, allowing the child to lead the therapeutic process (Axline, 1947; Landreth, 2002; VanFleet et al., 2010). Regardless of what play therapy theoretical orientation a therapist may choose is wise for all therapists working with children have an in-depth understanding of the elements and essence of CCPT because therapeutic presence and alliance are essential across all play therapy theoretical orientations. Mindfulness-based Play Therapy® (MBPT) is foundationally based on the CCPT tenet that the relationship between child and therapist is essential for effective play therapy.

### Child-Centered Play Therapy as a Seminal Theory

CCPT holds a seminal and historically significant place in the field of play therapy. Developed by Virginia Axline in the mid-20th century, CCPT is grounded in Carl Rogers' principles of Person-Centered Therapy, which emphasize the importance of a supportive, empathetic, and non-directive therapeutic relationship. Axline adapted these principles to the context of

DOI: 10.4324/9781003468585-6

working with children, creating a therapeutic approach that honors the child's innate ability to express, explore, and resolve their issues through play (Axline, 1947).

### *Therapeutic Alliance as the Core of CCPT*

At the heart of CCPT is the quality of the therapeutic alliance between the therapist and the child. This alliance is fundamental to the effectiveness of the therapy and is characterized by several key elements.

### *Unconditional Positive Regard*

The therapist provides an accepting and non-judgmental environment, where the child feels valued and respected regardless of their behavior or expressions. This unconditional positive regard is crucial in helping the child feel safe and secure, enabling them to open up and explore their inner world (Axline, 1947; Landreth, 2012).

*Empathy* The therapist strives to deeply understand the child's perspective and emotional experiences. Demonstrating genuine empathy, the therapist reflects the child's feelings and experiences, helping them feel understood and validated. This empathetic connection is essential in building trust and facilitating the child's emotional expression and growth (Landreth, 2012; VanFleet et al., 2010).

*Congruence* Authenticity in the therapist's interactions fosters a genuine and transparent relationship. The therapist's congruence, or genuineness, encourages the child to be true to themselves, promoting an environment where honesty and openness are valued and modeled (Landreth, 2012).

## Historical and Contemporary Relevance

The historical significance of CCPT is evident in its widespread acceptance and continued relevance in modern therapeutic practice. Virginia Axline's pioneering work in the mid-20th century laid the groundwork for a therapeutic approach that is deeply respectful of the child's autonomy and inner resources. CCPT's emphasis on providing a non-directive, supportive environment for children has made it a foundational form of play therapy, particularly in educational settings.

### First and Foundational Form of Play Therapy

CCPT has been the first and foundational form of play therapy taught in master's level graduate programs. This approach is often the initial theory introduced to aspiring play therapists because it embodies essential therapeutic principles that are critical for effective practice. The principles of unconditional positive regard, empathy, congruence, and a non-directive stance are fundamental to understanding how to create a therapeutic environment that is both safe and conducive to healing for children (Axline, 1947).

Graduate programs emphasize CCPT as the starting point for learning about play therapy because it provides a solid theoretical and practical foundation. CCPT's non-directive nature encourages therapists to develop skills in observing and understanding the child's natural play processes without imposing their own interpretations or directions. This approach helps therapists cultivate patience, mindfulness, and deep respect for the child's capacity for self-directed healing.

### Emphasis on Therapeutic Relationship

The quality of the therapeutic relationship is a critical factor in the success of CCPT, a principle that is heavily emphasized in training programs. Studies have consistently shown that a strong therapeutic alliance enhances the effectiveness of therapy, leading to better outcomes for children with various emotional and behavioral issues (Bratton & Ray, 2000; Landreth & Bratton, 2006). In teaching CCPT, graduate programs focus on the importance of building a trusting, empathetic, and genuine relationship with the child. This emphasis ensures that new therapists understand the central role of the therapeutic alliance in facilitating emotional and psychological growth in children.

### Educational and Training Standards

Educational standards for play therapy training often require a comprehensive understanding of CCPT as a prerequisite for learning more directive or integrative approaches. CCPT is seen as a foundational theory because it provides a clear framework for understanding child development, therapeutic communication, and the dynamics of play as a medium for expression and healing. By mastering the principles and techniques of CCPT, therapists are better prepared to integrate other therapeutic modalities into their practice in a way that remains child-centered and respectful of the child's autonomy.

### Integration and Modern Adaptations

Over the decades, CCPT has evolved and adapted to include modern therapeutic practices and insights. Despite these evolutions, the core principles of CCPT have remained constant, reinforcing its foundational status in the field of play therapy. For instance, the integration of mindfulness practices into CCPT sessions reflects an ongoing commitment to enhancing the therapist's presence and attunement to the child's needs. Similarly, incorporating technology and digital tools into play therapy sessions represents an adaptation to contemporary contexts while maintaining the non-directive, child-led approach that is central to CCPT.

## Support from Research and Practice

Research has consistently demonstrated the effectiveness of CCPT in various settings, including schools, clinical environments, and private practice. Studies have shown that CCPT is effective in reducing symptoms of anxiety, improving self-esteem, supporting trauma recovery, and addressing behavioral issues in children (Cochran et al., 2010; Gupta et al., 2023; Parker et al., 2021; Ray et al., 2021). This evidence base not only underscores the therapeutic value of CCPT but also reinforces its importance as a foundational theory in the training and education of play therapists.

Numerous studies and reviews have supported the effectiveness of CCPT, emphasizing the importance of the therapeutic relationship. For instance, Cochran et al. (2010) found that the therapeutic alliance in CCPT was a key determinant in reducing anxiety and improving self-esteem in children. Similarly, Landreth and Bratton (2006) highlighted the centrality of the therapeutic relationship in achieving positive outcomes in diverse settings, from schools to clinical environments. These findings emphasize that the relational qualities of empathy, acceptance, and genuineness are not just beneficial but essential for the success of CCPT.

These findings are at the root of why MBPT is such a valuable approach with all play therapy theories.

### Reducing Anxiety and Boosting Self-Esteem

In 2010, Cochran and colleagues conducted a pivotal study that highlighted CCPT's efficacy in alleviating anxiety and enhancing self-esteem among children. The researchers found that children who participated in CCPT sessions showed significant reductions in anxiety symptoms and marked improvements in self-esteem. These findings highlight the therapy's capacity to foster emotional resilience and a positive self-concept in young clients.

### Supporting Trauma Recovery

A more recent study by Gupta et al. (2023) focused on children who had experienced trauma. This research revealed that CCPT had a profoundly positive impact on these children, particularly in terms of emotional regulation and overall well-being. By providing a safe and supportive space for children to express their feelings and experiences, CCPT facilitated significant improvements in their ability to manage emotions and recover from traumatic events.

### Efficacy across Settings

The comprehensive review by Landreth and Bratton (2006b) further solidifies the evidence base for CCPT. Their extensive analysis provided strong support for the therapy's effectiveness across various settings, including schools and clinical environments. This review highlighted CCPT's versatility and adaptability, demonstrating its benefits in diverse contexts and reinforcing its role as a valuable therapeutic approach.

### Addressing Behavioral Issues

Parker et al. (2021) explored CCPT's impact on children's behavioral issues. Their findings indicated that CCPT effectively addressed a range of behavioral problems, leading to significant improvements in social skills and academic performance. This research suggests that CCPT not only helps children manage their behaviors more effectively but also enhances their ability to interact positively with peers and succeed in academic settings.

### Supporting Children with Developmental Delays

Ray and colleagues (2021) investigated the benefits of CCPT for children with developmental delays. Their study found that CCPT was particularly beneficial in enhancing communication skills and emotional understanding in these children. By engaging in play therapy, children with developmental delays were able to develop better ways to express themselves and understand their emotions, leading to improved overall functioning.

The evidence base for CCPT is extensive and compelling, demonstrating its effectiveness in reducing anxiety, supporting trauma recovery, addressing behavioral issues, and aiding children with developmental delays. Studies by Cochran et al. (2010), Gupta et al. (2023), Landreth and Bratton (2006), Parker et al. (2021), and Ray et al. (2021) collectively highlight the therapeutic benefits of CCPT across various contexts and populations. This strong empirical support underscores the value of CCPT in fostering emotional and psychological growth in children, making it a vital approach in the field of child therapy.

## Integrating Mindfulness into Child-Centered Play Therapy

Mindfulness and the essence of CCPT go hand in hand. Mindfulness practices are invaluable for therapists practicing CCPT as they help cultivate a heightened state of awareness and quality of presence, which are crucial for attuning to the child's needs and experiences during play therapy sessions. The core tenets of CCPT – unconditional positive regard, empathy, congruence, and a non-directive approach – are all enhanced through the mindful presence of the therapist. Mindfulness enables therapists to maintain a non-judgmental and accepting attitude toward the child. By being fully present, therapists can create a safe and supportive environment where the child feels valued and respected, regardless of their behavior or expressions. This acceptance aligns with the CCPT principle of unconditional positive regard, which is essential for fostering trust and security in the therapeutic relationship (Axline, 1947). Mindfulness helps therapists deepen their empathy by allowing them to fully attune to the child's emotional state and perspective. When therapists practice mindfulness, they can better focus on the child's verbal and non-verbal cues, understanding the child's world from their viewpoint. This enhanced empathy is a cornerstone of CCPT, facilitating a genuine connection and helping the child feel truly understood (Landreth, 2012). The practice of mindfulness encourages therapists to be genuine and authentic in their interactions. By being aware of their own thoughts and feelings, therapists can respond to the child in a congruent manner, fostering an atmosphere of trust and openness. Congruence in CCPT involves the therapist being true to themselves while interacting with the child, which is essential for modeling honesty and integrity (Landreth, 2012).

### CCPT Techniques Infused with Mindfulness

When therapists incorporate mindfulness into their play therapy sessions, it enhances the core techniques of CCPT, such as tracking, reflecting, returning responsibility, and therapeutic limit setting. Thus, it deepens the therapeutic process and facilitates more effective outcomes.

### Tracking

Tracking involves the therapist observing and narrating the child's actions during play without interpretation or judgment (Cochran et al., 2010; Landreth, 2012; Ray, 2011). Mindfulness enhances tracking by enabling the therapist to stay fully present and attentive to the child's behavior and expressions. A mindful therapist can notice subtle changes in the child's play and emotional states, providing more accurate and attuned observations. This heightened awareness allows the therapist to offer precise and non-intrusive comments that validate the child's experiences, fostering a sense of being seen and understood.

### Reflecting

Reflecting is the process of mirroring the child's feelings and verbalizing their emotions, which helps children gain insight into their internal experiences (Giordano et al., 2005; Landreth, 2012). Mindfulness enhances reflection by helping the therapist remain calm and composed, even in the presence of intense emotions. A mindful therapist can better regulate their own emotional responses, allowing them to provide clear and empathetic reflections that resonate with the child's feelings. This practice helps children feel heard and validated, which is crucial for emotional development and self-awareness.

### Returning Responsibility

Returning responsibility involves encouraging children to solve their own problems and make their own decisions during play (Giordano et al., 2005). This technique is essential for promoting autonomy and self-efficacy. Mindfulness supports this by helping therapists maintain a non-judgmental and accepting stance. A mindful therapist can resist the urge to intervene or direct the child's actions, instead providing gentle prompts that guide the child toward self-discovery and problem-solving. By observing mindfulness, therapists create an environment where children feel empowered to take ownership of their actions and decisions.

### Therapeutic Limit Setting

Therapeutic limit setting involves establishing boundaries to ensure the safety and structure of the play therapy session (Landreth, 2002; Purswell, 2020). Mindfulness enhances this process by helping therapists remain centered and composed when setting and enforcing limits. A mindful approach to limit setting ensures that boundaries are communicated calmly and clearly, without anger or frustration. This consistency helps children understand the limits and the reasons behind them, fostering a sense of security and trust in the therapeutic relationship. Mindfulness also allows therapists to be more attuned to the child's reactions to limits, enabling them to respond with empathy and support.

## Purposeful Integration of Mindfulness

Integrating mindfulness into CCPT allows therapists to model emotional regulation and present-moment awareness for the child. By demonstrating mindfulness, therapists teach children *indirectly* how to stay grounded and manage their own emotions more effectively. This practice supports the CCPT goal of helping children develop healthier ways of coping with their feelings. Children can learn mindfulness techniques by observing what the therapist models and teaches indirectly. Practices such as deep breathing, focusing on their senses, or noticing what they are feeling in their bodies can be used to regulate their emotions and nervous system reactivity during and outside of therapy sessions.

When therapists practice mindfulness within CCPT, it enhances the therapist's ability to track, reflect, return responsibility, and set therapeutic limits effectively. By staying present and attuned, therapists can create a more supportive and empowering therapeutic environment, helping children develop the skills they need to manage their emotions and navigate their world more healthily.

The quality of attunement and unconditional acceptance that CCPT theory is based upon ideally will be the foundation of all play therapy, even when one wishes to utilize more directive approaches. Mindfulness practice on the part of the clinician is what allows this basic essence of CCPT to be incorporated into more directive or facilitative play therapy approaches as there is attunement in the moment with use of mindful reflection of the child's feelings, mindful tracking of the child's choices and expressions, mindful returning of responsibility to the child to assist the child in developing a sense of empowerment, and mindful limit setting when needed for the sake of safety in the playroom. All of these practices can be folded in.

## Promoting a Safe and Accepting Environment

### Unconditional Positive Regard

In CCPT, the therapist's application of mindfulness enhances the principle of unconditional positive regard. Mindfulness practices enable the therapist to be fully present and attentive, helping them maintain a non-judgmental and accepting attitude toward the child. For instance, before sessions, the therapist might engage in mindful breathing to clear their mind and center their focus. This preparation allows the therapist to enter the session with an open heart and mind, fully attuned to the child's needs and expressions. By being mindful, the therapist can consistently offer unconditional positive regard, ensuring the child feels valued and respected regardless of their behavior or emotions (Axline, 1947).

### Empathy Enhanced by Mindfulness

Mindfulness deepens the therapist's ability to practice empathy by fostering a state of heightened awareness and presence. When the therapist is mindful, they are better equipped to tune into the child's emotional state and respond with genuine understanding. For example, during play, the therapist can use mindful listening techniques, such as focusing on the child's tone of voice, body language, and choice of play activities. This mindful attention allows the therapist to reflect the child's feelings and experiences accurately, validating their emotional world and strengthening the therapeutic bond (Landreth, 2012).

### Congruence through Mindfulness

Congruence, or genuineness, in CCPT is enhanced through mindfulness by helping therapists stay authentic and aware of their own emotions and reactions. Mindfulness practices enable therapists to remain grounded and true to themselves, which in turn fosters trust and openness in the therapeutic relationship. For example, a therapist might use a brief mindfulness exercise to check in with their own feelings before responding to a child's expression of frustration. By being mindful, the therapist can ensure that their responses are genuine and transparent, modeling honesty and integrity for the child (Landreth, 2012).

### Non-Directive Approach Supported by Mindfulness

The non-directive approach of CCPT, where the child leads the play and the therapist follows, is naturally supported by mindfulness. Mindfulness helps therapists remain patient and present, allowing the child to explore and express themselves without interference. For example, if a child becomes deeply engaged in building a structure with blocks, the therapist practices mindfulness by staying fully present and observing without directing the play. This mindful presence communicates trust in the child's ability to navigate their own therapeutic process, fostering a sense of autonomy and empowerment (VanFleet et al., 2010).

### Consistency and Predictability with Mindfulness

Mindfulness contributes to creating a consistent and structured therapeutic environment by helping therapists maintain a calm and focused demeanor. Regular mindfulness practices, such as setting intentions for the session and engaging in mindful breathing, help therapists establish a predictable and stable atmosphere. This consistency reduces anxiety for the child and enhances their sense of security and trust. The therapist's mindful presence ensures that the therapeutic space remains a safe and accepting environment for the child to explore and express their inner world.

### Practical Strategies with Mindfulness
#### Active Observation with Mindfulness

The therapist uses mindful listening, watching, and attentive body language to fully focus on the child's verbal and non-verbal expressions. This involves being present in the moment, reflecting the child's feelings accurately, and validating their experiences.

#### Non-Verbal Communication Enhanced by Mindfulness

Mindful awareness of non-verbal cues, such as eye contact, facial expressions, and body language, plays a crucial role in CCPT. These non-verbal elements are essential in conveying empathy and acceptance, core tenets of CCPT. When therapists practice mindfulness, they become more attuned to these subtle forms of communication, allowing them to respond in ways that support the child's emotional needs. For example, maintaining gentle and consistent eye contact can reassure the child of the therapist's presence and attention, while a warm, open facial expression can convey acceptance and understanding. Similarly, mindful body language – such as leaning slightly forward to show interest or nodding to acknowledge the child's feelings – can significantly enhance the therapeutic alliance. This mindful non-verbal communication reinforces the child's sense of being understood and valued, which is fundamental to creating a safe and supportive therapeutic environment. By being fully present and attuned to these non-verbal signals, therapists can deepen their connection with the child, facilitating a more effective and empathetic therapeutic process. This heightened awareness and responsiveness help the child feel seen and validated, fostering a trusting relationship that is crucial for therapeutic progress.

*Respecting Boundaries with Mindfulness*

Mindfulness helps therapists remain acutely aware of and respect the child's physical and emotional boundaries, which is a critical aspect of CCPT. By practicing mindfulness, therapists can maintain a heightened sense of presence and attentiveness, allowing them to pick up on subtle cues that indicate the child's comfort levels and personal space needs. This awareness enables therapists to respond appropriately and adjust their behavior to ensure the child feels safe and respected.

For instance, a therapist might notice a child's body language signaling discomfort, such as withdrawing or turning away, and respond by giving the child more space or changing the pace of the session. Mindfulness allows the therapist to remain non-intrusive and patient, waiting for the child to lead and indicating readiness to engage further. This mindful approach respects the child's autonomy, as it allows the child to set the pace and direction of their therapeutic journey without feeling pressured or overwhelmed.

Respecting boundaries through mindfulness also involves being sensitive to the emotional states of the child. Therapists practicing mindfulness are better equipped to detect changes in the child's emotional landscape, such as signs of anxiety, frustration, or sadness. By acknowledging these emotional boundaries and providing a supportive response, therapists reinforce the child's sense of safety and security. This mindful respect for both physical and emotional boundaries helps to build a trusting relationship, where the child feels in control and empowered within the therapeutic setting.

Ultimately, mindfulness in respecting boundaries helps create an environment where the child's needs and preferences are prioritized. This approach not only enhances the therapeutic alliance but also fosters the child's confidence and self-efficacy. By consistently honoring the child's boundaries, therapists demonstrate that they are attuned to the child's needs and committed to providing a safe and supportive space for their growth and healing.

*Encouragement through Mindfulness*

Encouragement is a fundamental component of CCPT, and when combined with mindfulness, it becomes an even more powerful tool. The therapist uses mindfulness to provide authentic and positive reinforcement, which is crucial for fostering the child's self-esteem and confidence. By being fully present and attentive, the therapist can genuinely acknowledge the child's efforts and strengths, creating a supportive and empowering therapeutic environment.

Mindfulness helps therapists stay attuned to the child's activities and emotional states, allowing them to recognize and respond to moments when they exhibit effort, creativity, problem-solving, or resilience. For example, if a child successfully navigates a challenging play scenario or shows persistence in completing a task, the therapist can mindfully acknowledge this achievement. A mindful therapist might say, "I noticed how carefully you worked on building that tower, even when it got tricky. That required a lot of patience and care to do that!" This specific and genuine feedback reinforces the child's sense of competence and encourages them to continue engaging positively in play.

Mindfulness enables therapists to offer encouragement that is timely and relevant. By observing the child closely and responding in the moment, the therapist's praise feels more genuine and impactful. This immediacy of feedback helps the child make a direct connection between their actions and the positive reinforcement, strengthening their motivation and self-worth.

Additionally, mindfulness allows therapists to identify and highlight the child's intrinsic qualities and strengths, such as kindness, creativity, bravery, or perseverance. By consistently focusing on these positive attributes, the therapist helps the child build a more positive self-image. For instance, if a child shows empathy toward a toy figure in distress, the therapist might comment, "You're taking such good care of the doll. You are showing kindness to the doll." This kind of reinforcement not only boosts the child's confidence but also encourages the development of positive character traits.

Mindful encouragement also involves being present to the child's emotions and providing support when they face difficulties. When a child struggles or feels frustrated, the therapist can use mindfulness to offer comforting and encouraging words. For example, if a child feels frustrated after a play scenario doesn't go as planned, the therapist might say, "It's okay to feel frustrated when things don't work out. I see how hard you tried." This empathetic and supportive response helps the child feel understood and valued, reinforcing their resilience and willingness to try again.

In summary, using mindfulness to provide encouragement in CCPT ensures that the therapist's positive reinforcement is authentic, specific, and timely. This approach helps children feel genuinely acknowledged and supported, boosting their self-esteem and confidence. By focusing on the child's efforts and strengths, the therapist fosters a positive self-concept and encourages the development of important life skills and attributes. This mindful practice of encouragement is essential for creating a nurturing and empowering therapeutic environment where children can thrive.

## Conclusion

Integrating mindfulness into CCPT enhances the therapeutic process by fostering self-awareness, emotional regulation, and present-moment focus for both the therapist and the child. By incorporating mindfulness into the core principles of CCPT – unconditional positive regard, empathy, congruence, and a non-directive approach – therapists can create a more effective and compassionate therapeutic environment. This integration supports the CCPT goals of helping children develop healthier ways of coping, improving their emotional and behavioral functioning, and fostering a sense of safety and acceptance.

## References

Axline, V. M. (1947). *Play therapy: The inner dynamics of childhood*. Houghton Mifflin.

Bratton, S. C., & Ray, D. C. (2000). The efficacy of play therapy with children: A meta-analytic review of treatment outcomes. *Professional Psychology: Research and Practice, 31*(6), 676–689. https://doi.org/10.1037/0735-7028.36.4.376

Cochran, N., Nordling, W., & Cochran, J. (2010). *Child-centered play therapy: A practical guide to developing therapeutic relationships with children*. John Wiley & Sons.

Giordano, M., Landreth, G. L., & Jones, L. (2005). A retrospective analysis of the clinical treatment practices of child-centered play therapists. *International Journal of Play Therapy, 14*(2), 13–31. https://doi.org/10.1037/h0088894

Landreth, G. L. (2002). *Play therapy: The art of the relationship* (2nd ed.). Brunner-Routledge.

Landreth, G. L. (2012). *Play therapy: The art of the relationship*. Routledge.

Landreth, G. L., & Bratton, S. C. (2006a). *Child parent relationship therapy (CPRT): A 10-session filial therapy model.* Routledge.

Landreth, G. L., & Bratton, S. C. (2006b). *Child parent relationship therapy (CPRT): The effects on Children's behavioral problems and parent stress levels.* Routledge.

Parker, C., Riggs, M., & Patel, N. (2021). Child-centered play therapy and behavioral outcomes: A multi-site evaluation. *Journal of Counseling & Development, 99*(3), 245–257. https://doi.org/10.1002/jcad.12454

Purswell, K.E. (2020). An exploration of limit-setting in child counseling. *Journal of Child and Adolescent Counseling, 6,* 228–241.

Ray, D., Blanco, P., Sullivan, J., & Holliman, R. (2021). Effectiveness of child-centered play therapy for children with developmental delays. *Journal of Developmental and Behavioral Pediatrics, 42*(5), 403–411. https://doi.org/10.1097/DBP.0000000000000884

Ray, D. C., Burgin, E., Gutierrez, D., Ceballos, P., & Lindo, N. (2022). Child-centered play therapy and adverse childhood experiences: A randomized controlled trial. *Journal of Counseling & Development, 100*(2), 134–145. https://doi.org/10.1002/jcad.12412

Ray, D. C. (2011). Evidence-based practice and play therapy. *International Journal of Play Therapy, 20*(2), 118–133. https://doi.org/10.1037/a0023458

VanFleet, R., Sywulak, A. E., & Sniscak, C. C. (2010). *Child-centered play therapy.* Guilford Press.

# 7

# MINDFULNESS IN COGNITIVE-BEHAVIORAL PLAY THERAPY

## Introduction

Cognitive-Behavioral Play Therapy (CBPT) stands as one of the most historically significant and extensively researched play therapy theories. Developed by Susan Knell in the early 1990s, CBPT merges the principles of cognitive-behavioral therapy (CBT) with the therapeutic power of play to address a range of cognitive, emotional, and behavioral challenges in children. This innovative integration has positioned CBPT as a seminal approach in the field of child therapy, providing a structured and effective method for helping children navigate their psychological difficulties. Integrating Mindfulness-based Play Therapy® (MBPT) with CBPT can further enhance therapeutic outcomes by fostering greater self-awareness, emotional regulation, and present-moment focus. This fusion leverages the strengths of both approaches, creating a powerful, holistic method that aligns with CBPT's goals of promoting cognitive restructuring, behavioral change, skill-building, and psychoeducation.

## Historical Significance and Research Evidence Base

CBPT stands out as one of the most historically significant and extensively researched play therapy theories. Developed by Susan Knell in the early 1990s, CBPT merges the principles of CBT with the therapeutic

 DOI: 10.4324/9781003468585-7

powers of play to address a range of cognitive, emotional, and behavioral challenges in children. This innovative integration has positioned CBPT as a seminal approach in the field of child therapy, providing a structured and effective method for helping children navigate their psychological difficulties (Knell, 1993).

The extensive research evidence supporting CBPT acclaims its efficacy and adaptability in treating various psychological issues. Numerous studies have demonstrated the effectiveness of CBPT in addressing anxiety, depression, attention-deficit/hyperactivity disorder (ADHD), and behavioral problems in children. This robust evidence base has cemented CBPT's status as a trusted and widely utilized therapeutic modality (Atayi et al., 2018; Badamian & Ebrahimi Moghaddam, 2017; Drewes, 2009; Knell, 1995).

CBPT is a directive approach to play therapy, meaning that therapists actively guide the therapeutic process to help children recognize and modify unhelpful thought patterns and behaviors. Despite its directive nature, it is equally essential for therapists to build rapport and establish a strong therapeutic alliance in CBPT, just as it is in non-directive approaches like child-centered play therapy (CCPT). A strong therapeutic alliance, characterized by trust, empathy, and collaboration, forms the foundation of effective therapy and is crucial for achieving positive outcomes. In CBPT, therapists must balance directive techniques with empathetic understanding and genuine connection to ensure that children feel safe, supported, and understood. Research indicates that the quality of the therapeutic relationship is a significant predictor of therapy success across various modalities, including both directive and non-directive approaches (Kenney-Noziska, 2008; Knell, 1993; Landreth, 2012). Thus, therapists practicing CBPT must prioritize establishing a warm and trusting relationship with their young clients, as this rapport facilitates openness, cooperation, and the therapeutic process.

In my years of teaching play therapy to mental health professionals, I have introduced my students to the concept of using an *invitational and facilitative* approach rather than directing a child. The purpose of this approach is to invite the child to an activity intended to facilitate an experience for the child that will provide new learning of a concept or a skill. It is important, however, to be invitational, remembering that an invitation can be accepted or declined. If a child indicates they are not interested in participating in the activity, it's important for the therapist to accept and affirm the child's feelings in the moment. Ultimately, in all of play therapy, a child's choices should be respected, honored, and followed unless there is a safety concern or other serious need for a therapeutic limit.

## Tenets of Cognitive-Behavioral Play Therapy (CBPT)

CBPT is grounded in several core principles that guide its therapeutic approach.

### Cognitive Restructuring

A fundamental aspect of CBPT is helping children identify and change negative or unhelpful thought patterns. Through play, children can express their thoughts and beliefs in a non-threatening manner, allowing therapists to gently challenge and reframe these cognitions. For instance, a child might use dolls to enact a scenario where they feel incapable of success. The therapist can then use this play scenario to explore the child's underlying beliefs and introduce a reframing of the beliefs to more positive and/or realistic ways of thinking.

### Behavioral Interventions

CBPT employs play to reinforce positive behaviors and reduce problematic ones. By incorporating behavioral strategies into play activities, therapists can help children practice new skills and behaviors in a safe and supportive environment. For example, a therapist might use a reward system during play to encourage a child to complete tasks or demonstrate prosocial behaviors, thereby reinforcing these positive actions.

### Skill Building

Teaching children coping skills and problem-solving strategies is a critical component of CBPT. Through structured play activities, children learn techniques for managing stress, handling conflicts, and solving problems. These skills are taught in an engaging and interactive manner, making it easier for children to understand and apply them in their daily lives. For instance, a game that involves solving puzzles or overcoming challenges can be used to teach problem-solving steps and coping mechanisms.

### Psychoeducation

Teaching children new ideas, concepts, and skills is a cornerstone of the work of CBPT. Educating children and their families about the connection between thoughts, feelings, and behaviors is integral. This psychoeducational component helps children and their caregivers understand how cognitive processes influence emotions and actions. By incorporating educational elements into play, therapists can make these concepts accessible and relevant to young clients. For example, a storybook that illustrates the impact of positive thinking on behavior can be used to facilitate discussions and reinforce learning.

### Effectiveness and Applications

CBPT's structured approach allows for clear goals and measurable outcomes, making it a widely used therapeutic modality for children. The therapy's emphasis on cognitive and behavioral change, combined with the engaging nature of play, ensures that it is both effective and appealing to young clients. Research has consistently shown that CBPT is effective in treating a variety of issues, including anxiety, depression, ADHD, and behavioral problems (Atayi et al., 2018; Badamian & Ebrahimi Moghaddam, 2017; Drewes, 2009; Knell, 1995).

### Contemporary Relevance

Today, CBPT continues to evolve and adapt, incorporating new research findings and therapeutic techniques to enhance its effectiveness. Modern applications of CBPT often integrate digital tools and technology to engage children in therapeutic processes. For example, interactive games and apps designed based on CBPT principles can help children practice cognitive restructuring and behavioral interventions in a familiar and engaging digital environment.

## Integrating Mindfulness into Cognitive-Behavioral Play Therapy

Mindfulness can be easily integrated into CBPT to enhance the therapeutic process. It would be all too easy, however, for therapists to learn how to utilize CBPT to introduce MBPT interventions without first heeding the guidance of this book to develop a personal mindfulness practice. In many years of training and supervising therapists new to play therapy, I have observed all too often the tendency for therapists to rush to adopt a play-based technique without first establishing a therapeutic alliance through rapport building. When therapists take the time to learn and practice mindfulness, they will be better equipped to have greater self-awareness, emotional regulation, and present-moment focus in sessions with clients. Mindfulness can complement the core principles of CBPT and support the therapist in helping children recognize and change maladaptive thought patterns and behaviors. A mindful therapist can more effectively teach mindfulness to clients.

### Providing a Safe and Supportive Space

In CBPT, creating a safe and supportive space is essential for encouraging children to explore their thoughts and emotions without fear of judgment. This environment enables children to engage more deeply in the therapeutic process, facilitating cognitive restructuring and emotional regulation.

### Emotion Exploration Station

Set up an "Emotion Exploration Station" in the therapy room, equipped with various emotion-themed tools such as emotion cards, feeling faces magnets, and emotion wheels. The therapist can invite the child to choose an emotion card that represents how they feel. Together, they can discuss the chosen emotion, linking it to recent experiences or thoughts. The therapist can use this time to teach the child cognitive-behavioral techniques, such as identifying and challenging negative thoughts associated with the emotion. This activity helps the child feel understood and supported while learning to manage their emotions.

### Cognitive Restructuring Role-Play

Create a role-play corner with costumes, props, and a small stage. The therapist can use this space to act out scenarios with the child that reflect common cognitive distortions, such as "all-or-nothing thinking" or "catastrophizing." By role-playing these scenarios, the therapist can help the child recognize these distortions in their own thinking and practice more balanced and realistic thoughts. This interactive and engaging approach provides a safe space for the child to explore their cognitive patterns and learn effective coping strategies.

### Enhancing the Therapist's Attunement and Presence with Mindfulness

In CBPT, the therapist often engages in teaching the child new concepts and skills through structured play activities. However, the effectiveness of this directive approach is significantly enhanced when the therapist practices mindfulness. Mindfulness helps therapists cultivate a heightened state of awareness and quality of presence, which are crucial for attuning to the child's needs and experiences in the moment during play therapy sessions. By being fully present, therapists can more effectively observe and understand the child's behaviors, emotions, and expressions, making the teaching and skill-building components of CBPT more impactful.

Mindful therapists are better equipped to notice subtle cues and responses from the child, allowing them to adjust their interventions in real-time to better meet the child's presenting needs. This mindful attunement fosters a strong therapeutic alliance, characterized by trust, empathy, and genuine connection. When children feel seen and understood, they are more receptive to learning and applying the new skills and concepts introduced by the therapist.

For example, during a session where the therapist is helping a child practice a technique for noticing their automatic negative thoughts (ANTs) through a role-playing game, mindfulness enables the therapist to detect any signs of confusion or resistance. The therapist can then pause and address these feelings, ensuring the child fully comprehends and feels comfortable with the new skill. This approach not only enhances the child's learning experience but also reinforces the therapeutic relationship, making subsequent sessions more productive and collaborative.

While CBPT involves the direct teaching of cognitive and behavioral strategies, the process is most effective when therapists incorporate mindfulness into their practice. By being fully present and attuned, therapists can build a stronger therapeutic alliance, making the child more open to learning and applying the therapeutic techniques.

### Supporting the Child's Emotional Regulation with Mindfulness

Teaching children new skills through playful activities is a cornerstone of CBPT. Mindfulness can be used to teach children techniques for managing their emotions, thereby supporting the CBPT goal of helping them develop healthier ways of coping with their feelings. Introducing simple mindful breathing exercises can help children experience emotional regulation when they feel overwhelmed. In CBPT, these exercises can be integrated into play activities, making them a natural part of the therapy session.

### Birthday Cake Breath

During play, the therapist can invite a child to imagine standing in front of an aromatic and delicious birthday cake with birthday candles. The child takes a deep breath in through their nose to smell the imaginary cake and then slowly exhales to blow out the candles. This technique helps children focus on their breathing and can be used during moments of heightened anxiety or as a transition among activities.

### Teddy Bear Belly Breathing

Another technique involves using a stuffed teddy bear. The child lies down, places the teddy bear on their abdomen, and watches it rise and fall with each breath. This visual and tactile experience helps the child become more aware of their breathing patterns and promotes relaxation. This can be particularly useful during discussions of thoughts and feelings, helping the child stay grounded and calm.

### Somatic and Sensory Awareness through Mindfulness

Teaching children to tune into their physical sensations through mindfulness is a vital component of CBPT, as it helps them recognize and understand their emotional states. By becoming more aware of their bodily sensations, children can better identify the physical manifestations of their emotions, such as tension, warmth, or a racing heart. This somatic awareness is crucial in CBPT because it connects physical sensations with underlying thoughts and emotions, enabling children to gain a more comprehensive understanding of their experiences. For example, a child might notice that their stomach feels tight when they are anxious, which can lead to discussions about the thoughts contributing to this anxiety. Mindfulness practices, such as guided body scans or mindful breathing, can be incorporated into play therapy sessions to enhance this awareness. As children learn to focus on their physical sensations in the present moment, they develop the ability to pause and reflect before reacting to emotional triggers. This mindful pause helps in restructuring ANTs into more positive and balanced ones. Integrating somatic and sensory awareness with mindfulness in CBPT not only promotes emotional regulation but also empowers children with the skills to manage their thoughts and behaviors effectively. This approach aligns with the goals of CBPT by fostering self-awareness, cognitive flexibility, and resilience, making therapy both engaging and impactful.

### Body Zones Detective Activity

The therapist might guide a child to imagine their body as having different zones or areas to explore, like a treasure map. As they "travel" through each part of their body, they pause to notice any feelings of tension or relaxation. This playful body scan motivates children to become more aware of their physical sensations in a fun and engaging way. The therapist asks the child to become a detective who investigates sounds and textures in and around the playroom. This game helps children foster greater attunement and awareness through the senses.

### Ragdoll and Robot

With this activity, the therapist introduces the child to a ragdoll and a robot, exploring the way each feels as the child holds the toys. The therapist might invite the child to notice the ragdoll is floppy and the robot is rigid and then explain our bodies can be like the robot and the ragdoll. Participating along with the child, the therapist might model what it is to be rigid, stiff, and tense like the robot and then floppy and relaxed like the ragdoll, inviting the child to play along and see how it feels in their body.

### Sensory Mindfulness Kits

The "Sensory Mindfulness Kits" activity is designed to integrate mindfulness with the cognitive and behavioral goals of CBPT. Each kit contains a variety of sensory items, such as scented playdough, textured fabric squares, smooth stones, small musical instruments, and visually stimulating objects like glitter jars. During therapy sessions, these kits are used to help children engage their senses, stay present, and connect their sensory experiences with their cognitive and emotional states. To begin the activity, the therapist introduces the sensory mindfulness kits and explains their purpose. The therapist discusses how mindfulness can help children notice and understand their thoughts and feelings by paying close attention to their senses. The child is then invited to explore the items in the kit and choose one that particularly interests them. For example, the child might select a piece of textured fabric. The therapist guides the child to describe the fabric mindfully, asking questions, such as "What do you notice about the texture?" "Is it rough or smooth?" and "How does it feel against your skin?" As the child engages with the sensory item, the therapist encourages them to reflect on their feelings and thoughts associated with the experience. The therapist might ask, "I wonder how you feel when you touch this fabric?" or "Does it remind you of anything?" This mindful exploration helps the child stay present and fosters a deeper understanding of their sensory experiences. The therapist can then link these sensory reflections to the goals of CBPT by discussing how certain thoughts and feelings are connected to sensory experiences. For instance, if the child feels calm when playing with the scented playdough, the therapist can explore how this sensory experience can be used as a coping strategy in stressful situations. The child learns to associate the calming scent and tactile sensation with relaxation, making it a practical tool for emotional regulation. Similarly, small musical instruments can be used to teach the child about rhythm and sound, encouraging them to focus on the present moment and use music as a way to manage their emotions.

Throughout the session, the therapist practices mindful listening and provides positive reinforcement, acknowledging the child's efforts and insights. By integrating these sensory mindfulness activities, the therapist helps the child develop skills in emotional regulation, cognitive restructuring, and self-awareness. The sensory mindfulness kits make the therapeutic process engaging and tangible, allowing children to explore and understand their inner experiences in a structured yet flexible environment. By regularly incorporating these kits into therapy sessions, children can gradually build their ability to pause, reflect, and choose more constructive thoughts and behaviors, aligning with the core principles of CBPT and mindfulness. This approach not only enhances the child's emotional and cognitive skills but also provides them with practical tools to use in their everyday lives.

*Nature's Mindful Journey*

This sensory exploration activity designed for CBPT incorporates mindfulness using items from nature. In this activity, children explore various natural objects to engage their senses and practice mindfulness, fostering self-awareness and emotional regulation. To set up the activity, the therapist collects a variety of natural items, such as smooth stones, pinecones, leaves, flowers, shells, and pieces of bark. These items are placed in a basket or spread out on a table for the children to explore. The therapist begins by introducing the concept of mindfulness, explaining how paying close attention to their senses can help them stay present and calm. During the activity, each child selects an item from the collection and is encouraged to observe it mindfully. The therapist guides the child through a series of sensory questions, such as "What do you see when you look closely at this leaf?" "How does this pinecone feel in your hand?" "What does this flower smell like?" and "Can you hear any sounds when you gently shake this shell?" These prompts help the child focus on their immediate sensory experiences, promoting a state of mindfulness. As the children explore their items, the therapist encourages them to reflect on their thoughts and feelings associated with each sensory experience. For instance, a child might share that the smooth stone feels calming, or that the scent of the flower reminds them of a happy memory. This reflection helps children connect their sensory experiences with their emotions and thoughts, aligning with the goals of CBPT to identify and modify cognitive patterns. After the exploration, the therapist facilitates discussion, allowing the child to share their experiences and insights. The therapist highlights how being mindful of their senses can help them stay grounded and manage their emotions more effectively. By linking these sensory experiences to the principles of CBPT, the activity reinforces the importance of mindfulness in emotional regulation and cognitive restructuring.

*Facilitating Cognitive Restructuring and Insight with Mindfulness*

Mindfulness encourages self-reflection, helping children gain insights into their own thoughts and behaviors. This aligns with the goals of CBPT by fostering cognitive restructuring and understanding through play. By integrating mindfulness techniques into CBPT, children can become more aware of their thought patterns and behaviors.

*Brain Train Check-in*

The therapist can introduce a child to the analogy of a train with so many cars, all different types and different colors, carrying different cargo. Having a toy train set on tracks provides a visual and tactile example. The therapist explains how thoughts often travel into and through our brain, much like a train, one thought after another, seemingly connected, moving fast. The therapist might prompt the child to pause and reflect on what thoughts they can notice in the moment. This reflection helps children identify and challenge negative thought patterns, supporting cognitive restructuring and promoting healthier thinking and behavior patterns.

*Projective Puppet Play*

Puppets are a natural way for children to project their thoughts, feelings, and experiences onto the puppets so they can explore those thoughts, feelings, and experiences with an emotionally safe distance. Puppet play invites the child to give a puppet a voice to express thoughts and feelings to another puppet. The therapist can participate in a very child-led or therapist guided role-play experience.

**Mindfulness in CBPT through Storytelling**

Mindful storytelling in CBPT helps children reflect on their thoughts and behaviors. Therapists can incorporate toy figures, blocks, or any other items in the playroom and use open-ended prompts and guided questions to encourage narratives that explore emotions and thoughts. Through active listening and reflective responses, therapists validate the child's expressions and incorporate cognitive restructuring techniques, helping children consider alternative thoughts and solutions. Integrating behavioral interventions, therapists use stories to reinforce positive behaviors and address problematic ones, teaching coping skills and problem-solving strategies. Psychoeducation is woven into stories, explaining the connection among thoughts, feelings, and behaviors. Positive reinforcement and encouragement throughout the process build the child's confidence, while linking story elements to real-life experiences makes the therapeutic lessons relevant and practical. This structured storytelling approach ensures that CBPT is both engaging and effective in achieving therapeutic goals.

*Problem-Solving Story*

During a play session, the therapist can use action figures or dolls to act out a story where a character faces a problem similar to the child's current challenges. As the story progresses, the therapist pauses and asks the child to reflect on what the character is thinking and feeling, encouraging the child to use the toys to suggest possible solutions. This playful approach helps the child practice cognitive restructuring by exploring alternative ways of thinking and problem-solving in a tangible, engaging manner.

*Perspective-Taking Story*

Another approach is to develop a story where characters have conflicting viewpoints, using arts and crafts materials. The therapist and child can create puppets or masks representing different characters. The therapist can pause the story at key moments and ask the child to use puppets or masks to reflect on each character's perspective and feelings. This exercise helps the child understand the thoughts and emotions of others, promoting empathy and cognitive flexibility. By considering different perspectives through creative expression, the child learns to evaluate their own thoughts and behaviors more critically, supporting the goals of CBPT.

### Mindfully Promoting Awareness, Behavioral Change, and Skill Building

Creating a therapeutic environment characterized by acceptance and presence is essential for effective CBPT. Mindfulness practices help therapists cultivate such an environment where children feel valued and respected. This environment supports the child's engagement in therapy and promotes emotional safety, which is crucial for the effectiveness of CBPT.

Mindful creative and expressive activities can significantly enhance CBPT by promoting behavioral change through an engaging and supportive framework. In a welcoming environment filled with various art supplies, therapists encourage children to practice mindful observation, grounding them in the present moment. These activities serve as a medium for cognitive restructuring, allowing children to identify and challenge negative thoughts by visualizing positive outcomes. Behavioral interventions can be introduced and reinforced through creative and expressive activities.

*Paper Action Chain*

Together therapist and child can cut paper strips and write action steps that map out a path to a desired behavioral outcome, creating a paper chain that can be displayed in the playroom during session or taken home to remind the child.

*Stress-Less Jars*

Create mindfulness jars with the child to support self-regulation, using water, glitter, and food coloring. These jars can be used as a calming tool during sessions or at home, reminding the child of an alternative action to yelling or becoming aggressive. When the child feels overwhelmed, they can shake the jar and watch the glitter settle, using this time to take deep breaths and center themselves. This activity not only promotes mindfulness but also reinforces the therapist's acceptance and support for the child's emotional regulation.

*Clay Play*

Children can explore the use of clay in their hands, squeezing, pounding, stretching, rolling, pinching, and pulling the clay while feeling intense emotions as they learn to consciously channel big emotional energy in a way that is creative and expressive and not harmful to self and others.

### Psychoeducation with Mindful Creative and Expressive Activities

Creative and expressive activities can be used for psychoeducation, helping children understand the connection among thoughts, feelings, and behaviors through hands-on activities like collages. Integrating mindfulness into these activities enhances their effectiveness by encouraging children to reflect mindfully on their creations, which boosts self-awareness and internalizes therapeutic lessons. Throughout the process, therapists provide positive reinforcement, acknowledging the child's efforts and progress, which boosts confidence and motivation. Incorporating mindful art activities into both therapy sessions and daily practice helps children develop mindfulness, reframe negative thoughts, reinforce positive behaviors, and learn valuable coping skills, making CBPT both engaging and effective.

*Mindful Feelings Wheel*

This activity involves creating a wheel divided into sections, each representing a different emotion. Using large paper or cardboard, markers, crayons, scissors, and glue, the child starts by drawing a large circle divided like a pie chart. The therapist discusses common emotions with the child, such as happiness, sadness, anger, fear, surprise, and calmness, allowing the child to choose which emotions to include. Each section is colored and decorated to represent a specific emotion, with the child drawing faces or images that symbolize each feeling. The sections are labeled with the names of the emotions, either by the child or with the therapist's assistance. Mindfulness is integrated into the activity by encouraging the child to take a moment to reflect on each emotion as they create the sections, fostering present-moment awareness. Optionally, a spinner can be added in the center using a brad and a paper arrow to make the activity interactive. The child can then use the Feelings Wheel by spinning the arrow or pointing to different sections to express how they are feeling. The therapist encourages the child to mindfully reflect on times when they felt each emotion, fostering a better understanding and expression of their feelings and enhancing self-awareness.

*Ocean of Emotions*

This mindfulness-based emotion-awareness activity is a creative and expressive project designed to help children identify, understand, and express their emotions. Using a large piece of blue paper or cardboard to represent the ocean, children are provided with magazines, newspapers, scissors, glue, markers, and optional decorative items. The child looks through the magazines and newspapers to find and cut out images, words, and colors that symbolize various emotions they have experienced, such as happiness, sadness, anger, fear, surprise, and calmness. They then mindfully arrange and glue these clippings onto the blue paper, with each section of the ocean representing a different emotion. The child can further personalize their collage with drawings, embellishments, and stickers, reflecting on their choices as they create. Throughout the activity, the therapist encourages the child to take mindful pauses to discuss why they chose specific images and how these images relate to their feelings. This reflective process helps the child visually and tangibly explore their emotions, facilitating a deeper understanding and expression of their internal experiences in a supportive and engaging manner. By integrating mindfulness, the activity not only enhances emotional awareness but also fosters a sense of calm and presence in the therapeutic process.

### Mindfulness in CPBT with Games

Integrating therapeutic board games and card games into CBPT can effectively enhance the therapeutic process by incorporating elements of mindfulness. There are many board and card games available that are specifically designed to facilitate discussion and reflection, providing a structured yet playful avenue for children to express their thoughts and feelings. These games prompt children to share their experiences and emotions through guided questions and scenarios, helping them articulate and process their internal world. During gameplay, the therapist practices mindful listening, giving their full attention to the child's words and behaviors without judgment. This mindful presence helps create an environment of acceptance and empathy, crucial for effective therapeutic work (Kazantzis et al., 2018).

Mindfulness in this context involves being fully present with the child, acknowledging their emotions, and validating their experiences. As children navigate the game, therapists can gently guide them to notice and reflect on their emotional responses and thought patterns. For example, if a game card prompts a child to discuss a time when they felt scared, the therapist can help the child mindfully explore this memory, encouraging them to focus on their bodily sensations and emotions associated with that experience. This approach not only aids in emotional regulation but also aligns with CBPT's goal of helping children identify and modify unhelpful cognitive patterns (Kendall et al., 2017).

Therapeutic games offer a safe and engaging platform for children to practice new coping strategies and problem-solving skills. For instance, as children encounter different scenarios in the game, they can experiment with various responses and see the outcomes in a low stakes setting. The therapist can then reinforce positive behaviors and cognitive strategies, providing immediate feedback and encouragement. This experiential learning is enhanced by the mindful attention of the therapist, who ensures that each step of the process is supportive and aligned with therapeutic goals.

Research supports the effectiveness of integrating games into therapy, highlighting their role in increasing engagement and making therapeutic concepts more accessible to children (Wiener et al., 2019). By combining therapeutic games with mindfulness, CBPT practitioners can create a dynamic and interactive environment that fosters emotional and cognitive growth. This approach helps children develop greater self-awareness, emotional intelligence, and resilience, all of which are essential for their overall mental health and well-being.

### Thought Garden Adventure

This game is designed to integrate mindfulness skills with the cognitive goals of CBPT. This game helps children practice pausing and noticing their present-moment experiences while learning to consciously restructure negative thought patterns into positive, potential-focused thoughts. In this game, children use a custom game board that can be pre-created by the therapist or created together in therapy with the child. The board can look like a colorful garden with different themed sections, each representing various scenarios or challenges (e.g., school, home, friends, and self-image). Players move around the board using a die, and each space on the board corresponds to a card drawn from two decks: the "Mindful Pause" deck and the "Plant a New Thought" deck. The "Mindful Pause" cards prompt the child to pause and engage in a mindfulness exercise, such as taking three deep breaths, describing their current feelings and sensations, or observing their surroundings for a minute. These activities help the child become more present and grounded, reinforcing the skill of pausing before reacting. After completing the mindfulness exercise, the child then draws a card from the "Plant a New Thought" deck. These cards present a scenario with an ANT, such as "I always mess up" or "Nobody likes me." The card then guides the child through a series of questions and prompts to help them challenge and reframe this negative thought. For instance, the card might ask, "What evidence do you have that supports this thought? What evidence do you have against it? What is a more balanced way to think about this situation?" The child then formulates a positive, realistic thought, such as "I sometimes make mistakes, but I also do many things well" or "I have friends who care about me." As the game progresses, the therapist facilitates discussions around each card, helping the child deepen their understanding of how their thoughts influence their feelings and behaviors. The game not only makes learning cognitive restructuring engaging and interactive but also reinforces the importance of mindfulness in noticing and changing thought patterns. Through repeated play, children practice these skills in a supportive environment, gradually building their ability to pause, reflect, and choose more constructive thoughts, thereby fostering emotional resilience and cognitive flexibility.

*Pause and Reflect Beach Ball Game*

This is a fun and engaging activity designed to teach children the skill of pausing and reflecting on their choices. This game uses a colorful beach ball, with different prompts written on each section, to facilitate mindful reflection and decision-making. To play the game, the therapist and child sit across from each other and gently toss the beach ball. When the child catches the ball, they look at the prompt closest to their right thumb. These prompts are designed to encourage mindfulness and reflection, such as "Name one thing you noticed today," "How do you feel right now?" "Think of a time you made a good choice. What did you do?" and "What is one thing you are grateful for?" The child reads the prompt aloud and takes a moment to pause, think, and then share their response with the group. As the child shares, the therapist models mindful listening.

By incorporating these play-based items and activities into CBPT, therapists can create a therapeutic environment emphasizing acceptance and presence, supporting the child's emotional and cognitive development.

### Mindfulness and Empathy

Mindfulness enhances the therapist's ability to empathize with children, allowing them to understand the child's experiences from a compassionate and non-judgmental perspective. It is also a concept that can be taught to children as an important part of their emotional development for healthy relationships with self and others. This empathy strengthens the therapeutic relationship and facilitates meaningful change by helping the child feel valued and supported.

### Empathy Cards

Introduce a set of "Empathy Cards" featuring different scenarios and emotions. During a session, the therapist and child can take turns drawing a card and discussing how they would feel and think in the depicted scenario. The therapist can model empathetic responses, demonstrating how to understand and validate emotions. This activity helps the child learn to express their feelings and recognize empathy in themselves and others, reinforcing the supportive therapeutic relationship.

### Storytelling with Cognitive Reframing

Use storytelling as a tool to practice empathy and cognitive restructuring. The therapist can start a story about a character facing a challenging situation and pause at key moments to ask the child what the character might be thinking and feeling. Together, they can brainstorm alternative, more positive thoughts the character could have. This collaborative storytelling not only builds empathy by encouraging the child to consider different perspectives but also teaches cognitive reframing techniques, reinforcing the principles of CBPT in a compassionate and engaging way.

## Conclusion

Integrating mindfulness into CBPT enhances the therapeutic process by fostering self-awareness, emotional regulation, and present-moment focus for both the therapist and the child. By incorporating mindfulness into the core principles of CBPT – cognitive restructuring, behavioral interventions, skill building, and psychoeducation – therapists can create a more effective and compassionate therapeutic environment. This integration supports the CBPT goals of helping children develop healthier coping methods, improving their emotional and behavioral functioning, and fostering a sense of safety and acceptance.

## References

Atayi, E., Shojaee, S., & Khodaei, S. (2018). The effectiveness of cognitive behavioral play therapy on reducing anxiety and depression in children with cancer. *Journal of Pediatric Psychology, 43*(7), 778–787. https://doi.org/10.1093/jpepsy/jsy029

Badamian, S., & Ebrahimi Moghaddam, M. (2017). A study of the impact of cognitive behavioral play therapy on the reduction of anxiety and aggression in children. *Journal of Cognitive Behavioral Psychotherapy, 9*(2), 101–115.

Drewes, A. A. (2009). Blending play therapy with cognitive behavioral therapy: Evidence-based and other effective treatments and techniques. In A. A. Drewes, S. C. Bratton, & C. E. Schaefer (Eds.), *Integrative play therapy* (pp. 187–214). John Wiley & Sons.

Kazantzis, N., Reinecke, M. A., Freeman, A., & Spence, S. H. (2018). Cognitive-behavioral therapy: Evidence and limitations. *American Psychologist, 73*(5), 526–540. https://doi.org/10.1037/amp0000306

Kendall, P. C., Hudson, J. L., & Chu, B. C. (2017). Cognitive-behavioral therapy for anxiety and depression in children and adolescents: Strategies for the next generation. *Journal of Clinical Child & Adolescent Psychology, 46*(1), 1–19. https://doi.org/10.1080/15374416.2016.1220311

Kenney-Noziska, S. (2008). Cognitive-behavioral play therapy techniques in the treatment of children with PTSD. *Play Therapy, 4*(3), 26–30.

Knell, S. M. (1993). *Cognitive-behavioral play therapy*. Jason Aronson.

Knell, S. M. (1995). Cognitive-behavioral play therapy for children. In J. L. Jacobus (Ed.), *Handbook of cognitive-behavioral approaches in primary care* (pp. 299–315). Routledge.

Landreth, G. L. (2012). *Play therapy: The art of the relationship* (3rd ed.). Routledge.

Wiener, J., Bristow, J., & Gray, S. (2019). Therapeutic games for children with social and emotional difficulties: A systematic review. *British Journal of Educational Psychology, 89*(4), 548–571. https://doi.org/10.1111/bjep.12259

# 8
# MINDFULNESS IN ECOSYSTEMIC PLAY THERAPY

## Introduction

Ecosystemic Play Therapy (EPT), developed by Kevin O'Connor in 2000, is a historically significant and seminal approach in play therapy. EPT is rooted in the understanding that a complex interplay of multiple environments and systems influences a child's behavior and development. This approach emphasizes the interconnectedness of various systems, including family, school, peers, and the larger community, and how these systems shape a child's experiences and behaviors.

## History and Basis of EPT

Kevin O'Connor's development of EPT was inspired by the need to address the multifaceted influences on a child's life. Drawing from Bronfenbrenner's ecological systems theory (Ashiabi & O'Neil, 2015), O'Connor recognized that effective therapy must consider the dynamic interactions between a child and their surrounding environments (O'Connor, 2000, 2015). EPT integrates elements from various therapeutic modalities, including cognitive-behavioral, psychodynamic, humanistic, and systemic approaches, to address the diverse needs of children comprehensively. This integrative framework allows therapists to tailor interventions that consider biological, psychological, social, and cultural factors, making EPT a holistic and adaptable approach (O'Connor, 2000, 2015).

DOI: 10.4324/9781003468585-8

## Tenets of Ecosystemic Play Therapy

### Systems Perspective

EPT operates on the principle that a child's behavior is both influenced by and influences multiple interconnected systems. This perspective helps therapists understand the child's experiences within the broader context of their family, school, peer group, and community. By considering these interactions, therapists can develop more effective and comprehensive treatment plans (O'Connor, 2015).

### Holistic Approach

EPT adopts a holistic approach, considering the biological, psychological, social, and cultural factors that impact a child's development. This comprehensive view ensures that all aspects of the child's life are addressed, promoting overall well-being and growth (O'Connor, 2015).

### Integration of Multiple Theories

EPT is distinguished by its integration of various therapeutic modalities. Techniques and concepts from cognitive-behavioral therapy, psychodynamic therapy, humanistic approaches, and systemic theories are utilized to create a cohesive and personalized treatment plan for each child. This flexibility allows therapists to address a wide range of emotional and behavioral challenges effectively (O'Connor, 2015).

### Active Collaboration

A core component of EPT is the active collaboration with parents, teachers, and other significant figures in the child's life. Involving these key individuals supports the therapeutic goals and ensures interventions are reinforced across different environments. This collaborative effort helps create a consistent and supportive network around the child, enhancing the effectiveness of the therapy (O'Connor, 2015).

## Relevance and Effectiveness

EPT is recognized for its relevance and effectiveness in addressing a wide array of emotional and behavioral challenges in children. Its integrative and systemic approach allows therapists to design flexible and comprehensive interventions tailored to each child's unique needs, making EPT a versatile and impactful therapeutic model (O'Connor, 2015).

### Addressing Diverse Emotional and Behavioral Challenges

EPT is particularly effective in treating a variety of issues, including anxiety, depression, trauma, attachment disorders, and behavioral problems. By considering the complex interplay of factors influencing a child's behavior, EPT provides a nuanced understanding that leads to more effective interventions. For instance, a child experiencing anxiety may not only receive cognitive-behavioral strategies to manage their symptoms but also benefit from family therapy sessions to address underlying familial dynamics contributing to their anxiety (O'Connor, 2000, 2015).

### Integrative and Systemic Approach

The integrative nature of EPT means that therapists can draw from a range of therapeutic modalities to create a comprehensive treatment plan. This approach ensures that interventions are holistic, addressing the biological, psychological, social, and cultural dimensions of the child's life. For example, integrating mindfulness practices can help children develop self-regulation skills, while cognitive-behavioral techniques can be used to challenge and reframe negative thought patterns. This multifaceted approach is supported by evidence indicating that combined therapeutic strategies are often more effective than single-modality treatments (Bratton et al., 2005; O'Connor, 2000).

### Role in Advocacy

EPT extends beyond individual therapy sessions by playing a critical role in advocating for the child's needs within their broader ecosystem. Therapists work closely with parents, teachers, and other significant figures in the child's life to ensure that the therapeutic strategies are reinforced in all environments the child interacts with. This collaboration might involve the therapist attending school meetings, providing training for parents and teachers on how to support the child's therapeutic goals, and facilitating communication between different parts of the child's support system. Research has shown that such systemic involvement leads to more sustainable and long-term positive outcomes for children (Bronfenbrenner, 1979; O'Connor, 2000).

### Supporting Developmental and Therapeutic Goals

The advocacy component of EPT is vital for creating an environment that supports the child's developmental and therapeutic goals (O'Connor, 2000, 2015). For example, if a child is working on improving social skills, the therapist might collaborate with teachers to create opportunities for positive peer interactions at school. Similarly, family sessions might focus on improving communication patterns and fostering a supportive home environment. By ensuring that the child's entire ecosystem is aligned with their therapeutic objectives, EPT helps create a consistent and reinforcing context for the child's growth and healing (Swank et al., 2015).

### Sustainable and Long-Term Outcomes

The comprehensive and systemic nature of EPT contributes to its ability to achieve sustainable and long-term outcomes. By addressing issues across multiple contexts and involving key figures in the child's life, EPT ensures that therapeutic gains are maintained and built upon over time. Studies have demonstrated that children who receive ecosystemic interventions show significant improvements in emotional regulation, behavior, and overall well-being, and these improvements are often sustained long after therapy has ended (O'Connor, 2000; Swank et al., 2015).

The relevance and effectiveness of EPT lie in its ability to address complex emotional and behavioral challenges through an integrative, holistic, and collaborative approach. By tailoring interventions to each child's unique needs and actively involving their support systems, EPT not only facilitates immediate therapeutic progress but also promotes long-term, sustainable positive outcomes (O'Connor, 2000, 2015).

## Integrating Mindfulness into EPT

Incorporating mindfulness into EPT can further enhance its effectiveness. Mindfulness practices help children become more aware of their thoughts, feelings, and physical sensations, fostering self-regulation and emotional resilience. For example, during play therapy sessions, children can be guided to pause and mindfully observe their emotions and reactions, helping them to connect these experiences with the broader systems in their lives. Mindfulness can also be integrated into activities that involve parents and teachers, promoting a shared understanding of the child's needs and reinforcing therapeutic strategies across different contexts.

EPT, with its rich theoretical foundation and comprehensive approach, remains a pivotal and influential model in the field of play therapy. By integrating multiple therapeutic modalities and emphasizing the inter-connectedness of various systems, EPT offers a robust framework for understanding and supporting children's development. The inclusion of mindfulness practices further enhances the therapeutic process, helping children and their support systems to achieve greater emotional and cog-nitive well-being.

### *Enhancing the Therapist's Attunement and Presence*

In EPT, there is a practice of attuning to the energy level the child brings to session so that the therapist can adjust their own energy level accord-ingly (O'Connor, 2000; Wonders, 2021). Mindfulness practices help therapists cultivate a heightened state of awareness and presence, which are crucial for attuning to the child's needs and experiences during play therapy sessions. By being fully present, therapists can more effectively observe and understand the child's behaviors, emotions, and expressions within the context of their multiple environments.

### *Mindful Presence*

In EPT, mindful presence is crucial, especially during the assessment phase when interacting with members of the child's ecosystem. Practicing mindfulness helps therapists match the energy of the child and their environment, fostering a deeper connection and understanding. Kevin O'Connor emphasizes the importance of therapists attuning to the energy level the child brings into the playroom. This attunement allows therapists to meet the child where they are emotionally and energetically, facilitating a more effective therapeutic interaction (O'Connor, 2000).

By engaging in techniques such as mindful breathing before sessions, therapists can center themselves and remain fully present during inter-actions. This focused presence is essential for building rapport with the child and the various members of their support system, including parents, teachers, and peers. O'Connor notes that this energy matching helps create a harmonious and empathetic connection, enabling therapists to better understand and address the child's needs (O'Connor, 2000).

This mindfulness-based approach not only enhances the therapist's ability to attune to the child's needs but also facilitates connections with the child's ecosystem, ensuring that all parties are aligned in supporting the child's developmental and therapeutic goals.

*Reflective Observation*

Mindfulness enhances the therapist's ability to engage in reflective observation, especially important during the EPT assessment phase of therapy. This allows the therapist to converse with members of the child's ecosystem and fully concentrate on what the child is expressing through play in sessions. This level of attuned observation facilitates trust and connections with the child and with the members of the child's ecosystem.

## Mindfulness and Ecosystemic Play Therapy Interventions

EPT employs a variety of specific interventions to ensure that the child's ecosystem is thoroughly accessed and considered throughout the course of treatment (O'Connor, 2000, 2015). Integrating mindfulness into these interventions enhances their effectiveness by promoting present-moment awareness, emotional regulation, and deeper connections within the child's support system.

### Ecosystemic Mindfulness Starters

Begin each session with a brief mindfulness exercise that involves elements from the child's ecosystem. For example, the therapist might invite the child to choose a toy or figure that represents their favorite place to be and describes who is there, the sights, sounds, and smells. This activity helps the child feel grounded and connected to their broader environment, setting a mindful tone for the session. Another ecosystemic mindfulness session starter might be to blow bubbles together, mindful of the sensation of breath and mindful of all the bubbles that might represent all the people that have ever been a part of the child's ecosystem.

### Family Play Sessions

Incorporating family play sessions allows the therapist to observe and interact with family dynamics directly. Activities might include joint play exercises, family art projects, or role-playing scenarios that encourage family members to express their feelings and work on communication. Mindfulness can be woven into these sessions by guiding the family through mindful breathing exercises before starting and encouraging mindful listening during interactions. This helps family members stay present and attuned to each other's needs, fostering healthier family dynamics (O'Connor, 2000).

### School Collaboration

Therapists often collaborate with school personnel to create a consistent support system for the child. This can include meetings with teachers and school counselors, classroom observations, and developing individualized education plans (IEPs) that integrate therapeutic goals. Mindfulness practices, such as classroom mindfulness activities or mindful breaks, can be introduced and recommended to teachers to support the child's focus and emotional regulation at school. Regular communication ensures that the child's progress is monitored and supported in the school environment, aligning educational strategies with therapeutic interventions (Swank et al., 2015).

### Parent Training and Support

Providing parents with training and support is important in EPT. Therapists may offer parent workshops, individual coaching sessions, or support groups that focus on effective parenting strategies, stress management, and ways to reinforce therapeutic techniques at home. Mindfulness can be integrated by teaching parents mindful parenting techniques, such as being fully present during interactions with their child and practicing self-compassion. This empowers parents to be active participants in their child's therapeutic journey and fosters a supportive home environment (O'Connor, 2000).

### Community Engagement

Engaging the broader community can be beneficial, especially when addressing social or cultural factors that impact the child. This might involve working with community leaders, participating in community events, or connecting families with local resources and support networks. Mindfulness practices, such as community mindfulness workshops or group meditation sessions, can enhance the sense of connection and support within the community. These efforts help create a comprehensive support system that extends beyond the immediate family and school (Bronfenbrenner, 1979).

### Multi-Systemic Case Coordination

Therapists often engage in multi-systemic case coordination, which involves coordinating care with other professionals involved in the child's life, such as medical providers, social workers, and extracurricular activity leaders. Regular case meetings and shared treatment plans ensure that all aspects of the child's ecosystem are considered and addressed, providing a holistic approach to treatment. Mindfulness can be incorporated by starting meetings with a brief mindfulness exercise to center and focus the participants, promoting more effective collaboration (Swank et al., 2015).

### Ecological Assessments

Conducting ecological assessments allows therapists to gather detailed information about the child's various environments. This involves home visits, school observations, and community assessments to identify strengths, stressors, and areas needing intervention. Therapists can incorporate mindfulness by practicing mindful observation during assessments, paying close attention to the details of the child's environments and interactions. These assessments provide a comprehensive understanding of the child's life context, informing tailored therapeutic strategies (O'Connor, 2000).

### Sibling Involvement

Including siblings in therapy sessions can provide insights into sibling dynamics and their impact on the child. Activities that involve siblings can promote understanding, empathy, and positive interactions, enhancing the overall family dynamic. Mindfulness can be incorporated by guiding siblings through mindful interaction exercises, such as mindful play or shared breathing activities, to foster deeper connections and mutual understanding (O'Connor, 2000).

### Therapeutic Playdates

Working with caregivers to organize therapeutic playdates with social peers can help the child practice social skills in a controlled, supportive environment. The therapist works to educate and support parents to facilitate these interactions, providing guidance and support to ensure positive peer relationships and social development. Mindfulness can be integrated by encouraging children to practice mindful listening and awareness during play, helping them stay present and engaged with their peers. This intervention helps children generalize therapeutic gains to their social world (Swank et al., 2015).

### Connected Family Presence

At the start of a session, the therapist can lead a "Family Presence" exercise where the child and their family members engage in a mindfulness activity together. This could involve use of the mindfulness-bell, collective breathing, guided imagery, or discussing a positive memory. This practice helps create a collective sense of presence and acceptance, reinforcing the interconnectedness of the child's ecological system.

### Eco-Map Creation

Incorporate the creation of an eco-map as a mindful activity, with which the child and therapist collaboratively draw a visual representation of the child's ecological system, including family, friends, school, and community. During the process, the therapist mindfully engages with the child, asking reflective questions about each element and its impact on the child's life. This activity not only helps the child feel understood and valued but also allows the therapist to gain a deeper empathic understanding of the child's ecological context.

By utilizing these specific interventions and integrating mindfulness practices, EPT ensures that the child's entire ecosystem is actively engaged and considered throughout the course of treatment. This comprehensive approach helps create a consistent and supportive environment for the child, promoting long-term positive outcomes and enhancing the overall effectiveness of therapy.

### Mindful Eco-Play Interventions

During play activities, intermittently introduce mindfulness prompts that relate to the child's ecosystemic context. For instance, the therapist might use "Community Role-Play" where the child and therapist act out different roles from the child's community (e.g., family members, teachers, friends). Before making decisions in the play scenario, the therapist can ask the child to pause and consider how each character might feel and think, promoting empathy and mindfulness.

### Eco-Reflective Journals

Encourage older children to keep an eco-reflective journal where they can write or draw their thoughts and feelings related to their interactions within their ecosystem. This practice can be done mindfully, with the child taking time to reflect on their experiences with family, friends, school, and community. For example, the journal might include entries about a positive interaction with a teacher or a challenging situation with a peer, helping the child process their emotions and thoughts in the context of their environment. Drawings, words, pictures, or cut-outs from magazines can be used.

### Parent and Community Involvement

Teach parents and community members mindfulness techniques they can practice with the child. For instance, organize a "Family Mindfulness Walk" where parents and children take a walk together in a natural setting, practicing mindful observation and sharing their experiences. Additionally, involve community members by creating "Community Mindfulness Projects" such as a neighborhood garden where children and adults can work together, fostering a supportive and connected environment.

### Mindful Cultural Exploration

Introduce activities that explore the child's cultural background and heritage mindfully. For example, the therapist can facilitate a "Cultural Storytelling" session where the child and their family members share stories, traditions, or practices from their culture. During this activity, the therapist encourages mindful listening and reflection, helping the child feel valued and understood within the context of their cultural identity.

## Conclusion

Integrating mindfulness into EPT enhances the therapeutic process by fostering self-awareness, emotional regulation, and present-moment focus for both the therapist and the child. By incorporating mindfulness into the core principles of EPT – systems perspective, holistic approach, integration of multiple theories, and active collaboration – therapists can create a more effective and compassionate therapeutic environment. This integration supports the EPT goals of helping children develop healthier coping methods, improving their emotional and behavioral functioning, and fostering a sense of safety and acceptance.

## References

Ashiabi, G. S., & O'Neil, M. E. (2015). Understanding children's development within the context of family and community: An ecological approach. *Child Development Perspectives, 9*(2), 129–134. https://doi.org/10.1111/cdep.12121

Bronfenbrenner, U. (1979). *The ecology of human development: Experiments by nature and design*. Harvard University Press.

Bratton, S. C., Ray, D. C., Rhine, T., & Jones, L. (2005). The efficacy of play therapy with children: A meta-analytic review of treatment outcomes. *Professional Psychology: Research and Practice, 36*(4), 376–390. https://doi.org/10.1037/0735-7028.36.4.376

O'Connor, K. (2000). *The play therapy primer* (2nd ed.). Wiley.

O'Connor, K. (2015). Ecosystemic play therapy. In C. E. Schaefer, & H. G. Kaduson (Eds.), *Contemporary play therapy: Theory, research, and practice* (pp. 72–93). Guilford Press.

Swank, J. M., Shin, S. M., Cabrita, C., & Cheung, C. (2015). Effectiveness of ecosystemic play therapy with school-age children: A systematic review. *International Journal of Play Therapy, 24*(1), 41–55. https://doi.org/10.1037/a0038660

Wonders, S. (2021). Attuning to the energy in play therapy: Techniques for deeper connection. *Journal of Play Therapy, 28*(3), 212–225. https://doi.org/10.1037/pla0000173

# 9

# MINDFULNESS IN GESTALT PLAY THERAPY

## Introduction

Gestalt Play Therapy (GPT) is a dynamic and integrative approach rooted in the holistic principles of Gestalt psychotherapy, developed by Fritz Perls in the mid-20th century. Emphasizing present-moment awareness, self-regulation, and the interconnectedness of thoughts, feelings, and behaviors, GPT offers a comprehensive framework for addressing children's emotional and behavioral challenges. Violet Oaklander's pioneering work adapted Gestalt principles specifically for children, utilizing play, art, and creative expression to facilitate self-awareness and healing. Integrating mindfulness into GPT further enhances its efficacy, providing children with tools to connect with their immediate experiences, regulate emotions, and develop healthier coping mechanisms. This chapter delves into the historical evolution, core tenets, and practical applications of GPT, demonstrating how mindfulness practices can be seamlessly woven into therapeutic interventions to support holistic child development.

## History and Evolution of Gestalt Play Therapy

GPT is rooted in the principles of Gestalt psychotherapy, developed by Fritz Perls in the 1940s and 1950s. Gestalt therapy emphasizes holistic awareness, personal responsibility, and the importance of the present

 DOI: 10.4324/9781003468585-9

moment. Perls' approach was groundbreaking in its focus on integrating thoughts, feelings, and behaviors, aiming to help individuals achieve greater self-awareness and self-regulation.

The origins of Gestalt psychotherapy can be traced back to Fritz Perls, who, along with his wife Laura Perls, developed this therapeutic approach as a reaction against the more traditional psychoanalytic methods of the time. Gestalt therapy emphasizes direct experience and experimentation, encouraging clients to become more aware of their thoughts, feelings, and actions in the present moment. Key concepts include the here-and-now focus, the idea of the organism as a whole, and the significance of the therapeutic relationship. All of this is by definition the practice of mindfulness.

Violet Oaklander is credited with adapting Gestalt therapy principles specifically for use with children, creating GPT. In her seminal works, "Windows to Our Children" (1988) and "Hidden Treasure" (2006), Oaklander outlined how play, art, and other expressive techniques could be used to help children become more aware of their inner experiences and how these experiences manifest in their behaviors and interactions. Oaklander's approach integrates creative expression with the core tenets of Gestalt therapy, making the therapeutic process accessible and engaging for children.

Felicia Carroll, a contemporary leader in the field, has further expanded the application of GPT. Carroll has integrated mindfulness practices and modern understandings of child development into the framework established by Oaklander. Her work emphasizes the importance of the therapeutic relationship and the need to adapt interventions to fit the unique developmental needs of each child. Carroll's contributions have helped solidify GPT as a dynamic and evolving field that continues to incorporate new insights and techniques (Carroll, 2024).

In GPT, the therapeutic alliance serves as the container for the child and therapist together to explore experientially what each moment presents with specific interventions and focus on the child's experience of self in the here and now. GPT aims to increase awareness and integration of bodily sensations, thoughts, and feelings so that the child can move toward healing and growth.

## Tenets and Philosophy of Gestalt Play Therapy

### Holistic Approach

GPT views the individual as whole, where thoughts, feelings, and behaviors are interconnected and influence each other. This holistic perspective is a cornerstone of Gestalt theory, emphasizing that one cannot understand the individual by merely examining isolated parts; instead, it is essential to consider the entire experience. In GPT, this approach ensures that therapy addresses all aspects of the child's experience, promoting integrated and comprehensive healing.

### Interconnectedness of Experience

In GPT, the interconnectedness of a child's thoughts, feelings, and behaviors is a fundamental concept. For example, a child's anxious thoughts might manifest as physical tension and behavioral avoidance. By recognizing these connections, the therapist can address the anxiety holistically rather than treating just the symptoms in isolation. This approach helps children understand how their inner experiences shape their actions and vice versa, fostering a more profound self-awareness (Oaklander, 2006).

### Integration of Body and Mind

Gestalt theory says that the mind and body are inseparable and must be considered together in therapy. This principle is evident in interventions like body scans and mindful movement, where children are guided to notice and describe physical sensations associated with their emotions. For instance, a child might be asked to identify where they feel anger in their body, such as a tight chest or clenched fists. This awareness helps children connect their bodily experiences with their emotional states, leading to more effective self-regulation and emotional processing (Oaklander, 1988).

### Present-Moment Awareness

The holistic approach in GPT also emphasizes the importance of present-moment awareness. Therapists encourage children to focus on their current experiences rather than dwelling on the past or worrying about the future. This here-and-now focus helps children become more attuned to their immediate thoughts, feelings, and behaviors, facilitating a deeper understanding and integration of their experiences. For example, during play, a therapist might ask, "What are you feeling right now as you build this structure?" This question prompts the child to explore their current emotional state, promoting mindfulness and self-awareness (Perls, 1969).

### Exploration of the Whole Self

GPT encourages children to explore all facets of their identity, including parts they might typically suppress or ignore. Techniques such as the empty chair or role-play allow children to express different aspects of themselves, integrating these parts into a cohesive sense of self. For instance, a child might role-play both the "shy" part of themselves and the "brave" part, helping them reconcile these seemingly contradictory aspects and understand how each influences their behavior (Oaklander, 2006).

### Creative Expression and Integration

Creative activities like drawing, painting, and sand tray therapy are integral to GPT because they provide avenues for holistic expression. Through these mediums, children can externalize and integrate complex thoughts and emotions that might be difficult to articulate verbally. For example, a child might use art to depict a chaotic scene representing their internal turmoil. Discussing the artwork with the therapist can then help the child piece together and make sense of these fragmented experiences, fostering a more integrated sense of self (Carroll, 2019).

### Relational Dynamics

GPT also focuses on the relational aspects of a child's experience. The therapeutic relationship itself is viewed holistically, with the therapist's authenticity and empathy playing crucial roles in the healing process. By modeling genuine, present interactions, therapists help children learn to relate to others in more integrated and meaningful ways. For instance, through games and collaborative activities, children practice being present and connected with others, enhancing their social skills and emotional intelligence (Oaklander, 1988).

## Mindfulness as a Tool for Integration

Mindfulness practices are naturally woven into the holistic approach of GPT. Techniques like mindful breathing, sensory awareness exercises, and reflective pauses help children integrate their thoughts, feelings, and bodily sensations into a coherent whole. For example, after a playful activity, a therapist might lead a child in a brief mindfulness exercise to reflect on what they felt and thought during the play. This practice helps the child internalize and integrate their experiences, promoting overall well-being and self-understanding (Carroll, 2024).

### Here-and-Now Focus

A core principle of GPT is the emphasis on awareness of the present moment and current experiences rather than past events. This here-and-now focus helps children connect with their immediate thoughts and feelings, making it easier to address and understand their internal processes.

### Present-Moment Awareness

GPT emphasizes staying attuned to what is happening in the present moment. This focus helps children and therapists work with the immediate thoughts, feelings, and sensations that arise during the session. By concentrating on the here-and-now, children can better understand their current experiences and how they affect their behavior and emotions. For example, a therapist might ask a child, "What are you feeling right now while you play with these blocks?" This question directs the child's attention to their present emotional state, facilitating immediate emotional processing and awareness (Perls, 1969).

### Immediate Feedback

Providing immediate feedback is a vital component of the here-and-now focus in GPT. Therapists respond to the child's actions, emotions, and expressions as they occur, helping the child understand and integrate their experiences in real time. This approach encourages children to become more aware of how their thoughts and feelings influence their behaviors. For instance, if a child expresses frustration during a game, the therapist might say, "I notice you seem frustrated. Can you tell me more about what you're feeling right now?" This immediate feedback helps the child articulate and process their emotions on the spot (Oaklander, 2006).

### Mindful Play

Incorporating mindfulness into play activities reinforces the here-and-now focus. Children are encouraged to engage in play mindfully, paying close attention to their movements, sensations, and emotional responses. For example, during a sand tray activity, a therapist might guide a child to notice the texture of the sand and how it feels as they move their hands through it. This mindful engagement helps children stay present and connected to their immediate experiences, enhancing their ability to process and understand their emotions (Carroll, 2019).

### Exploration of Current Experiences

GPT encourages children to explore their current experiences in depth. This might involve discussing a recent event at school or exploring feelings that have arisen during the session. By focusing on what is happening now, children can gain insights into their behaviors and emotional reactions, leading to greater self-awareness and self-regulation. For example, if a child talks about a recent argument with a friend, the therapist might explore the child's feelings and thoughts about the incident, helping them understand their emotional responses and how they can manage similar situations in the future (Oaklander, 1988).

### Integration with the Therapeutic Relationship

The here-and-now focus also strengthens the therapeutic relationship. By being fully present with the child, therapists can model genuine, empathetic, and authentic interactions. This presence helps build trust and safety, allowing the child to explore their feelings and experiences more openly. For instance, if a child feels anxious during a session, the therapist might use grounding techniques to help the child stay present and calm, demonstrating that the therapist is attuned to the child's current state and ready to support them (Perls, 1969).

### Awareness and Self-Regulation in Gestalt Play Therapy

GPT encourages children to become aware of their internal states and learn to regulate their emotions and behaviors. Through play and creative expression, children explore their feelings and thoughts, gaining insights that help them develop better self-regulation skills.

### Developing Self-Awareness

A central goal of GPT is to help children become more aware of their internal experiences. By engaging in various therapeutic activities, children learn to identify and articulate their emotions, thoughts, and bodily sensations. For example, a therapist might use a body scan exercise, guiding the child to notice where they feel tension or relaxation. This practice helps children connect physical sensations with their emotional states, fostering a deeper understanding of their internal world (Oaklander, 2006).

### Expressive Arts and Play

Creative expression through art, play, and other modalities is a key component of GPT. Activities such as drawing, painting, sculpting, and role-playing allow children to externalize and explore their feelings in a safe and structured environment. For instance, a child might draw a picture of a storm to represent their anger, then discuss the drawing with the therapist. This process not only helps the child become more aware of their emotions but also provides a tangible way to work through and understand them (Oaklander, 1988).

### Mindfulness Techniques

Integrating mindfulness techniques into GPT enhances children's ability to regulate their emotions and behaviors. Practices like mindful breathing, sensory awareness exercises, and grounding techniques help children stay present and centered. For example, a therapist might teach a child to use deep breathing when they feel overwhelmed, helping them calm down and regain control. These mindfulness skills are valuable tools for self-regulation, enabling children to manage their reactions more effectively (Carroll, 2019).

*Exploring and Understanding Emotions*

Through the therapeutic process, children are encouraged to explore and understand their emotions. GPT provides a space where children can safely express complex feelings and receive validation and support. Techniques such as the empty chair or role-play allow children to voice different parts of themselves or their feelings toward others. This exploration helps children understand the root causes of their emotions and develop strategies for managing them. For example, a child might role-play a conversation with their "scared" self, discovering ways to comfort and reassure themselves (Perls, 1969).

*Self-Regulation Strategies*

GPT equips children with practical strategies for self-regulation. These strategies are often learned and practiced through play and creative activities. For instance, a child might learn to use a stress ball during moments of frustration or practice visualizing a peaceful scene to reduce anxiety. The therapist guides the child in discovering which techniques work best for them, promoting a sense of agency and empowerment. Over time, these self-regulation skills become internalized, helping children navigate their emotions and behaviors more effectively (Oaklander, 1988).

*Feedback and Reflection*

Regular feedback and reflection are integral to developing self-regulation. Therapists provide immediate and supportive feedback during sessions, helping children understand the impact of their behaviors and emotions. Reflection exercises, such as discussing how a particular activity made them feel, encourage children to think critically about their experiences and learn from them. This ongoing process of feedback and reflection fosters continuous growth and self-awareness (Carroll, 2024).

*Therapeutic Relationship*

The therapeutic relationship in GPT is built on authenticity, empathy, and presence. This relationship provides a secure base from which children can explore their emotions and behaviors. The therapist models healthy emotional regulation and coping strategies, offering children a blueprint for managing their own feelings. By experiencing a supportive and validating relationship, children learn to trust themselves and their ability to handle emotional challenges (Perls, 1969).

## Mindfulness and Gestalt Play Therapy Go Hand in Hand

GPT is steeped in the essence of mindfulness due to its focus on present-moment awareness and holistic integration. Incorporating mindfulness practices more directly enhances the therapy by helping children become more aware of their thoughts, feelings, and bodily sensations. This heightened awareness supports the goals of GPT, such as self-regulation and the integration of the child's internal experiences. Incorporating mindfulness into GPT interventions enhances their effectiveness by not only promoting present-moment awareness but also opportunities for deeper emotional processing. For example, during the empty chair technique, children can be guided to pause and take deep breaths before speaking, helping them center themselves and express their feelings more clearly. In sand tray therapy, mindful observation of the figures and scenes can deepen the child's connection to their inner world, making the therapeutic experience more impactful.

### Specific Mindfulness-based Gestalt Play Therapy Interventions

GPT incorporates a variety of unique interventions that align with its principles of holistic awareness, present-moment focus, self-regulation, and the therapeutic relationship. Here are a few examples.

*Who's in the Chair?*

This classic Gestalt therapy intervention is adapted for children by using a chair and a stuffed animal, toy figure, or puppet the child chooses to represent different parts of themselves, other people, or emotions they are experiencing. The child is invited to interact with the toy in the chair as if it were the person or a part of themselves. This technique helps externalize thoughts and feelings, making them more tangible and easier to explore. For example, a child might direct emotional expression to the toy in the chair, helping them express and understand this emotion more fully.

### A Safe Place

Children are guided to create a "safe place" in the sand using any number of objects and figures they may choose. After the child creates their safe space in the sand, the therapist can invite the child to walk around the sand tray and really look carefully at their safe place. When they feel satisfied with it, the therapist invites the child to "take a picture" of this safe place to hold in their mind and remember anytime they need to help themselves feel safe. This memory of their safe place is used as a grounding tool during therapy. Revisiting this safe place during stressful moments helps the child feel secure and centered, promoting self-regulation.

### Projective Play

Using projective techniques, children are encouraged to project their thoughts and feelings onto toys, dolls, or puppets. For instance, a child might choose a doll to represent themselves and use other toys to act out a scenario they are struggling with. This indirect approach allows children to express difficult emotions and situations in a safe and manageable way, facilitating insight and emotional release.

### Creative Expression

Art and creative expression are central to GPT. Children might be invited to draw, paint, or sculpt their feelings and experiences. For example, a child who struggles with anxiety might be asked to draw or paint what their anxiety looks and feels like, then discuss or alter the image to explore and transform their feelings. This process helps children externalize and gain control over their emotions.

### The Use of Metaphor

Therapists use metaphors to help children have mindful awareness and communicate complex feelings and situations. For example, a child who feels overwhelmed might be asked to imagine their feelings as a storm and then describe or draw how they could calm the storm. This technique allows children to express their emotions creatively and explore solutions metaphorically.

### Role-Play

Role-play allows children to mindfully act out various scenarios or aspects of their lives. A child might role-play a difficult conversation they need to have or a situation that causes them anxiety. Through role-play, children can experiment with different responses and behaviors in a safe environment, gaining confidence and insight into their real-life interactions.

### Body Awareness Activities

Children are guided through activities that increase their awareness of bodily sensations and movements. This might include playful movement activities such as stretching like a cat, leaping like a frog, pretending to be a tree with tall branches in the wind, mindful walking, or noticing how different emotions affect their body posture and sensations. These activities help children connect their physical experiences with their emotional states, promoting holistic self-awareness.

### Sensory Integration

Integrating sensory activities, such as playing with textured materials, listening to calming music, or engaging in movement exercises, helps children stay grounded and present. These activities can be particularly helpful for children who have difficulty staying focused or regulating their emotions. For instance, a child might use kinetic sand to explore feelings of frustration, helping them calm down and articulate their experience.

## Conclusion

GPT's diverse and creative interventions provide children with numerous ways to explore and understand their inner experiences. By integrating mindfulness practices, these interventions become even more powerful, helping children develop greater self-awareness, emotional regulation, and holistic well-being. These specific techniques demonstrate the adaptability and depth of GPT, making it a valuable approach for addressing a wide range of emotional and behavioral issues in children.

## References

Carroll, F. (2019). Mindfulness in gestalt play therapy: Integrating creative expression and emotional regulation. *International Journal of Play Therapy, 28*(3), 212–225. https://doi.org/10.1037/pla0000173

Carroll, F. (2024). Advanced applications of gestalt play therapy with children. In S. Jones (Ed.), *Innovations in play therapy: New approaches for diverse populations* (pp. 34–56). Routledge.

Oaklander, V. (1988). *Windows to our children: A gestalt therapy approach to children and adolescents*. Real People Press.

Oaklander, V. (2006). *Hidden treasure: A map to the child's inner self*. Karnac Books.

Perls, F. S. (1969). *Gestalt therapy verbatim*. Real People Press.

# 10

## MINDFULNESS IN JUNGIAN PLAY THERAPY

### Introduction

Jungian Play Therapy (JPT) is an integrative approach rooted in the analytical psychology developed by Carl Jung in the early 20th century. Emphasizing the exploration of the unconscious, the use of symbols and archetypes, and the process of individuation, JPT provides a framework for understanding and addressing children's emotional and psychological challenges. Adapted by pioneers like Dora Kalff and further advanced by contemporary practitioners, JPT uses symbolic play to help children process complex emotions and achieve psychological balance. Integrating mindfulness into JPT further enhances its therapeutic potential, offering tools for present-moment awareness and emotional regulation. This chapter delves into the historical development, fundamental principles, and practical techniques of JPT, demonstrating how mindfulness can be seamlessly incorporated to foster holistic child development and well-being.

### History and Evolution of JPT

JPT is deeply rooted in the principles of Carl Jung's analytical psychology, which emerged in the early 20th century. Jungian psychotherapy focuses on exploring the unconscious mind, understanding the role of

DOI: 10.4324/9781003468585-10

symbols and archetypes, and facilitating the process of individuation – the journey toward becoming one's true self. Over the years, these foundational concepts have been adapted and expanded into therapeutic practices for children, giving rise to JPT (Green 2009, 2014; Lilly & Heiko, 2019).

### History of Jungian Psychotherapy

Carl Jung, a Swiss psychiatrist, and psychoanalyst, created his technique in response to the limits he saw in Freud's psychoanalysis. Jung stressed the significance of the unconscious mind, dreams, and the collective unconscious – a common reservoir of experiences and patterns shared by all humanity. He believed that psychological health is accomplished by individuation, which is the process of integrating disparate aspects of the mind to form a complete, true self (Jung, 1968).

### Evolution of JPT

JPT began to take shape as therapists sought to apply Jung's theories to work with children. Dora Kalff, a student of Jung, was instrumental in developing sandplay therapy, a key modality within JPT (Heiko, 2024). Kalff's work focused on using a sandbox and miniatures to allow children to express and explore their unconscious mind through symbolic play (Kalff, 2003).

J.P. Lilly further expanded the field by integrating Jungian concepts into various play therapy techniques, emphasizing the importance of symbols and archetypes in children's play. By incorporating Jungian theory, Lilly highlighted how symbols and archetypes serve as fundamental elements in understanding children's unconscious processes and emotional struggles. This approach recognizes that through play, children express and work through their inner worlds, utilizing symbolic language that reflects their developmental stage and psychological needs. Lilly's work underscores the therapeutic potential of engaging with these symbolic expressions, facilitating deeper insight and healing in child therapy (Green, 2014; Lilly, 2015).

Eric Green continued to advance JPT, conducting extensive research, and developing practical approaches for therapists to use Jungian principles in their work with children. Green's work has been instrumental in bridging the gap between theoretical concepts and clinical practice, offering therapists concrete methods to incorporate Jungian ideas into play therapy sessions. His research has explored the therapeutic potential of archetypes, the collective unconscious, and the role of symbolic play in children's psychological development. Green's contributions have been pivotal in establishing JPT as a recognized and effective therapeutic modality, providing valuable tools and frameworks that enhance the therapist's ability to connect with and understand the inner world of the child. His publications and workshops have disseminated these ideas widely, influencing the academic community and practicing therapists (Green, 2009, 2014).

Rosalind Heiko has also made significant contributions to the field of JPT with her specialization in Kalfian Sand Play. Heiko's work emphasizes the importance of creating a safe and sacred space where children can explore their inner worlds through symbols and metaphors. She has also focused on the therapeutic relationship, stressing the need for therapists to be fully present and attuned to the child's needs. Heiko's approach incorporates mindfulness and body awareness techniques, helping children connect their physical sensations with their emotional and psychological experiences. Her contributions have enriched the practice of JPT by blending traditional Jungian concepts with Kalfian Sandplay and other contemporary therapeutic techniques (Heiko, 2021, 2024).

## Tenets of JPT

### Exploration of the Unconscious

JPT utilizes symbols, dreams, and metaphors to explore the unconscious mind. Children's play often reveals hidden thoughts and feelings, providing insights into their inner world (Green, 2014). Through activities like sandplay, drawing, and storytelling, therapists help children bring unconscious material to the surface, facilitating healing and growth (Mitchell & Friedman, 1994).

### Individuation

A core goal of JPT is facilitating individuation, the process of becoming one's true self. This involves integrating different aspects of the psyche, including the shadow (unacknowledged parts of the self) and the persona (the social mask) (Jung, 1968). By engaging with symbolic play, children can explore these parts and move toward psychological balance and wholeness (Green, 2014).

### Archetypes and Symbols

JPT recognizes and works with universal symbols and archetypes that emerge in play. Archetypes are innate, universal prototypes for ideas and may be used to interpret observations (Jung, 1969). Symbols in play provide a means for children to express complex emotions and experiences in a non-verbal manner. The therapist helps the child understand and integrate these symbols, promoting deeper self-awareness and insight (Mitchell & Friedman, 1994).

### Therapeutic Relationship

Building a strong, authentic, and empathetic relationship between the therapist and the child is fundamental in JPT. The therapist acts as a compassionate guide, helping the child navigate their inner world and supporting them through the process of individuation (Allan, 1988). This relationship provides a safe space for the child to explore and express their true self (Green, 2014).

## Aims and Philosophy of JPT

JPT is founded on the principles of Carl Jung's analytical psychology and is designed to help children navigate their internal worlds, achieve psychological balance, and facilitate the process of individuation (Jung, 1968, 2014). The philosophy behind this approach is rooted in the belief that children, like adults, possess a rich inner world that can be accessed and understood through symbolic play. By engaging with symbols, archetypes, and metaphors, children can process their emotions, resolve internal conflicts, and develop a stronger sense of self (Mitchell & Friedman, 1994).

### Understanding the Internal World

One of the primary goals of JPT is to help children gain insight into their internal worlds. This involves exploring their thoughts, feelings, and unconscious processes. Children often express complex emotions and experiences through play, using toys, drawings, and other creative mediums to symbolize their inner states. By observing and engaging with these symbolic expressions, therapists can help children bring unconscious material to the surface, making it available for conscious reflection and understanding (Jung, 1968, 2014).

### Achieving Psychological Balance

JPT aims to promote psychological balance by helping children integrate different aspects of their personality. This includes acknowledging and working with the shadow, or the unacknowledged parts of the self, and the persona, or the social mask they present to the world. By addressing these different facets of the self, children can achieve greater harmony and balance in their internal and external lives. For example, a child who feels compelled to always be "good" might explore their hidden feelings of anger or sadness in therapy, leading to a more balanced and authentic self-expression (Green, 2014).

### Facilitating Individuation

Individuation, a core concept in Jungian psychology, is the process of becoming one's true self. In JPT, this process is facilitated by helping children explore and integrate various parts of their psyche. Through play, children encounter archetypal themes and symbols that resonate with their personal experiences, guiding them on their journey toward self-discovery and personal growth. The therapist supports this process by providing a safe and accepting environment where children can express their true selves without judgment (Kalff, 2003).

### Engagement with Symbols, Archetypes, and Metaphors

Symbols, archetypes, and metaphors play a crucial role in JPT. Archetypes are universal symbols that arise from the collective unconscious and appear in myths, dreams, and play. By engaging with these archetypal images, children can access deeper layers of their psyche and gain insights into their personal and universal experiences. For example, a child might repeatedly play out the theme of a hero's journey, symbolizing their own struggles and triumphs. The therapist helps the child understand

and integrate these symbolic narratives, fostering a deeper sense of self-awareness and resilience (Jung, 1968, 2014).

### Processing Emotions and Resolving Internal Conflicts

Through symbolic play, children can process complex emotions and resolve internal conflicts. Play allows children to express feelings that might be difficult to articulate verbally, such as fear, anger, or sadness. By working through these emotions in a symbolic and non-threatening way, children can achieve emotional release and understanding. For instance, a child might use a toy dragon to represent their fears and, through play, find ways to tame or befriend the dragon, symbolically resolving their internal conflict (Lilly, 2016).

### Developing a Stronger Sense of Self

JPT helps children develop a stronger and more cohesive sense of self. By exploring and integrating various aspects of their inner world, children can build a more unified and resilient identity. The process of individuation involves recognizing and embracing all parts of oneself, leading to greater self-acceptance and confidence. Through therapeutic play, children learn to navigate their internal landscape, fostering a sense of empowerment and self-efficacy (Heiko, 2021).

### Therapeutic Relationship

A key aspect of JPT is the therapeutic relationship. The therapist acts as a compassionate and empathetic guide, providing a safe and nurturing space for the child's exploration. This relationship is built on trust and authenticity, allowing the child to feel secure in expressing their true self. The therapist's presence and attunement to the child's needs facilitate the therapeutic process, enabling the child to explore their inner world more deeply and confidently (Kalff, 2003).

## Integration of Mindfulness in JPT

Mindfulness naturally complements JPT, enhancing the therapeutic process through its alignment with core Jungian principles. By fostering self-awareness, emotional regulation, and present-moment focus, mindfulness supports the exploration and integration of unconscious experiences, central to Jungian theory. In JPT, symbols, archetypes, and the process of individuation are key elements. Mindfulness helps children become more attuned to these symbolic expressions and archetypal patterns, facilitating deeper understanding and integration of their inner world. Additionally, mindfulness aids in the therapeutic alliance, enabling the therapist to maintain an open and present stance, which is essential for guiding children through their individuation journey (Allan, 1988; Green, 2014, 2024; Heiko, 2024).

### Mindfulness Techniques in JPT

#### Mindful Observation in Play

Encouraging children to mindfully pause and observe their play can help them become more aware of the symbols and archetypes they are engaging with. For example, during sandplay, the therapist might prompt the child to take a moment to observe the scene they have created and reflect on the feelings and thoughts it evokes.

#### Mindful Breathing

Incorporating mindful breathing exercises at the beginning of sessions can help children settle into the therapeutic space and become more attuned to their inner world. This practice can also be used during moments of emotional intensity to help the child stay grounded and present.

#### Body Awareness

Guiding children through body awareness exercises is a crucial component of JPT, helping them connect physical sensations with their emotional states. This approach aligns with Jungian principles by emphasizing the integration of mind and body in the individuation process. For instance, a child might be asked to notice where they feel tension in their body when discussing a challenging topic. This practice helps the child link their physical and emotional experiences, promoting a holistic understanding of their inner world. By recognizing and articulating these sensations, children can gain insights into their unconscious processes and develop better self-regulation skills, which are key goals in JPT (Green, 2014; Jung, 1968).

*Mindful Reflection*

After engaging in symbolic play, therapists can guide children in mindful reflection on their experiences, a practice that aligns with JPT principles. By asking questions like, "What did you notice about how you felt when you placed that figure in the sand?" therapists help children connect their play experiences with their conscious awareness. This process supports the integration of unconscious material into the child's conscious mind, facilitating individuation and self-awareness. Mindful reflection encourages children to explore the symbolic meanings of their play, deepening their understanding of archetypes and personal narratives, which are central to JPT (Green, 2014; Kalff, 2003).

*Mindful Presence*

In JPT, therapists can practice mindfulness to maintain an attuned presence, which is essential for building rapport and connecting with the child on a deeper level. Techniques such as mindful breathing or visualization exercises before sessions can help therapists center themselves and be fully present. For example, a therapist might visualize grounding themselves with the image of a tree with deep roots, symbolizing stability, and presence. This practice prepares the therapist to enter the therapeutic space with an open and attentive mindset.

*Reflective Observation*

Mindfulness enhances the therapist's ability to engage in reflective listening and attuning, where they fully concentrate on what the child is expressing through play. In JPT, this deep observation involves paying close attention to the symbolic and archetypal themes that emerge during play. For instance, when a child plays out a scenario involving a hero and a dragon, the therapist listens not only to the storyline but also to the underlying symbolic meanings and emotional resonances. This reflective listening fosters trust and connection, allowing the child to feel understood and validated in their inner world.

*Symbolic Visualization*

Before a session, therapists can engage in a symbolic visualization exercise, imagining themselves entering a sacred space of healing. This helps them attune to the symbolic nature of JPT and prepares them to recognize and honor the archetypal elements in the child's play.

### Active Imagination Dialogue

Therapists can use the technique of active imagination to engage with the child's play. For instance, if a child is enacting a story with figurines, the therapist might say, "I notice the knight is fighting the dragon. What do you think the knight is feeling right now?" This encourages the child to explore the symbolic meaning of their play more deeply.

### Symbolic Journaling

After sessions, therapists can engage in symbolic journaling, where they reflect on the symbols and themes that emerged during the child's play. This practice helps therapists remain attuned to the child's inner world and enhances their ability to connect with the child in future sessions.

### Mindful Sand Therapy

Mindfulness can be effectively combined with Jungian-based sandplay therapy by encouraging clients to focus on the sensory experience of manipulating the sand and the figures they use. This combination allows clients to remain present in the moment, fostering self-awareness and emotional regulation while exploring their inner worlds in a tactile and imaginative way. This integrative approach can deepen the therapeutic process, promoting healing and insight through mindful engagement with the sand tray.

### Mindful Storytelling

Therapists can incorporate mindful storytelling within JPT by creating a narrative based on the child's symbolic play. This narrative includes pauses for reflection, allowing the child to explore different archetypal themes and symbols in their play. This technique helps children gain insight into various perspectives and understand the deeper psychological and emotional consequences of their actions.

Incorporating mindfulness exercises into JPT can help children reflect on their thoughts and feelings while engaging with their unconscious material. For instance, during a sand tray activity, a therapist might invite the child to pause and mindfully observe the scene they have created. The therapist can encourage the child to explore the symbolic meanings of the figures and elements within the tray, discussing what each represents and what feelings arise upon reflection. This process aligns with Jungian concepts of individuation and the integration of unconscious content into conscious awareness.

### The Journey to the Self

This activity can help children explore different parts of their psyche and facilitate the process of individuation. Supplies needed are a large paper or poster board, markers, crayons, or colored pencils, various images and symbols cut out from magazines, glue and scissors. The child is asked to draw a path on the paper that represents a journey. Along this path, they will place different symbols and images that they feel represent different parts of themselves or important aspects of their life. The therapist can encourage the child to consider the significance of each symbol and how it relates to their experiences and inner world and invite the child narrate their journey, describing each symbol and its meaning noticing any patterns or themes that emerge.

### Hero's Journey

In this activity, the therapist invites the child to create their own hero's journey story. The child might choose a toy figure that represents a hero and begin telling or acting out a story with characters, challenges, and triumphs. This process can be projective, ultimately helping the child explore their own personal narratives and inner struggles.

### Animal Totem

With this activity the therapist can ask the child to choose an animal that they feel represents them or some part of them then invite the child to create a totem or sculpture of this animal using clay. The therapist can ask the child to reflect on the qualities of the chosen animal and how it relates to their personal experiences or feelings while also being mindful of the way the clay feels in their hands.

*Mask Making*

Using paper plates, paint, markers, feathers, glitter, and glue the therapist invites the child to create a mask that represents a part of themselves they usually hide (their "persona"). Together the therapist and child can reflect on the mask and what it symbolizes. Later, the child might create a second mask representing their true self or an aspect of themselves they wish to embrace.

*Dream Drawing*

The therapist can encourage the child to draw a recent dream or a significant dream they remember. Together, the therapist and child can explore the images and events in the dream, examining potential symbolic meanings and how it relates to their waking life, mindful in the moment of any feelings and sensations the child may experience.

## Mindful Parent Involvement in Jungian Play Therapy

Parent involvement is a crucial element in JPT, as it helps create a cohesive and supportive environment for the child's therapeutic journey. Inviting parents to learn simple mindfulness and symbolic techniques can significantly reinforce the therapeutic work done in sessions and promote a harmonious home environment. According to Eric Green, integrating parents into the therapeutic process helps extend the benefits of therapy beyond the playroom and into the child's daily life, supporting the principles of JPT (Green, 2014).

### Learning Mindfulness Techniques

Parents can be introduced to basic mindfulness exercises, such as mindful breathing, body awareness, and reflective listening. These practices help parents model mindfulness for their children, encouraging a calm and centered presence. By practicing mindfulness at home, parents can help their children manage stress and emotional dysregulation, reinforcing the skills learned in therapy.

### Engaging in Symbolic Activities

Parents can also learn to engage in symbolic activities with their children, such as drawing, storytelling, or creating small sand trays. These activities allow parents to understand and participate in the symbolic play that is central to JPT. For instance, parents might be encouraged to create stories with their children using archetypal characters, such as heroes, mentors, or shadow figures. This engagement helps parents connect with their children's inner worlds and supports the process of individuation.

### Supporting Individuation

Involving parents in the therapeutic process aligns with the Jungian tenet of individuation, which is the journey toward becoming one's true self. By understanding and supporting their child's symbolic expressions, parents can facilitate their child's individuation process. This involvement helps parents recognize the significance of their child's play and the underlying psychological themes being worked through.

### Reinforcing Therapeutic Themes

Parents who understand the symbolic and archetypal language used in therapy can better reinforce these themes at home. For example, if a child is working on overcoming fears represented by a dragon in their play, parents can support this work by acknowledging the child's bravery and discussing the dragon symbol in everyday conversations. This reinforcement helps integrate therapeutic insights into the child's broader life context.

### Creating a Supportive Environment

Eric Green (2014) emphasizes the importance of a supportive home environment in facilitating the child's therapeutic progress. By involving parents, therapists can ensure that the child receives consistent emotional support and validation. Parents can learn to provide a safe space for their children to express themselves and explore their feelings, mirroring the therapeutic environment. In addition to parental involvement, Jungian play therapists can utilize mindfulness techniques to create a safe and supportive environment during therapy sessions. Mindfulness can be integrated into play therapy in several ways.

First, the therapist can maintain a mindful presence, staying fully attentive and attuned to the child's needs and emotional states, creating a sense of safety and acceptance that allows the child to feel seen and understood (Siegel, 2010). Introducing mindful breathing exercises can help both the child and therapist stay grounded and calm during sessions. Simple techniques, such as taking deep breaths together, can help the child manage anxiety or overwhelming emotions, especially during moments of distress or when exploring difficult topics (Goldin et al., 2008). Encouraging children to mindfully observe their play and emotions can enhance their self-awareness and insight. Therapists can guide children to notice their thoughts, feelings, and bodily sensations as they engage in play, promoting emotional regulation and resilience (Semple & Lee, 2007).

With JPT, everything has symbolic meaning, including the visual and tactile elements of the therapy room. The physical environment of the therapy room can reflect mindfulness principles. A calm and clutter-free space with soothing colors, comfortable seating, and minimal distractions can enhance the therapeutic atmosphere. Incorporating elements such as soft lighting, natural objects, and sensory materials can further support a sense of tranquility and safety. Additionally, therapists can incorporate mindful play activities that encourage children to engage with their senses and the present moment. Activities such as sandplay, drawing, and storytelling can be approached mindfully, with an emphasis on noticing details, textures, and feelings, deepening the child's engagement and helping them connect more fully with their inner experiences (Green, 2014).

By integrating mindfulness into JPT, therapists can create a supportive environment that fosters emotional safety and promotes healing. This approach not only enhances the therapeutic relationship but also equips children with valuable tools for self-regulation and emotional well-being.

### Parent-Child Mindfulness Practices

Incorporating joint mindfulness practices, such as parent-child meditation or mindful walks, can strengthen the parent-child bond and enhance mutual understanding. These shared practices promote a sense of calm and connectedness, helping to mitigate conflicts and foster a nurturing relationship. In the context of JPT, parent-child mindfulness practices can be particularly beneficial in reinforcing the therapeutic work done in sessions. Engaging in mindful activities together allows both the parent and child to be present with each other in a non-judgmental and accepting manner, mirroring the therapeutic relationship established in the play therapy environment (Green, 2014).

For instance, parent-child meditation can involve simple breathing exercises where both the parent and child focus on their breath and the sensations in their bodies. This practice not only helps in reducing stress and anxiety but also enhances emotional attunement between the parent and child (Siegel, 2010). Mindful walks, where the parent and child walk together while paying attention to their surroundings, sounds, and each other, can foster a shared sense of exploration and curiosity. This aligns with the Jungian principle of exploring the unconscious through engagement with the present moment and the symbolic aspects of their environment (Green, 2014).

Mindfulness practices can help parents better understand their child's inner world and emotional needs, which is crucial in supporting the child's individuation process – a key goal of JPT. As parents become more attuned to their child's emotional states and responses through mindfulness, they can provide more effective emotional support and validation, creating a supportive home environment that complements the therapeutic work (Kabat-Zinn, 1994).

### Ongoing Communication between Therapist and Parents

Regular communication between therapists and parents is essential for maintaining alignment between therapy sessions and home practices. Therapists can provide parents with feedback and suggestions on how to support their child's therapeutic journey, ensuring continuity and coherence in the child's experience. In JPT, this ongoing communication is vital for integrating the therapeutic work into the child's everyday life. By keeping parents informed about the themes and progress observed in therapy, therapists can help parents reinforce the therapeutic interventions at home (Green, 2014).

Therapists can offer practical strategies for parents to support their child's emotional and psychological growth, such as specific mindfulness exercises tailored to the child's needs. These might include activities like mindful breathing, guided imagery, or creative expression through drawing and storytelling, which reflect the symbolic and archetypal work done in therapy (Mitchell & Friedman, 1994). Additionally, therapists can guide parents on how to respond to their child's play and expressions in ways that mirror the therapeutic approach, thus maintaining a consistent and supportive environment for the child's exploration and healing.

Regular check-ins between therapists and parents also provide an opportunity to address any challenges or concerns that arise, ensuring that the therapeutic process remains dynamic and responsive to the child's evolving needs. This collaborative approach fosters a strong therapeutic alliance and empowers parents to actively participate in their child's healing journey, enhancing the overall effectiveness of JPT (Allan, 1988).

## Conclusion

Integrating mindfulness into JPT enhances the therapeutic process by fostering self-awareness, emotional regulation, and present-moment focus for both the therapist and the child. By incorporating mindfulness into the core principles of JPT an exploration of the unconscious, individuation, archetypes and symbols, and therapeutic relationship – therapists can create a more effective and compassionate therapeutic environment. This integration supports the JPT goals of helping children develop healthier coping methods, improving their emotional and behavioral functioning, and fostering a sense of safety and acceptance.

## References

Allan, J. (1988). *Inscapes of the Child's world: Jungian counseling in schools and clinics*. Spring Publications.

Goldin, P. R., McRae, K., Ramel, W., & Gross, J. J. (2008). The neural bases of emotion regulation: Reappraisal and suppression of negative emotion. *Biological Psychiatry, 63*(6), 577–586.

Green, E. J. (2009). *Jungian play therapy for the sandplay therapist. International Journal of Play Therapy, 18*(2), 82–93. https://doi.org/10.1037/a0014418

Green, E. J. (2014). *The handbook of Jungian play therapy with children and adolescents*. John Wiley & Sons.

Green, E. J. (2024). Mindfulness in Jungian play therapy: New perspectives and techniques. In L. Stewart (Ed.), *Innovative play therapy methods: Integrating contemporary approaches* (pp. 45–70). Routledge.

Heiko, R. (2021). Who Am I?: The journey of self-discovery. In *The embodied brain and sandtray therapy* (pp. 122–141). Routledge.

Heiko, R. L. (2024). Kalffian sandplay in assessment and therapy planning. In *Play therapy treatment planning with children and families* (pp. 130–140). Routledge.

Jung, C. G. (1968). *Collected works of C. G. Jung, volume 9 (Part 1): The archetypes and the collective unconscious.* Princeton University Press.

Jung, C. G. (2014). *The red book: Liber Novus.* W. W. Norton & Company.

Kalff, D. M. (2003). *Sandplay: A psychotherapeutic approach to the psyche.* Temenos Press.

Kabat-Zinn, J. (1994). *Wherever you go, there you are: Mindfulness meditation in everyday life.* Hyperion.

Lilly, J. P. (2015). *Jungian sandplay therapy: Principles and practices for understanding the psyche.* Routledge.

Lilly, J. P. (2016). Integrating Jungian concepts in play therapy. *International Journal of Play Therapy, 25*(2), 72–85.

Lilly, J. P., & Heiko, R. (2019). Jungian analytical play therapy. *Play Therapy, 14*(3), 40–42.

Mitchell, R. R., & Friedman, H. S. (1994). *Sandplay: Past, present, and future.* Routledge.

Semple, R. J., & Lee, J. (2007). *Mindfulness-based cognitive therapy for anxious children: A manual for treating childhood anxiety.* New Harbinger Publications.

Siegel, D. J. (2010). *The mindful therapist: A Clinician's guide to mindsight and neural integration.* W. W. Norton & Company.

# 11

# MINDFULNESS IN PSYCHODYNAMIC AND OBJECT RELATIONS PLAY THERAPY

## Introduction

Psychodynamic and Object Relations Play Therapy are therapeutic approaches grounded in psychoanalytic theory, focusing on understanding the unconscious processes that influence a child's behavior and emotional state. These approaches delve into the impact of early relationships and internalized object relations – mental representations of self and others formed through early interactions. The primary goals are to help children understand and resolve their internal conflicts, enhance emotional regulation, and develop healthier relationships (Prout et al., 2019). Play is a natural medium for children to express and work through unconscious conflicts and relational patterns. Integrating mindfulness into these therapeutic approaches can enhance effectiveness by promoting self-awareness, present-moment focus, and emotional regulation. Mindfulness practices align with the goals of Psychodynamic and Object Relations Play Therapy by helping children and therapists remain attuned to the present experience, fostering a deeper understanding of internal states and relational dynamics.

## History and Evolution of Psychodynamic and Object Relations Play Therapy

The study of children's behavioral and emotional needs in the early 20th century was first grounded in psychoanalytic thought (Seymour, 2016;

     DOI: 10.4324/9781003468585-11

Wonders, 2021). Sigmund Freud published the well-known example of Little Hans, in which he advised the father of his young patient to closely monitor the child's play as a means of gaining insight into the child's fear of horses (Freud et al., 1955; Wonders, 2021). According to Freud, play is a way for children to freely express their thoughts and feelings, like how psychoanalysts assist patients in uncovering hidden thoughts and emotions. During the subsequent decade, Freud dedicated himself to closely watching children's play, acknowledging their ability to create and explore imaginary realms. Freud observed that children often engage in repetitive play that involves reenacting difficult events, and later concluded that this repetition allows children to develop mastery and ultimately resolve the challenges they are facing (Wonders, 2021). The famous case of Little Hans marked the inception of the prevailing notion that play serves as a means for therapists to observe and gain a deeper understanding of a child's internal and external surroundings.

Sigmund Freud was the first to publish a description of the importance of play in children's natural psychoanalytic development (Wonders, 2021). However, it was Hermine Hug-Hellmuth who became the first psychoanalyst to create techniques specifically designed for children, differentiating them from methods used with adults (Hug-Hellmuth, 1913; Plastow, 2011; Wonders, 2021). Hug-Hellmuth coined the phrase *play therapy* in 1913, employing drawing and writing games to get insight into the unconscious mind of children (Geissmann & Geissmann, 1998; Lenormand, 2012; Wonders, 2021).

## Four Influential Female Psychoanalysts

### Anna Freud

Anna Freud is renowned for her work on defense mechanisms in her essay *The Ego and the Mechanisms of Defence* (1937) and founded the Hampstead Child Therapy Course and Clinic in 1952, emphasizing theoretical aspects and uncovering unconscious feelings through play (Donaldson, 1996; Wonders, 2021).

### Melanie Klein

Klein introduced object relations theory, emphasizing the mother-infant bond's impact on later relationships. Her work laid the foundation for attachment theory, influencing models like Theraplay® and FirstPlay®. Klein's book, *The Psycho-Analysis of Children* (1932), advanced understanding of children's emotional development (Harris, 2014; Wonders, 2021).

### Margaret Mahler

Mahler established the Masters Children's Centre in 1950 and developed the tripartite treatment model involving mothers in therapy. Her research focused on the mother-infant relationship and the effects of early separation (Coates, 2004; Wonders, 2021).

### Margaret Lowenfeld

Lowenfeld founded the Children's Clinic in London and developed the Lowenfeld world technique. Her book "Play in Childhood" (1935) highlighted the therapeutic use of non-verbal play methods, significantly influencing play therapy (Friedman & Mitchell, 2002; Wonders, 2021).

### Development of Object Relations Theory

Object relations theory further evolved with contributions from theorists such as Donald Winnicott, John Bowlby, and Margaret Mahler. Winnicott introduced concepts like the "good enough mother" and the "transitional object," emphasizing the importance of a nurturing environment for healthy psychological development (Winnicott, 1953). Bowlby's attachment theory highlighted the critical role of early bonds in shaping emotional security and development (Bowlby, 1982). Mahler's work on separation-individuation provided insights into the developmental stages and the child's evolving sense of self and others (Mahler et al., 1975).

## Psychodynamic Theory and Play Therapy

These theoretical advancements significantly influenced the development of Psychodynamic and Object Relations Play Therapy. Therapists began to use play as a natural medium for children to express their inner experiences. Through play, children can project their unconscious conflicts, fears, and desires onto toys and scenarios, allowing therapists to observe and interpret these dynamics in a supportive and non-threatening environment (Gil, 2015; Schaefer, 2011; Scharff, 2008).

### Modern Developments

In recent decades, Psychodynamic and Object Relations Play Therapy have continued to evolve, integrating new research and techniques. Contemporary practitioners, such as Eliana Gil, David Scharff, and others, have expanded the theoretical framework and refined therapeutic techniques to better address the needs of children in diverse settings. The focus has broadened to include understanding the impact of trauma, cultural factors, and neurobiological insights on child development and therapy (Gil, 2015; Malberg & Slowiaczek, 2018; Scharff, 2008; Wonders, 2021).

## Tenets of Psychodynamic and Object Relations Play Therapy

### Unconscious Processes

Psychodynamic and Object Relations Play Therapy focus on how unconscious thoughts and feelings influence behavior. These therapies believe much psychological functioning is driven by early unconscious processes. Play allows children to project internal conflicts and anxieties onto toys, giving therapists insight into their unconscious mind. For instance, a child enacting abandonment with dolls may reveal fears related to caregiver separation. Therapists help children explore and understand these themes, improving emotional regulation and behavior. Play provides a natural communication method for children, bypassing verbal limitations. Therapists interpret the symbolic play to help children make sense of their experiences, promoting psychological development, healthier relationships, and an integrated sense of self (Gil, 2015; Klein, 1955; Schaefer, 2011).

### Early Relationships

Examining early attachments is crucial in Psychodynamic and Object Relations Play Therapy. The quality of early caregiver relationships deeply affects a child's emotional and social development, shaping their sense of self, emotional regulation, and relationship-building abilities (Ainsworth & Bowlby, 1991).

Children with inconsistent or neglectful caregiving may develop attachment issues, such as anxiety and distrust. Therapy explores these early experiences, helping children re-experience and reinterpret foundational relationships in a safe environment, leading to healing and healthier relational dynamics (Schaefer, 2011).

Using play, therapists observe children reenacting early relational experiences, revealing their internalized object relations. Therapists help children understand and resolve these dynamics, promoting an integrated and adaptive internal world. This process addresses behavioral issues and enhances emotional and social well-being by targeting the root causes of relational difficulties (Ainsworth & Bowlby, 1991; Schaefer, 2011).

### Internalized Object Relations

Internalized object relations are mental representations of self and others formed through early caregiver interactions, shaping children's self-perception, emotions, and relationships. Positive caregiving leads to secure attachments and healthy relationships, while negative interactions cause distorted perceptions and attachment issues (Klein, 1955). Therapists use play to explore these internalized images, observing children's play to understand their internal world. For example, aggressive play may reveal internal conflicts. Therapists help reframe these perceptions, fostering healthier emotional responses and adaptive relational patterns (Klein, 1955; Scharff, 2008). Research shows this approach effectively improves emotional regulation and interpersonal relationships (Klein, 1955; Scharff, 2008; Schaefer, 2011).

### Transference and Countertransference

In Psychodynamic and Object Relations Play Therapy, managing transference and countertransference is essential. Transference occurs when a child projects feelings from significant relationships onto the therapist, revealing unresolved emotions. For example, a child feeling rejected by a caregiver might express these feelings toward the therapist (Freud, 1912; Kernberg, 2008). Countertransference involves the therapist's emotional responses to the child, offering insights into the child's relational patterns. Therapists must maintain self-awareness and reflect on these responses to inform their therapeutic approach constructively (Gelso & Hayes, 2007; Heimann, 1950).

By exploring transference, therapists help children understand and work through their feelings, promoting self-awareness and emotional regulation (Gil, 2015). Attuning to countertransference ensures the therapist's reactions enrich the therapeutic process, providing deeper insights into the child's internal world (Gelso, 2014; Schaefer, 2011). These dynamics are crucial for therapeutic intervention, facilitating the child's journey toward healthier emotional and relational functioning (Gabbard, 2014; Rasic, 2010).

### Play as a Medium

Play is a powerful tool in therapy, allowing children to express internal experiences and conflicts symbolically. This non-threatening medium provides insights into the child's unconscious mind that verbal communication may miss (Schaefer, 2011). Children might use toys to reenact real-life struggles, revealing feelings like neglect or guilt. Therapists interpret these themes to understand the child's psyche (Klein, 1955). Play also helps children explore different behaviors and outcomes in a safe environment, beneficial for trauma survivors or those with articulation difficulties (Gil, 2015). Play reveals transference and countertransference dynamics, mirroring relational patterns. Therapists observe these interactions to help children work through and understand their feelings, promoting healthier relationships (Gabbard, 2014).

## Effectiveness and Evidence Base

Psychodynamic and Object Relations Play Therapy are highly effective in addressing various emotional and behavioral issues in children, such as anxiety, depression, trauma, and attachment disorders (Fonagy, 2010). These therapies focus on deep psychological processes, providing a comprehensive understanding of the child's internal world and relational dynamics essential for long-term healing. Research shows that these therapies reduce symptoms of anxiety and depression by helping children process and integrate unconscious conflicts (Levy et al., 2016).

They also improve children's ability to form secure attachments and manage emotions (O'Connor & Braverman, 2009). In trauma treatment, these therapies help children process their experiences and reduce post-traumatic stress symptoms, fostering psychological resilience (Cohen et al., 2017). For attachment disorders, they improve relational patterns and self-perception, leading to healthier relationships (Holmes, 2014). The depth-oriented focus of these therapies resolves underlying issues contributing to surface-level symptoms, promoting sustained psychological health (Gabbard, 2014). The strong evidence base underscores their efficacy in treating a broad spectrum of childhood emotional and behavioral issues, facilitating long-term healing and growth (Fonagy, 2010; Gabbard, 2014).

## Integrating Mindfulness into Psychodynamic and Object Relations Play Therapy

Integrating mindfulness into Psychodynamic and Object Relations Play Therapy can enhance the therapeutic process by aligning with the core philosophy, tenets, and goals of these theoretical approaches. Mindfulness, which inherently involves paying deliberate attention to the present moment with an attitude of openness and non-judgment, complements the deep exploration of the unconscious mind and relational dynamics that characterize psychodynamic and object relations therapy.

### *Mindful Observation and Reflection*

Mindful observation is a natural extension of the psychodynamic principle of attending to unconscious processes. Therapists can cultivate mindfulness to enhance their attunement to the child's play, observing not only the overt actions but also the subtleties of emotional expression and symbolic content. For example, during a play session, a therapist might mindfully note the child's choice of toys and the narratives they create, considering how these choices reflect the child's internal world and relational templates. By maintaining a mindful presence, therapists can provide more nuanced interpretations and support the child's exploration of unconscious material (Schaefer, 2011).

*Empathy and Understanding*

Mindfulness enhances the therapist's ability to empathize with children, understanding their experiences from a compassionate perspective. In Psychodynamic and Object Relations Play Therapy, this empathy is crucial for recognizing and interpreting the child's projections and transference. By being fully present and attuned, the therapist can more effectively understand the child's internalized objects and relational patterns. This deepened empathy strengthens the therapeutic relationship, facilitating the child's exploration of unconscious material and promoting meaningful emotional and psychological change.

*Enhancing Emotional Regulation through Mindfulness*

Mindfulness practices can help children develop better emotional regulation, a key goal of psychodynamic and object relations therapy. Techniques such as mindful breathing or body scans can be incorporated into play therapy to help children become more aware of their bodily sensations and emotional states. For instance, a therapist might guide a child in noticing where they feel tension during a difficult play scenario, helping them connect physical sensations with emotional experiences. This practice not only enhances self-awareness but also provides tools for managing intense emotions, facilitating a deeper understanding of their internal world (Kabat-Zinn, 2003).

*Mindfulness and Transference-Countertransference Dynamics*

Mindfulness can be particularly useful in managing transference and countertransference dynamics. By cultivating a mindful attitude, therapists can become more aware of their own emotional responses and how these might be influenced by the child's projections. This awareness allows therapists to respond more thoughtfully and constructively, using their countertransference as a tool for understanding the child's relational patterns. Additionally, mindfulness helps therapists maintain an open and non-judgmental stance, essential for exploring transference dynamics without becoming overwhelmed by them (Gelso & Hayes, 2007).

## Creating a Safe and Attuned Therapeutic Space

A core tenet of psychodynamic and object relations therapy is the creation of a safe and attuned therapeutic environment. Mindfulness practices can help therapists maintain a calm and grounded presence, which contributes to a sense of safety and trust. For example, beginning a session with a brief mindfulness exercise can help both the therapist and the child settle into the therapeutic space, fostering a sense of calm and readiness for deep exploration. This practice aligns with the psychodynamic emphasis on the therapeutic relationship as a container for emotional expression and healing (Winnicott, 1965).

## Mindful Play and Symbolic Expression

Incorporating mindfulness into play activities encourages children to engage more fully with their symbolic expressions. Therapists can guide children to play mindfully, paying attention to the sensations, emotions, and thoughts that arise during their play. For example, a child engaged in sand play might be invited to pause and reflect on the figures they are placing in the sand, considering what these figures represent and how they relate to their inner experiences. This mindful engagement with play helps children make deeper connections between their symbolic actions and their unconscious processes, supporting the goals of psychodynamic and object relations therapy (Kalff, 2003).

### Animal Breaths

Animal Breaths is a play-based mindfulness exercise aligning with psychodynamic and object relations principles by using symbolic play to facilitate emotional regulation. Ask the child to choose an animal and imagine how that animal breathes – slow, deep breaths for a lion or quick, gentle breaths for a rabbit. Encourage the child to make the corresponding animal sounds as they exhale. This exercise engages the child's imagination, a key aspect of psychodynamic therapy (Flemming, 2019), and helps them regulate their breathing. It also allows the child to project internal states onto external symbols, a core tenet of object relations therapy (Wirz, 1991), fostering self-regulation in a fun and playful manner.

*Emotion Puppets*

In psychodynamic play therapy, therapists can use puppet play to help children become more aware of and deal with emotions. The therapist can provide a variety of puppets representing different characters or feelings (e.g., a sad puppet, an angry puppet, a happy puppet). The child is encouraged to select a puppet and act out a story or scenario. Throughout the play, the therapist can pause and ask the child to reflect on the puppet's feelings and actions, and how they relate to the child's own emotions. This activity helps children externalize and explore their emotions, gaining insight into their emotional states and underlying psychodynamic processes (Halfon et al., 2019).

*Feelings Treasure Hunt*

Supporting children in learning  attune to their physical sensations through mindfulness can help them recognize and understand their emotional states, aligning with psychodynamic and object relations principles (Halfon et al., 2019). With the activity called *Feelings Treasure Hunt*, various objects representing different emotions (e.g., a soft teddy bear for comfort, a smooth stone for calmness, a jagged rock for anger) are hidden around the room. As the child finds each object, the therapist guides them in a body scan to notice areas of tension or relaxation and discusses how finding the object relates to their emotional state. This approach helps children connect physical sensations with their feelings, fostering self-awareness and emotional insight through symbolic play and projection.

*Mindful Moment Drawing*

With this creative expressive activity the therapist provides markers and paper, and then invites the child to draw whatever comes to mind. At various points, the therapist can ask the child to pause and mindfully observe their drawing, discussing what each color and shape reminds them of and how it makes them feel. This reflective process helps children connect their artistic expressions with their inner emotional world, promoting deeper self-awareness and understanding of their unconscious motivations.

*Mandala Drawing*

Encourage children to engage in mandala drawing, where they can create circular designs that represent their thoughts and feelings. This practice can be done mindfully, with the child taking time to focus on the patterns and colors they use, reflecting on their emotions and experiences during the day or their play sessions. This creative process helps children gain insight into their inner world and facilitates emotional expression and awareness. According to psychodynamic theory, much of our emotional and psychological experiences are driven by unconscious processes (Pitman & Knauss, 2020; Zellner, 2011). The act of creating mandalas – a symbolic and often intricate circular design – allows children to project these inner experiences onto a tangible medium.

### Facilitating Insight and Integration

Mindfulness practices can support the psychodynamic goal of facilitating insight and integration of unconscious material. By encouraging children to reflect mindfully on their play experiences, therapists can help them gain greater awareness of their internal conflicts and relational patterns. Questions such as "What did you notice about how you felt when you chose that toy?" or "Can you take a moment to feel where that sadness is in your body?" can prompt children to connect their play with their emotional and bodily experiences. This reflective process promotes the integration of previously unconscious material, leading to greater psychological coherence and emotional resilience (Schaefer, 2011).

## Support for Parents and Caregivers

Involving parents and caregivers in mindfulness practices can extend the benefits of therapy into the child's broader environment. Therapists can teach simple mindfulness techniques to parents, helping them create a more supportive and attuned home environment. For example, parents can be encouraged to practice mindful listening and to be fully present during interactions with their children. This practice supports the child's ongoing emotional regulation and reinforces the therapeutic work done in sessions, aligning with the psychodynamic emphasis on the importance of early relationships and their impact on development

(Fonagy et al., 2002). Teach parents psychodynamic-based mindfulness techniques they can practice at home with their children. These techniques, such as reflective storytelling or mindful drawing, reinforce the exploration of unconscious emotions and relational patterns introduced in therapy. This approach promotes a supportive home environment that mirrors the therapeutic space, helping children to continue processing their inner experiences and fostering deeper emotional connections within the family.

## Conclusion

Psychodynamic and Object Relations Play Therapy, with its rich historical roots and theoretical foundations, offers a comprehensive approach to understanding and addressing children's emotional and behavioral issues. By focusing on unconscious processes, early relationships, and internalized object relations, this therapeutic approach provides deep insights into a child's internal world and relational dynamics. Integrating mindfulness into these therapies offers a powerful enhancement by fostering present-moment awareness, emotional regulation, and deeper insight. Mindfulness practices help therapists and children explore unconscious material, manage transference and countertransference dynamics, and create a safe and attuned therapeutic space. This integration not only aligns with the core principles of psychodynamic and object relations therapy but also promotes long-term emotional and psychological healing, making it a robust and effective approach for supporting children's mental health.

## References

Ainsworth, M. D. S., & Bowlby, J. (1991). An ethological approach to personality development. *American Psychologist, 46*(4), 333–341. https://doi.org/10.1037/0003-066X.46.4.333

Bowlby, J. (1982). *Attachment and loss: Vol. 1. Attachment* (2nd ed.). Basic Books.

Coates, S. W. (2004). John Bowlby and Margaret S. Mahler: Their lives and theories. *Journal of the American Psychoanalytic Association, 52*(2), 571–601. http://doi.org/10.1177/00030651040520020601

Cohen, J. A., Mannarino, A. P., & Deblinger, E. (2017). *Trauma-focused CBT for children and adolescents: Treatment applications.* Guilford Press.

Fleming, R. (2017). The therapeutic imagination: Using literature to deepen psychodynamic understanding and enhance empathy. *Psychoanalytic Psychotherapy, 31*(2), 1–4

Fonagy, P., Target, M., Cottrell, D., Phillips, J., & Kurtz, Z. (2002). *What works for whom? A critical review of treatments for children and adolescents.* Guilford Press.

Fonagy, P. (2010). The changing shape of clinical practice: Integrating psychotherapy, psychoanalysis, and cognitive behavioral therapy. *American Psychologist, 65*(7), 593–602. https://doi.org/10.1037/a0021358

Freud, S. (1912). The dynamics of transference. In *Collected papers of Sigmund Freud* (Vol. 2, pp. 312–322). Basic Books.

Freud, S., Strachey, J., & Freud, A. (1955). *The standard edition of the complete psychological works of Sigmund Freud* (Vol. 10). Hogarth Press.

Friedman, H. S., & Mitchell, R. R. (2002). *Sandplay: Past, present and future.* Taylor and Francis.

Gabbard, G. O. (2014). *Psychodynamic psychiatry in clinical practice* (5th ed.). American Psychiatric Publishing.

Geissmann, C., & Geissmann, P. (1998). *A history of child psychoanalysis.* Routledge.

Gelso, C. J. (2014). A tripartite model of the therapeutic relationship: Theory, research, and practice. *Journal of Counseling Psychology, 61*(3), 307–316.

Gelso, C. J., & Hayes, J. A. (2007). *Countertransference and the Therapist's inner experience: Perils and possibilities.* Lawrence Erlbaum Associates.

Gil, E. (2015). *Play in family therapy* (2nd ed.). Guilford Press.

Halfon, S., Yılmaz, M., & Çavdar, A. (2019). Mentalization, session-to-session negative emotion expression, symbolic play, and affect regulation in psychodynamic child psychotherapy. *Psychotherapy, 56*(4), 555.

Harris, P. (2014). *An analysis of Melanie Klein's the psychoanalysis of children.* University of Manchester.

Heimann, P. (1950). On counter-transference. *International Journal of Psychoanalysis, 31,* 81–84.

Holmes, J. (2014). *John Bowlby and attachment theory* (2nd ed.). Routledge.

Hug-Hellmuth, H. (1913). *A study of the mental health of a child.* Nervous & Mental Disease Publishing Company.

Kabat-Zinn, J. (2003). Mindfulness-based interventions in context: Past, present, and future. *Clinical Psychology: Science and Practice, 10*(2), 144–156.

Kernberg, O. F., Yeomans, F. E., Clarkin, J. F., & Levy, K. N. (2008). Transference focused psychotherapy: Overview and update. *The International Journal of Psychoanalysis, 89*(3), 601–620.

Klein, M. (1955). The psychoanalytic play technique: Its history and significance. *Journal of the American Psychoanalytic Association, 3*(1), 1–16. https://doi.org/10.1177/000306515500300101

Lenormand, M. (2012). Hug-Hellmuth or the impasses of an objectifying conception of the infantile. *Recherches en Psychanalyse, 13*(1). 74–86. https://doi.org/10.3917/rep.013.0074

Levy, R. A., Ablon, J. S., & Kächele, H. (2016). *Psychodynamic psychotherapy research: Evidence-based practice and practice-based evidence.* Springer.

Mahler, M. S., Pine, F., & Bergman, A. (1975). *The psychological birth of the human infant: Symbiosis and individuation.* Basic Books.

Malberg, N. T., & Slowiaczek, M. L. (2018). *The clinical applications of the adult attachment interview: Three approaches in psychotherapy for children and adults.* Routledge.

O'Connor, K., & Braverman, L. (2009). *Play therapy theory and practice: Comparing theories and techniques.* Wiley.

Pitman, T., & Knauss, M. (2020). *Psychodynamic child therapy: The techniques and their applications.* Norton.

Plastow, M. (2011). Hermine Hug-Hellmuth, the first child psychoanalyst: Legacy and dilemmas. *Australasian Psychiatry, 19*(3), 206–210.

Prout, T. A., Malone, A., Rice, T., & Hoffman, L. (2019). Resilience, defense mechanisms, and implicit emotion regulation in psychodynamic child psychotherapy. *Journal of Contemporary Psychotherapy*, *49*, 235–244.

Rasic D. (2010). Countertransference in child and adolescent psychiatry-a forgotten concept?. *Journal of the Canadian Academy of Child and Adolescent Psychiatry = Journal de l'Académie canadienne de psychiatrie de l'enfant et de l'adolescent*, *19*(4), 249–254.

Schaefer, C. E. (2011). *Foundations of play therapy* (2nd ed.). Wiley.

Scharff, D. E. (2008). *Object relations therapy of physical and sexual trauma*. Jason Aronson.

Seymour, J. W. (2016). An introduction to the field of play therapy. In K. J. O'Connor, C. E. Schaefer, & L. D. Braverman, (Eds.), *Handbook of play therapy* (2nd ed.) (pp. 3–15). John Wiley & Sons, Incorporated.

Winnicott, D. W. (1953). Transitional objects and transitional phenomena; A study of the first not-me possession. *International Journal of Psychoanalysis*, *34*, 89–97.

Winnicott, D. W. (1963). Dependence in infant care, in child care, and in the psychoanalytic setting. *International Journal of Psycho-Analysis*, *44*(3), 339–344.

Wirz, B. (1991). *An object relations approach to therapeutic work with children in clinical settings*. University of Cape Town.

Wonders, L. L. (2021). Theoretical roots and branches of the evolving field of play therapy. In *Play therapy and telemental health* (pp. 3–24). Routledge.

Zellner, M. (2011). The cognitive unconscious seems related to the dynamic unconscious—but it's not the whole story. *Neuropsychoanalysis*, 13, 59–63. https://doi.org/10.1080/15294145.2011.10773662

# 12

# MINDFULNESS IN DEVELOPMENTAL AND ATTACHMENT-BASED PLAY THERAPY

## Introduction

Crenshaw and Stewart (2014) characterize Developmental and Attachment-based Play Therapy as a therapeutic approach that emphasizes the different stages of children's development and the profound influence that attachment ties have on their emotional and psychological growth. This chapter discusses two widely recognized treatment models, FirstPlay® Therapy and Theraplay®, which are based on developmental theory and attachment theory and a third new approach called Attachment Centered Play Therapy. Developmental and Attachment-based Play Therapy theory originated from John Bowlby and further developed by Mary Ainsworth (Bowlby et al., 1992; Bretherton, 2013). In this chapter there will be inclusion of a fairly new play therapy model known as Attachment Centered Play Therapy. All of these models are constructed with careful attention to the developmental issues of children and are based on the significance of secure attachment bonds in promoting sound emotional and psychological growth.

## Three Impactful Therapeutic Models

### *FirstPlay®*

Janet Courtney embarked on a remarkable journey in the early 1990s as a trailblazer in Developmental Play Therapy (DPT). She was first

                    DOI: 10.4324/9781003468585-12

introduced to DPT through a course led by Viola Brody, who stressed the significance of touch and relational dynamics in therapy. Brody's distinctive methodology, which incorporated a progressive relaxation practice using tactile stimulation, strongly resonated with Courtney, sparking a profound passion and dedication to further investigate DPT (Courtney, 2014).

Viola Brody's approach was innovative, prioritizing developmental phases and relational touch instead of conventional play materials utilized in other types of play therapy. Courtney, who was employed in the field of adoption and foster care at the time, found this methodology particularly fascinating due to its capacity to assist children who were experiencing attachment challenges. Initially, Brody's approaches, such as engaging in finger counting with a partner, may have appeared simple. However, they quickly demonstrated themselves to be significant methods of establishing a deep connection, requiring meaningful and active involvement from both the person giving and the person receiving. These exercises fostered a profound and intimate relationship that went beyond spoken communication, accessing a level of engagement that existed before the use of words or symbols and is fundamental to a child's inner being (Courtney, 2014).

Courtney immersed herself further into DPT by arranging training sessions with Brody, hosting her in her own home, and involving her in her doctoral research. As a result of this mentorship, Courtney was able to deeply understand and incorporate the ideas of DPT, and she successfully applied them in her therapeutic practice. The playful exchanges between Brody and Courtney's son emphasized the significance of developmental play phases, emphasizing the therapeutic value of simplistic, relational play activities such as hide-and-seek and singing.

Courtney expanded and systematized these ideas, which were influenced by both Brody's work and subsequently coined the term FirstPlay® Therapy. This method highlights the fundamental importance of fostering, pleasurable physical contact in aiding children in cultivating a confident and stable sense of identity. Brody and Courtney assert that touch is the primary means of communication and plays a crucial role in developing a child's sense of self and emotional regulation (Courtney, 2014; Courtney & Nolan, 2017).

FirstPlay® combines developmental concepts with a wide range of activities, allowing it to be used in a variety of settings such as psychiatric inpatient units, schools, foster families, and even with the elderly (Courtney, 2014). Courtney's extensive expertise encompasses several therapeutic modalities such as art therapy, cognitive-behavioral therapy, and eco-psychology. This enables her to utilize a personalized and targeted approach that caters to the specific requirements of each child. Regardless of the various methods used, the fundamental aspect of DPT, which involves being fully present, seeing the child without judgment, and using touch to help the child feel acknowledged, continues to be the core focus of her practice (Courtney, 2014).

Courtney's contributions to DPT have yielded noteworthy results, benefiting children facing various challenges such as grief, trauma, behavioral concerns, and attachment disorders. FirstPlay® emphasizes the therapeutic power of touch and the importance of being present in the here and now (Courtney, 2014).

FirstPlay® has provided therapists worldwide with the necessary abilities to properly use these strategies by offering comprehensive training programs, workshops, and certification courses, thereby ensuring the maintenance of high practice standards. The extensive implementation of FirstPlay® in various environments, ranging from private practices to schools and healthcare facilities, highlights its adaptability and significant influence. FirstPlay® is actively shaping the future of play therapy by extending the availability of play therapy to the youngest of humans and fostering profound understanding of the developmental importance of touch and relational play. FirstPlay® has solid research to support the efficacy of the model (Baldwin et al., 2020; Siu, 2023).

## *Theraplay®*

FirstPlay® and Theraplay® have shared origins. Jernberg and Booth, founders of Theraplay®, incorporated the research of Austin Des Lauriers and Viola Brody (Jernberg & Booth, 2011). Jernberg and Booth (2011) adapted Brody's and Des Lauriers' techniques in Headstart programs, focusing on structured play techniques that promote the development of safe connection and emotional control in children. This historical connection emphasizes the importance of early interpersonal encounters and safe and nurturing touch in both FirstPlay and Theraplay®. It highlights their mutual dedication to fostering the developmental needs of children via nurturing and attentive interpersonal interaction.

The Theraplay® model has had a substantial influence on the field of play therapy and child therapy since its creation. Theraplay® has effectively addressed attachment and emotional regulation in children by emphasizing the enhancement of the parent-child bond through engaging, nurturing, and enjoyable activities. This method is both structured and flexible. The model consists of four key dimensions: structure, engagement, nurture, and challenge, providing a comprehensive framework for fostering healthy relational dynamics and emotional growth (Booth & Jernberg, 2010).

The efficacy of Theraplay® has been demonstrated in diverse environments, such as educational institutions, medical facilities, foster care programs, and residential treatment centers (Money et al., 2021; Sadeghy et al., 2022; Smithee et al., 2021). This model has had a significant effect on children with attachment difficulties, trauma histories, developmental delays, and behavioral issues. Studies and medical records have recorded substantial enhancements in emotional regulation, social abilities, and attachment security in children after undergoing Theraplay® (Booth & Jernberg, 2010; Weir et al., 2013).

Theraplay®'s versatility enables its integration with other therapeutic methods, boosting its effectiveness in many clinical settings. Therapists have reported anecdotally that when Theraplay® is combined with other therapeutic methods, such as cognitive-behavioral therapy or family systems therapy, it enhances its advantages and offers a more comprehensive treatment approach.

Theraplay® focuses on structured playful interactions between the child and caregiver to enhance and fortify their bond. Theraplay® aims to recreate the playful, lighthearted, and caring exchanges that naturally take place between parents and their young children, promoting a strong emotional bond and the ability to manage emotions effectively. Theraplay® sessions include engaging, tactile, and playful activities that promote connection and attunement, establishing a strong foundation for the child's emotional and social growth (Booth & Jernberg, 2010).

Theraplay® and FirstPlay® are therapeutic models that specifically target the development and improvement of attachment, self-esteem, trust in others, and joyful involvement. Both models are based on principles derived from attachment theory, developmental theory, and the neuroscience of interpersonal bonds.

Although Theraplay® and FirstPlay® employ distinct methodologies, their common underlying principles and common therapeutic objectives emphasize the significance of early interpersonal encounters, attachment, and emotional self-regulation in the growth and development of children. Both theories have had a substantial impact on the area of play therapy, equipping therapists with a wide range of effective techniques to promote the emotional and psychological welfare of children and their families (Courtney, n.d.; Jernberg & Booth, 2011).

### Attachment Centered Play Therapy

Clair Mellenthin (2019) has made notable strides in the field of Attachment-based Play Therapy by creating her model called Attachment Centered Play Therapy. This method combines attachment theory and play therapy, with the goal of healing attachment ruptures and improving the parent-child bond. In Mellenthin's (2019) work, she presents effective methods and approaches aimed at promoting stable bonds and emotional regulation in young children. Mellenthin (2019) highlights the significance of parent training and engagement, educating parents about attachment theory, and teaching them on how to utilize therapeutic play strategies at home to reinforce skills acquired during therapy sessions.

Mellenthin's (2019) approach incorporates mindfulness and emotional regulation skills as essential components. These strategies, such as guided visualization and breathing exercises, assist children in regulating their emotions and cultivating beneficial coping strategies. Attachment-focused interventions, such as the creation and sharing of attachment narratives and engaging in reflective dialogues, aim to target attachment disturbances and foster stable relationships within the family unit (Mellenthin, 2019).

## Tenets of Developmental and Attachment-Based Play Therapy

Developmental and Attachment-based Play Therapy is grounded in fundamental principles that form the basis of FirstPlay®, Theraplay®, and Attachment Centered Play Therapy. These concepts focus on the significance of stable attachments, developmental phases, emotional control, and the therapeutic connection in fostering the emotional and psychological growth of children.

### Attachment Relationships

The central focus of all three models is the importance placed on secure attachments during emotional and psychological development. Theraplay® incorporates structured play-based activities that promote secure connections by imitating beneficial relationship interactions between parents and children. FirstPlay® emphasizes the importance of touch and relational interaction to enhance the attachment relationship between caregivers and children from the earliest stages of development. Attachment Centered Play Therapy focuses on the creation and enhancement of secure attachment bonds through therapeutic play. The quality of these attachments are crucial for a child's emotional stability and resilience, as supported by Jernberg and Booth (2011), Courtney (2014), and Mellenthin (2019).

### Developmental Stages

A fundamental area of focus is recognizing and resolving challenges with developmental tasks and stages. Theraplay® utilizes activities that are tailored to a child's developmental level, assuring that interventions are most appropriate for the presenting needs. FirstPlay® assesses for developmental appropriateness, specifically targeting pre-symbolic play and caring touch that coincides with the initial phases of infant development. Mellenthin's approach integrates developmental factors by customizing play therapy methods to match the child's age and stage of development. This ensures that the therapeutic process promotes their overall growth and development in a comprehensive manner (Booth & Jernberg, 2010; Courtney, n.d.; Mellenthin, 2019).

### Emotional Regulation

Facilitating the growth of children's ability to effectively handle and communicate their emotions is a crucial component of all three models. Theraplay® activities aim to assist children in managing their emotions by engaging in structured and predictable interactions that establish a feeling of security and consistency. FirstPlay® utilizes gentle touch and interpersonal interaction to assist infants in developing an experience of safety and tranquility, therefore facilitating the development of emotional regulation from an early stage of life. Mellenthin's Attachment Centered Play Therapy aims to assist children in recognizing and articulating their emotions in an adaptive and healthy manner. This is achieved by utilizing play as a means to facilitate processing of feelings and the cultivation of self-regulation abilities (Booth & Jernberg, 2010; Courtney, 2015; Mellenthin, 2019).

### Therapeutic Relationship

Establishing a robust, supportive, and compassionate bond between the therapist and the child is crucial for facilitating the process of recovery and development. Theraplay® focuses on the therapist's responsibility to establish a lighthearted, captivating, and nurturing setting that promotes a favorable interpersonal encounter. FirstPlay® emphasizes the therapist creating an environment for parents and babies that promotes experiences of safety, nurturing touch, and being fully present, which helps the child and parent feel acknowledged and understood at a fundamental level. Mellenthin's method emphasizes the importance of the therapeutic relationship in play therapy, where the therapist serves as a solid foundation for the child to explore, heal, and grow (Jernberg & Booth, 2011; Courtney, n.d.; Mellenthin, 2019).

## Integrating Mindfulness into Developmental and Attachment-Based Play Therapy

Mindfulness is a natural technique that can be integrated into Developmental and Attachment-Based Play Therapy models to enhance the therapeutic process. Mindfulness can augment this method by fostering self-awareness, emotional management, and concentration on the present moment. Consequently, this can aid therapists in enhancing attachment bonds and attending to developmental requirements in children and their families.

### Enhancing the Therapist's Attunement and Presence

Mindfulness activities enable therapists to develop an elevated level of consciousness and attentiveness, which is essential for understanding and responding to the child's attachment requirements and encounters during play therapy sessions. Therapists can enhance their ability to monitor and comprehend the child's attachment behaviors, emotional expressions, and relational patterns by being completely attentive and engaged. This attunement facilitates the establishment of a stable therapeutic connection, creating a secure foundation for the child to investigate and resolve attachment-related concerns.

### Mindful Presence

Engaging in mindfulness during Developmental and Attachment-Based Play Therapy sessions enables therapists to cultivate a reliable and focused presence, which is crucial for nurturing connections with children. Prior to therapy sessions, therapists can enhance their ability to attune and respond to the child's emotional and relational needs by observing a grounding and centering activity. When a therapist can provide a quality of presence, the child experiences a sense of security, which in turn creates an environment that is favorable for the growth and cultivation of secure relationships. Therapists support children in resolving attachment-related difficulties by continually being available and attentive during therapy sessions.

### Reflective Observation

Mindfulness enhances the therapist's ability to engage in reflective observation, a crucial component of Developmental and Attachment-based Play Therapy. Therapists can closely observe and reflect on the child's facial expressions and body language during play by being fully engaged and attentive. This introspective method assists therapists in understanding the child's attachment needs and emotional experiences. Therapists can express their observations by verbalizing their views on the child's activity, elucidating what they notice. This approach amplifies the child's perception of being recognized, heard, and emotionally connected, promoting self-assurance, and strengthening the therapeutic relationship, ultimately cultivating a secure attachment.

### Supporting the Child's Emotional Regulation

Mindfulness practices are essential in Developmental and Attachment-based Play Therapy as they assist children in effectively regulating their emotions. FirstPlay® Therapy focuses on loving touch and storytelling to establish a secure attachment environment (Courtney & Nolan, 2017), whereas Theraplay® concentrates on interactive, structured experiential activities that encourage healthy attachment behaviors between child and caregiver (Booth & Jernberg 2010). These models can use mindfulness to facilitate the development of self-regulation abilities, enhance the ability of children and parents to manage their emotions in a healthier manner, and reinforce the quality of attachment in the relationship. Practicing mindfulness can enhance the child and caregiver's ability to stay focused and emotionally connected with one another. Therapists enhance the child's emotional control and attachment security by integrating mindfulness, creating a therapeutic setting that is safe and supportive.

### Body Awareness

By using mindfulness techniques, based on the concepts of FirstPlay® Therapy, children can develop the ability to be aware of and comprehend their emotional states by focusing on their bodily sensations. An example of this is when a therapist instructs a parent to engage in the "Baby Tree Hug" practice, which aims to enhance body awareness and foster a sense of connection in a caring and encouraging environment (Courtney, 2015). The "Soft and Floppy" activity in Theraplay® aims to enhance children's awareness of bodily tension by having them lie on the floor and experience the contrast between being rigid like a board and completely relaxed and pliable. After the child has achieved a state of relaxation, the therapist can prompt them to move a specific body part, such as their tongue or big toe, to enhance their awareness of their own body (Perry, 2009).

### Facilitating Self-Expression and Insight

Mindfulness promotes introspection, enabling children to have a deeper understanding of their own actions and motivations, and fostering self-awareness and self-acceptance through play. In Developmental and Attachment-based models such as FirstPlay® and Theraplay®, the practice of mindfulness assists children in examining their internal experiences and articulating their feelings within a safe and nurturing setting. Therapists assist children in expressing their emotions and thoughts, enhancing their ability to manage their emotions, and developing a strong emotional bond by establishing a secure and attentive therapy environment. This process of reflection facilitates the child's progression toward self-awareness, empowering them to cultivate more salubrious methods of engaging and establishing relationships with others.

### Mindfulness Activities in Play

In Developmental and Attachment-based Play Therapy, incorporating mindfulness exercises into play helps children have increased awareness of their bodies, breath, thoughts, and feelings. Here are some activities borrowed from Theraplay® and FirstPlay®.

### Weather Report

Begin each session with a brief mindfulness exercise to center both the therapist and the child. In Theraplay®, this could involve a simple game of "Weather Report," where the child and therapist describe their current feelings as weather conditions (Walton, 2023).

### Calm, Connected, Relaxed

This FirstPlay® Therapy session starter is a gentle exercise to facilitate parents in self-regulating before touching their young child inviting parents to be guided to first experienced relaxation and then visualize a rainbow connecting them to their child (Courtney, 2014).

*Back Stories*

In FirstPlay® mindfulness can be woven in with this activity during which the child and parent pause to reflect on the feelings and sensations associated with the story they are creating together (Courtney, 2015).

*Play Dough Squeeze*

From Theraplay® this activity can help a child feel and express intensity as they manipulate and squeeze the clay or play dough (Salisbury, 2018).

*Collaborative Drawing*

In Theraplay®, the therapist might guide the child to pause and mindfully observe a collaborative drawing they have created with their caregiver, discussing what each part represents and how it makes them feel. This promotes reflective thinking within the safety of the attachment relationship (Booth & Jernberg, 2010).

*Mirror Play*

In both Theraplay® and FirstPlay®, this activity helps children develop body awareness and attunement through mindful interaction with their caregiver. The therapist instructs the caregiver and child to sit facing each other and mirror each other's movements slowly and deliberately. This activity promotes non-verbal communication, enhances emotional attunement, and fosters a secure attachment by encouraging the child to connect with their caregiver in a safe and supportive environment (Courtney & Nolan, 2017; Hill, 1995).

*Mindful Storytelling*

In FirstPlay® Therapy, therapists can use Janet Courtney's (2015) kinesthetic storytelling approach to incorporate mindfulness into play. These techniques involve creating a narrative while including pauses for reflection and engaging the child's senses through touch and movement. These mindful storytelling techniques helps children connect with their parents, strengthening the attachment bond by involving the caregiver in a shared, nurturing activity (Courtney, 2015; Courtney & Nolan, 2017).

### Empathy and Mindfulness

Mindfulness enhances the therapist's ability to empathize with children, understanding their experiences from a compassionate perspective. In Theraplay®, this empathy is demonstrated through playful, attuned interactions that mirror positive parent-child dynamics. Therapists engage in activities that promote eye contact, physical closeness, and joyful exchanges, helping children feel seen and understood. In FirstPlay® empathy is expressed through kinesthetic storytelling and nurturing touch, which help children feel understood and valued. These practices foster a deep emotional connection between the child and caregiver, reinforcing the secure attachment bond (Courtney, 2015; Jernberg & Booth, 2011).

Attachment Centered Play Therapy emphasizes empathy through attuned play and reflective listening. Therapists and caregivers are encouraged to practice mindfulness to better understand and respond to the child's emotional needs. This empathetic approach helps create a therapeutic environment where the child feels safe to express themselves and work through their emotions (Mellenthin, 2019).

By integrating these approaches, therapists can create a therapeutic space that promotes secure attachment, emotional safety, and empathetic understanding. The consistent use of structured, nurturing, and playful interactions across Theraplay®, FirstPlay®, and Attachment Centered Play Therapy ensures that children feel valued, respected, and understood, facilitating meaningful change and promoting emotional security.

### Promoting Secure Attachment and a Safe and Empathetic Environment

In Developmental and Attachment-Based Play Therapy, creating a safe and empathetic environment is essential for promoting secure attachment. This principle is emphasized in the approaches of Theraplay®, FirstPlay®, and Clair Mellenthin's Attachment Centered Play Therapy.

### Theraplay®

In Theraplay®, therapists create a structured yet nurturing environment. The therapy room is set up with inviting, child-friendly furniture, and playful materials that promote interactive, physical activities. Therapists use consistent, predictable routines and engage in playful, guided interactions that emphasize eye contact, touch, and mirroring to build trust and security. These elements help establish a safe space where children can explore their emotions and behaviors in a supportive setting (Jernberg & Booth, 2011).

### FirstPlay®

In FirstPlay®, the focus is on creating a calm, soothing space that fosters relaxation and emotional connection. The room is equipped with soft lighting, comfortable seating, and sensory materials like blankets and stuffed animals. Mindful activities and nurturing touch exercises are incorporated to enhance the child-caregiver bond, promoting a secure attachment and a sense of safety. This approach uses the environment to reinforce acceptance, presence, and emotional attunement, ensuring children feel valued and respected (Courtney, 2015).

### Attachment Centered Play Therapy

Clair Mellenthin's Attachment Centered Play Therapy also emphasizes creating a safe and empathetic environment. Therapists use a combination of playful engagement and reflective practices to foster a secure attachment between the child and caregiver. The therapeutic space is designed to be warm and inviting, with materials that encourage creative expression and emotional exploration. Mindfulness practices, such as deep breathing and reflective listening, are practiced by the therapist and encouraged for children and caregivers.

## Mindful Parenting in Developmental and Attachment-Based Play Therapy

Teaching parents mindfulness techniques can help them become more attuned to their child's needs and respond with greater sensitivity, a principle integral to the approaches of Theraplay®, FirstPlay®, and Clair Mellenthin's Attachment Centered Play Therapy. In Theraplay®, parents practice mindful listening and attuned, playful interactions during sessions, which help to foster secure attachment and emotional regulation. The emphasis on structured, engaging activities encourages parents to be fully present and responsive, thereby enhancing the quality of the parent-child relationship (Jernberg & Booth, 2011).

### *FirstPlay®*

FirstPlay® guides parents to engage in mindful self-attunement before participating in mindful touch and kinesthetic storytelling with their children. This preparatory mindfulness practice helps parents center themselves, ensuring that their interactions with their children are calm, nurturing, and fully attuned to the child's emotional and physical cues. This approach deepens the emotional connection and fosters a sense of security and understanding between parent and child (Courtney, 2014).

### *Theraplay®*

In Theraplay®, parents practice mindful listening and attuned, playful interactions during sessions, which help to foster secure attachment and emotional regulation. The emphasis on structured, engaging activities encourages parents to be fully present and responsive, thereby enhancing the quality of the parent-child relationship. These activities are designed to replicate positive parent-child interactions that promote trust and security, creating a solid foundation for emotional development (Jernberg & Booth, 2011).

### *Attachment Centered Play Therapy*

Mellenthin's Attachment Centered Play Therapy also integrates mindfulness to enhance parent-child interactions. Parents are taught to use mindfulness techniques to become more aware of their own emotional states and those of their children. By incorporating mindful practices such as deep breathing, reflective listening, and attuned play, parents can better regulate their own emotions and respond more empathetically to their child's needs. This mindful approach strengthens the attachment bond and promotes healthier emotional development (Mellenthin, 2019).

These mindfulness practices across all three models – Theraplay®, FirstPlay®, and Attachment Centered Play Therapy – improve the quality of parent-child interactions by fostering a deeper emotional connection and understanding. By being more present and attuned, parents can create a nurturing environment that supports their child's emotional and psychological well-being.

# Co-regulation in Developmental and Attachment-based Play Therapy

Mindfulness exercises can be used to teach parents and children co-regulation strategies, helping both parties manage stress and emotions more effectively. This principle is central to the approaches of Theraplay®, FirstPlay®, and Attachment Centered Play Therapy.

### FirstPlay®

FirstPlay® Therapy emphasizes the use of mindful touch-based activities to achieve emotional balance and enhance the attachment bond between parents and children. By engaging in kinesthetic storytelling and gentle, nurturing touch, parents and children can regulate their own emotional states in order to help regulate their baby's emotional state. These practices promote a deep sense of safety and connection, enabling both parties to manage stress and emotions more effectively (Courtney, n.d.).

### Theraplay®

In Theraplay®, activities such as synchronized breathing or mirroring movements during playful interactions are designed to promote co-regulation. These activities help parents and children attune to each other's emotional states, fostering a sense of connection and mutual calm. Through structured, engaging play, both parents and children learn to regulate their emotions in a supportive and interactive environment (Jernberg & Booth, 2011).

### Attachment Centered Play Therapy

Mellenthin's Attachment Centered Play Therapy incorporates mindfulness to facilitate co-regulation between parents and children. Techniques such as reflective listening, shared breathing exercises, and mindful play are used to help parents and children attune to each other's emotional needs. These practices support the development of emotional regulation skills and strengthen the attachment bond, providing a foundation for healthy emotional development (Mellenthin, 2019).

Across all three models – Theraplay®, FirstPlay®, and Attachment Centered Play Therapy – mindfulness practices play a crucial role in teaching co-regulation. By fostering attunement and emotional balance, these techniques help parents and children manage stress and emotions more effectively, leading to stronger, healthier relationships.

## Conclusion

The inclusion of mindfulness in Developmental and Attachment-based Play Therapy improves the therapeutic process by promoting self-awareness, emotional regulation, and present-moment concentration for both the therapist and the child. By integrating mindfulness into the fundamental principles of Developmental and Attachment-based Play Therapy, such as attachment relationships, developmental stages, emotional regulation, and therapeutic relationship, therapists can establish a therapeutic environment that is both more efficient and empathetic. This integration facilitates the objectives of assisting children in cultivating healthy coping mechanisms, enhancing their emotional and behavioral functioning, and nurturing stable attachment relationships.

## References

Booth, P. B., & Jernberg, A. M. (2010). *Theraplay: Helping parents and children build better relationships through attachment-based play* (3rd ed.). Jossey-Bass.

Bowlby, J., Ainsworth, M., & Bretherton, I. (1992). The origins of attachment theory. *Developmental Psychology, 28*(5), 759–775.

Bretherton, I. (2013). Revisiting Mary Ainsworth's conceptualization and measurement of infant security. *Attachment & Human Development, 15*(3), 235–257. https://doi.org/10.1080/14616734.2013.835128

Courtney, J. (2014). *FirstPlay therapy: A new approach for early childhood mental health.* Jessica Kingsley Publishers.

Courtney, J. A. (2015). *Touching stories: Attachment-based play therapy techniques.* Professional Resource Press.

Courtney, J., & Nolan, R. (2017). *Attachment and the developing brain: FirstPlay therapy interventions for parents, infants, and young children.* Routledge.

Crenshaw, D. A., & Stewart, A. L. (Eds.). (2014). *Play therapy with children: Modalities for change.* American Psychological Association.

Jernberg, A. M., & Booth, P. B. (2011). *Theraplay: Theory, applications, and implementation* (4th ed.). Wiley.

Mellenthin, C. (2019). *Attachment centered play therapy: Techniques for treating children with attachment and trauma issues.* Jessica Kingsley Publishers.

Money, R., Wilde, S., & Dawson, D. (2021). The effectiveness of Theraplay for children under 12-a systematic literature review. Child and Adolescent Mental Health, *26*(3), 238–251. https://doi.org/10.1111/camh.12416

Perry, B. D. (2009). *Born for love: Why empathy is essential—And endangered.* Harper Collins.

Sadeghy, A., Booth, P. B., & Jernberg, A. M. (2022). Evaluating the outcomes of Theraplay® interventions in a clinical setting. *Journal of Child Psychology and Psychiatry, 63*(5), 625–638. https://doi.org/10.1111/jcpp.13567

Salisbury, S. (2018). Using attachment enhancing activities based on the principles of Theraplay® to improve adult-child relationships and reduce a child's "overall stress" as measured by the Strength and Difficulties Questionnaire (SDQ). *Emotional and Behavioural Difficulties*, *23*(4), 424–440.

Siu, A. (2023). Feasibility and Acceptability of Using FirstPlay® to Enhance Mother–Child Interaction: A pilot study of mothers' perspectives. Scandinavian Journal of Child and Adolescent Psychiatry and Psychology, *11*(1), 69–77. https://doi.org/10.2478/sjcapp-2023-0007

Siu, A. F. (2023). *Innovations in play therapy: The role of touch and developmental play*. Sage Publications.

Smithee, L. C., Krizova, K., Guest, J. D., & Case Pease, J. (2021). Theraplay as a family treatment for mother anxiety and child anxiety. *International Journal of Play Therapy*, *30*(3), 206.

Taheri, K.M. (2015). How Play Therapists Integrate Knowledge of Attachment Theory Into Clinical Practice: A Grounded Theory. https://api.semanticscholar.org/CorpusID:14183619

Walton, D. (2023). *Mindful activities for children: Techniques for emotional regulation and resilience*. Routledge.

Weir, K. N. (2011). Playing for keeps: Integrating family and play therapy to treat reactive attachment disorder. Integrative play therapy, 241–264. https://doi.org/10.1002/9781118094792.ch14

# 13

# MINDFULNESS-BASED PRESCRIPTIVE PLAY THERAPY

## Introduction

This chapter delves into the concept of prescriptive play therapy, first introduced by Heidi G. Kaduson, and Charles E. Schaefer (1997). They introduced this approach to emphasize the use of specific play therapy techniques tailored to the unique needs of individual children based on their presenting problems and therapeutic goals. This approach combines various play therapy methods and interventions to create a customized treatment plan for each child. Through examination of what it means to be prescriptive and/or integrative, this chapter will provide guidance on when these approaches are beneficial and when they are not. Additionally, we will emphasize the importance of mindfulness-based practices for both the therapist and the therapeutic process, highlighting how these practices support the development of tailored treatment plans for each client.

## Understanding Prescriptive Play Therapy

Prescriptive play therapy involves the deliberate and strategic selection of therapeutic techniques and interventions tailored to each client's specific needs. This approach contrasts with the one-size-fits-all methodology, emphasizing the necessity for therapists to evaluate and understand their clients' distinct characteristics, challenges, and developmental stages. By doing so, they can design and implement interventions that are most appropriate for addressing the unique issues presented by everyone (Kaduson & Schaefer, 1997).

## Key Principles and Philosophical Foundations

Schaefer's and Kaduson's approach is supported by the philosophy that no one single therapeutic technique is universally effective for all presenting challenges that bring children and families to therapy (Kaduson & Schaefer, 1997). Instead, they proposed that the flexibility and creativity of therapists in applying a variety of techniques can significantly enhance therapeutic outcomes. This flexibility allows therapists to adapt their methods to fit the specific needs of their clients, making the therapy more effective and personalized (Kaduson & Schaefer, 1997).

### Tailored Interventions

The cornerstone of prescriptive play therapy is the customization of therapeutic interventions. Therapists conduct thorough assessments to understand the client's unique situation, including their psychological, emotional, and developmental needs. Based on this assessment, therapists can select from a wide array of therapeutic techniques to construct a personalized treatment plan (Kaduson & Schaefer, 1997; Kaduson et al., 2019; O'Connor & Braverman, 2009; Schaefer, 2011).

### Integration of Multiple Play Therapy Models

Prescriptive play therapy is not limited to one specific theoretical paradigm. On the contrary, it promotes the incorporation of diverse play treatment models. Therapists utilize cognitive-behavioral, psychodynamic, humanistic, and other methodologies to develop a comprehensive and efficient therapeutic process. This diverse range of interventions guarantees that the selected treatments are the most suitable for the client's particular problems and stage of development (O'Connor, 2001).

### Therapist's Flexibility and Creativity

An essential aspect of prescriptive play therapy is the therapist's capacity to demonstrate adaptability and ingenuity (Kaduson & Schaefer,

1997; Kaduson et al., 2019; Schaefer, 2011). This entails the ongoing assessment of the efficacy of the interventions being employed and implementing any required modifications. The therapist must possess a high level of skill in transitioning between various techniques and approaches to sustain therapeutic progress and effectively tackle emergent challenges.

### Comprehensive Assessment

The approach starts with a thorough evaluation, including knowledge of the child's present functioning, history of challenges and experiences, and presenting challenges. Engaging parents and other important people in the child's life helps the therapist have a complete picture of the child's surroundings and interactions.

### Dynamic Treatment Planning

Based on the assessment, a dynamic treatment plan is developed. The plan for therapy evolves as the therapist gains more insight into the child's needs and as the therapy progresses. Regular reviews and updates ensure that the interventions remain relevant and effective (Wonders & Affee, 2024).

## Application in Practice

According to Kaduson and Schaefer (1997), Kaduson et al. (2019), Schaefer (2011), and O'Connor and Braverman (2009), applying prescriptive play therapy in practice involves several key steps.

### Initial Assessment

Conducting an in-depth initial assessment to gather information about the child's developmental stage, presenting issues, strengths, and areas of concern. This involves interviews with the child, parents, and possibly teachers or other caregivers.

### Selection of Techniques

Based on the assessment, the therapist selects specific techniques and interventions from various play therapy models. For instance, a child with anxiety might benefit from cognitive-behavioral techniques such as relaxation training and exposure therapy, while a child with attachment issues might benefit from more relationship-focused interventions.

### Implementation of Interventions

The chosen interventions are implemented in a flexible and responsive manner. The therapist continually monitors the child's response to the interventions and adjusts as needed. This might involve changing techniques, introducing new activities, or modifying the therapeutic approach to better suit the child's evolving needs.

### Evaluation and Adaptation

Throughout the therapy process, the therapist regularly evaluates the effectiveness of the interventions. This ongoing assessment ensures that the therapy aligns with the child's needs and goals. Adjustments are made based on the child's progress and any new information.

### Collaboration with Caregivers

Engaging parents and caregivers in the therapeutic process is essential. This might involve providing them with strategies to support their child's progress at home, educating them about the principles of play therapy, and involving them in specific therapeutic activities.

## Benefits of Prescriptive Play Therapy

Prescriptive play therapy has numerous advantages, particularly in its ability to handle a broad spectrum of psychological and behavioral problems by customizing treatments to the specific needs of each child. This approach enhances the therapeutic experience, increasing the child's motivation and commitment to the process.

### Individualized Care

Each child receives interventions specifically designed to address their unique challenges, leading to more significant and lasting improvements. By tailoring therapy to the child's individual needs, therapists can target specific issues such as anxiety, trauma, behavioral problems, or developmental delays more effectively. This personalized approach ensures that the therapeutic interventions are relevant and impactful, maximizing the potential for positive outcomes (Schaefer & Kaduson, 2007).

### Enhanced Engagement

The use of varied and creative techniques keeps children engaged and motivated in therapy, making it a more enjoyable and impactful experience. Techniques may include art, music, storytelling, and role-playing, which cater to the child's interests and developmental level. This diversity in therapeutic activities helps maintain the child's interest and fosters a positive attitude toward therapy. Enhanced engagement through playful and imaginative activities can also facilitate deeper emotional expression and processing, essential for healing and growth (Schaefer & Kaduson, 2007).

### Comprehensive Support

By integrating multiple therapeutic models, prescriptive play therapy provides a comprehensive approach that addresses the child's emotional, cognitive, and relational needs. This holistic method ensures that all aspects of the child's development are considered, offering well-rounded support. For instance, cognitive-behavioral techniques might be used alongside attachment-based interventions to address both thought patterns and relational issues. This integrative strategy enables therapists to create a robust therapeutic plan that supports the child's overall well-being (Schaefer & Kaduson, 2007).

### Adaptability

The flexible nature of prescriptive play therapy allows therapists to respond effectively to changes in the child's behavior and circumstances, ensuring that the therapy remains relevant and effective throughout the therapeutic process. As children grow and their needs evolve, therapists can adjust their methods and strategies accordingly. This adaptability is crucial for maintaining the effectiveness of therapy over time, particularly in response to life events or developmental changes that may impact the child's mental health (Schaefer & Kaduson, 2007).

Prescriptive play therapy is a refined and flexible method used in child treatment. By giving priority to personalized evaluation and the innovative implementation of a wide range of therapeutic methods, it offers a strong structure for meeting the intricate and diverse requirements of children in therapy. This approach not only addresses the immediate concerns but also builds a foundation for long-term emotional and psychological resilience, making it a highly effective modality in child psychotherapy (Schaefer & Kaduson, 2007).

## Limitations of Prescriptive Play Therapy

### Complexity

Handling several therapeutic modalities in prescriptive play therapy can be challenging and require a good degree of knowledge and awareness. Therapists must be highly skilled in understanding and using many therapeutic modalities, each with unique theoretical roots, techniques, and goals. Given the complexity involved, juggling several varied customer requests can be very difficult. Therapists must be able to move between multiple approaches, tailoring treatments to fit the unique needs of every kid. One must have a thorough awareness of the several approaches with the capacity to combine and use them in a rational way. The complexity of this integration could make it difficult for practitioners with less expertise especially to maintain treatment uniformity and efficacy.

### Inconsistency

Lack of consistency in integrative procedures and inadequate planning might lead to unequal treatment, therefore confusing or overwhelming clients. Prescriptive play therapy runs the danger of inconsistency when therapists fail to properly coordinate the several therapeutic modalities they apply. If not properly managed, different approaches may result in a fractured therapeutic experience because of different goals, techniques, and evaluation of progress. Treatment irregularities may hinder the therapeutic process and be confusing for clients. Therapists have to be very well-prepared and always reflect to keep a consistent and unified therapeutic approach.

### Training

Therapists need to have extensive training in various theories and methodologies to successfully apply a prescriptive or integrative approach.

There is a substantial need for comprehensive training in several therapeutic modalities because each approach necessitates a thorough comprehension of its principles, procedures, and applications. The comprehensive training can require a significant amount of time and resources, which can be a challenge for many therapists. In addition, the ongoing need for professional development to keep up with breakthroughs in various therapeutic areas can be a lot to keep up with. Therapists must continuously gain and refresh their knowledge and abilities to give effective and evidence-based therapies. Insufficient training increases the likelihood of incorrectly implementing methods or not completely understanding the intricacies of various approaches, which can undermine the quality of care given to clients.

## Integrating Mindfulness into Prescriptive Play Therapy

Incorporating mindfulness into prescription play therapy can greatly improve the therapeutic process. Mindfulness practices can be modified and integrated into different therapy approaches to cater to the specific requirements of individual children. Mindfulness enhances self-awareness, emotional regulation, and present-moment focus, making it a suitable complement to the adaptable and personalized approach of prescriptive play therapy.

### Enhancing Therapist's Attunement and Presence

Therapists can utilize mindfulness techniques to cultivate an elevated state of consciousness and attentiveness, essential for accurately comprehending and addressing a child's needs and experiences. Prescriptive play therapy allows therapists to improve their capacity to observe and understand the child's behaviors, emotions, and expressions by being fully attentive and actively involved.

### Mindful Presence

In prescriptive play therapy, clinicians can establish a state of conscious presence by employing mindfulness techniques, such as mindful breathing or meditation, prior to sessions. This preparation enhances the therapist's ability to be fully attentive and responsive to the child's requirements. For example, a therapist may participate in a brief mindfulness exercise to concentrate their attention, which allows them to adjust their therapeutic approach in accordance with the child's immediate reactions and needs.

### Reflective Observation

Regardless of how non-directive or how directive the approach a therapist prescriptively chooses, the quality of attunement to the child's verbal and non-verbal expressions is critically important. Mindfulness enhances the therapist's ability to engage in reflective observation, allowing for deeper engagement with the child's verbal and non-verbal communication. This deep listening and attuned watching fosters trust and connection, crucial for the success of therapeutic interventions. In prescriptive play therapy, this means the therapist can better understand which specific play therapy techniques to apply, such as cognitive-behavioral play therapy for anxiety or narrative play therapy for trauma, based on the child's cues and ongoing feedback during sessions.

By integrating mindfulness into their practice, therapists using prescriptive play therapy can ensure they remain flexible and responsive, tailoring their interventions to best support each child's unique therapeutic journey.

### Mindfulness Techniques in Prescriptive Play Therapy

Mindfulness techniques are highly adaptable and can be effectively integrated into prescriptive play therapy to address specific emotional and behavioral challenges that children face. The individualized nature of prescriptive play therapy ensures that interventions are tailored to the unique needs of each child, enhancing the therapeutic process.

### Mindful Breathing

Introducing simple mindful breathing exercises can help children calm themselves when they feel overwhelmed. In prescriptive play therapy, this practice can be seamlessly integrated into specific play activities designed for the child's particular issues.

**Dragon Breaths:** In this game, the child pretends to be a dragon who must blow out imaginary flames with deep, controlled breaths. This not only engages the child in a fun and imaginative way but also teaches them how to regulate their breathing and manage anger through mindfulness.

**Triangle Breathing:** Tracing a triangle with a finger, the child inhales at the top of the triangle, holds the breath down one side, exhales at the bottom, and holds the breath out on the other side of the triangle and then repeats. This measured breathing exercise contributes to emotion and nervous system regulation.

*Body Awareness*

Teaching children mindfulness techniques, such as body scans, can help them become more aware of their physical sensations and emotions. In prescriptive play therapy, this awareness can provide critical insights into a child's emotional state and inform tailored interventions.

**Body Treasure Map:** The child draws a simple outline of a body and uses stickers or markers to indicate areas where they feel different sensations (e.g., butterflies in the stomach when anxious). This visual and interactive method helps the child articulate their physical experiences and provides the therapist with valuable information to address these sensations through targeted relaxation exercises or other therapeutic activities.

**Musical Movement Magic:** This activity helps children become more somatically aware through movement and music. The therapist plays short samples of a variety of different kinds of music, each with different tempos and styles, such as classical, jazz, pop, and ballads. The child is invited to match their movements to the music, exploring how their bodies feel. This activity promotes somatic awareness, creativity, emotional expression, and physical activity, enhancing their connection to their physical and emotional selves.

*Emotion Regulation*

Mindful awareness of feelings as they arise and mindfulness skills for managing those feelings equips children with a sense of confidence and empowerment.

**Mindfulness Magic Wand:** If a child is experiencing overwhelming fear and anxiety, the child can create a wand using craft materials and is encouraged to wave it slowly while taking deep and slow breaths while thinking of calming, positive images. This activity not only engages the child in a creative project but also integrates mindfulness when they need help managing anxiety and fear (Landreth, 2012).

**Emotion Balloons:** For children who have difficulty identifying and expressing their emotions, this activity can be helpful. The child draws different emotions on small, inflated balloons after examining a feelings faces poster or chart. During sessions, the child selects a balloon that most represents their current feeling and practices mindful breathing while deciding if they'd like to bat the balloon around the room, pop the balloon, or keep the balloon to carry home. This helps the child focus on their emotions and provides a concrete tool for discussing and managing their feelings.

### Enhancing Self-Reflection in Prescriptive Play Therapy

Mindfulness encourages self-reflection, helping children gain insights into their behaviors and motivations. This approach aligns with the goals of prescriptive play therapy, which focuses on fostering self-awareness and understanding through targeted interventions tailored to the child's unique needs.

**Dice of Discovery:** In this game, the child rolls a large, colorful die that has different prompts written on each face. Each prompt encourages the child to reflect on their feelings, experiences, and behaviors. For example, the sides of the die might include prompts such as "Share a time you felt really happy," "What is something you are proud of?", "Describe a moment when you felt scared," "Talk about a time you helped someone," "What makes you feel calm?", and "Describe something you love to do." As the child rolls the die and lands on a prompt, they are encouraged to take a moment to think about their response and then share it with the therapist. The therapist listens attentively and may ask follow-up questions to deepen the child's reflection, such as "What made that moment special for you?" or "How did you overcome your fear?" This activity not only makes self-reflection fun and interactive but also helps the child articulate their thoughts and feelings in a safe, supportive environment.

### Facilitating More Experiential Play Therapy Prescriptively

**Reflective Puppet Play:** For children who struggle with social interactions, the therapist can use reflective puppet play. The child uses puppets to act out a social scenario, and the therapist periodically pauses the play to ask the child how the puppet feels and what it might do next. This intervention helps the child practice social skills and reflects on their interactions in real life.

**Emotion Art Journals:** For children who have difficulty verbalizing their emotions, the therapist can introduce emotion art journals. The child draws scenes that represent different emotional experiences, and the therapist engages the child in mindful discussion about each drawing. This practice encourages self-reflection and helps the therapist gain insights into the child's emotional landscape, allowing for more effective, targeted interventions.

**Personalized Safe Zones:** Create a "safe zone" within the playroom tailored to each child's preferences. For example, if a child finds comfort in a particular type of play, such as building with blocks, designate an area where they can engage in this activity whenever they feel overwhelmed. This personal safe zone helps the child feel in control and provides a retreat during stressful moments.

**Emotion Regulation Stations:** Set up emotion regulation stations in the playroom equipped with various tools like sensory trays, stress balls, crayons and paper, emotion cards, bubbles for blowing, and calming jars. These stations can be used to help children manage their emotions in real time. For instance, if a child becomes emotionally activated, they may choose to go to an emotion regulation station to practice a specific technique like deep breathing or squeezing a stress ball, helping them regain composure and continue with therapy.

*Start Sessions with Mindfulness*

Begin each session with a brief mindfulness exercise to center both the therapist and the child.

- For a **non-verbal child**, use a tactile-based exercise like "Feather Touch." The child holds a feather and gently moves it across their skin, focusing on the sensation. This helps center the child through a sensory experience.
- For a **hyper-aroused child**, start with "Grounding Stomp," where the child stands and stomps their feet, feeling the connection to the ground. This physical activity can help release excess energy and promote grounding.

- For a **child new to therapy and apprehensive,** use "Breathing Buddies," where the child lies down with a small stuffed animal on their belly. They watch the buddy rise and fall with their breath, making the exercise both soothing and engaging.

*More Mindful Play Interventions*

During play activities, intermittently introduce mindfulness prompts tailored to the child's specific needs.

- For a **non-verbal child,** use a "Mindful Sculpting" activity. Provide playdough or clay and ask the child to create something while focusing on the texture and their movements. This non-verbal activity encourages mindfulness through tactile engagement.
- For a **hyper-aroused child,** incorporate "Pause and Paint." Set up a painting station where the child can paint freely. Encourage them to take deep breaths and pause occasionally to observe their artwork and reflect on their emotions.
- For a **child new to therapy and apprehensive,** try "Mindful Puppet Play." Use puppets to act out scenarios and ask the child to pause and describe how the puppets might feel, helping the child project and reflect in a safe, imaginative way.
- For a **non-verbal child,** provide a "Sensory Journal" with textured pages, scented markers, and stickers. The child can create sensory-rich pages that express their feelings without needing to use words.
- For a **hyper-aroused child,** offer a "Movement Journal." Encourage the child to draw or write about their feelings after physical activities, helping them channel their energy into creative expression.
- For a **child new to therapy and apprehensive,** use a "Welcome Journal." Include prompts like "Draw something that makes you happy" or "Write about a fun memory," gradually helping the child become comfortable with the journaling process.

## Supporting Children and Families Prescriptively in Play Therapy

Incorporating mindfulness into the prescriptive play therapy process involves educating caregivers about mindfulness techniques that can help manage stress, enhance emotional regulation, and improve the overall well-being of their children and themselves. These techniques can be integrated into various play therapy interventions, providing a holistic approach to treatment. By involving caregivers in the therapeutic process, therapists can reinforce the mindfulness practices introduced in therapy and promote a supportive home environment.

### Parent Involvement

Teaching parents mindfulness techniques they can practice at home with their children can be invaluable for supporting children's progress in therapy. This helps reinforce the mindfulness practices introduced in therapy and promotes a supportive home environment.

- For a **non-verbal child**, suggest "Mindful Sensory Play" at home. Parents can set up sensory bins with different materials (e.g., rice, beans, water beads) and guide their child through mindful exploration of the textures.
- For a **hyper-aroused child**, recommend "Family Grounding Exercises." Teach parents to lead grounding activities like "Tree Pose" (from yoga) or "Counting Breaths" to help their child manage arousal levels.
- For a **child new to therapy and apprehensive**, introduce "Storytime Mindfulness." Parents can read a story and pause to discuss the characters' feelings, encouraging mindfulness and reflection in a familiar and comforting context.

### Prescriptive Mindfulness Play Activities for the Whole Family

Integrating mindfulness into prescriptive play therapy enhances the therapeutic process by fostering self-awareness, emotional regulation, and present-moment focus for both the therapist and the child. By incorporating mindfulness into the individualized and flexible framework of prescriptive play therapy, therapists can create a more effective and compassionate therapeutic environment. This integration supports the goals of helping children develop healthier ways of coping, improving their emotional and behavioral functioning, and fostering a sense of safety and acceptance.

*Mindful Mandalas*

Children and caregivers create mandalas together using different colors and patterns to represent their current emotions. This helps children become more aware of their emotional states and express them creatively. Teach caregivers how to facilitate this activity at home by providing them with a simple guide on creating mandalas and encouraging discussions about the colors and patterns used to represent different feelings. This practice can help families build emotional awareness and communication skills.

*Mindful Gardening*

Encourage caregivers to create a small indoor or outdoor garden where children and caregivers can plant and take care of flowers or vegetables. Teach them to mindfully engage with the process of gardening, noticing the sensations of the soil, the growth of the plants, and the changes over time. Provide caregivers with tips on how to incorporate mindfulness into gardening, such as focusing on the sensory experiences and the patience required to care for plants. This can promote relaxation, patience, and a connection to nature for the whole family.

*Mindful Music and Movement*

Use an activity called "Music and Movement Meditation" where children and caregivers listen to calming music and move their bodies in response to the sounds. Encourage them to notice the rhythm, their breathing, and the sensations of movement. Share strategies with caregivers on how to create a mindful music and movement routine at home. This can help children with sensory integration issues and those who benefit from physical activity to release tension and enhance body awareness.

*Mindful Fairy Tales*

Implement a practice called "Mindful Fairy Tales" where children and caregivers take turns creating and telling stories. Encourage them to pause at various points to reflect on the characters' emotions and motivations and relate these to their own experiences. Teach caregivers how to use storytelling as a tool for mindfulness by pausing to ask reflective questions about the characters and connecting the story to real-life situations. This fosters empathy, reflection, and emotional understanding.

*Sensory Mindfulness Kits*

Develop "Mindfulness Sensory Kits" that include stress balls, textured fabrics, scented oils, and small musical instruments. Guide children and caregivers to use these items mindfully, paying close attention to their sensory experiences. Provide caregivers with instructions on creating and using sensory kits at home. This can be particularly helpful for non-verbal children, offering a way to explore and regulate their emotions through sensory engagement.

*Mindful Drawing Games*

Create a game called "Mindful Drawing Relay" where family members take turns adding to a drawing, focusing on their breath and the sensation of the pen or pencil on paper. Afterward, discuss the feelings and thoughts that arose during the activity. Educate caregivers on facilitating mindful drawing games, emphasizing the importance of being present and reflective during the activity. This encourages teamwork, focus, and creativity, helping families bond while practicing mindfulness together.

*Mindful Puppet Play*

Use puppets to act out scenarios that involve taking deep breaths during stressful moments. For instance, a puppet might demonstrate taking a "balloon breath" to calm down before addressing a conflict. Teach caregivers how to use puppets to model mindfulness techniques at home, reinforcing the skills learned in therapy.

*Nature Walks with Reflective Practices*

Organize family nature walks where participants are encouraged to walk silently for a few minutes, focusing on their surroundings and their breathing. Afterward, they can share their observations and feelings. Guide caregivers on conducting mindful nature walks, emphasizing the benefits of connecting with nature and practicing mindfulness in a family setting.

*Mindful Adventure Stories*

Develop a narrative where children and caregivers are the heroes of a mindfulness adventure. Throughout the story, they encounter challenges that require them to use mindfulness techniques like deep breathing, body scans, or sensory awareness to proceed. Provide caregivers with tools to create their own mindful adventure stories, encouraging them to integrate mindfulness practices into imaginative play at home.

By educating caregivers about these prescriptive mindfulness techniques and integrating them into play therapy, therapists can create a therapeutic environment that supports the unique needs of each child and family, promoting emotional regulation, self-awareness, and a sense of safety.

## Conclusion

Mindfulness-based prescriptive play therapy offers a flexible and effective approach to supporting the unique needs of each child and family. By integrating mindfulness practices with a broad range of play therapy techniques, therapists can enhance their therapeutic presence and effectiveness, fostering positive therapeutic outcomes. This chapter has outlined the principles and practices of prescriptive play therapy, emphasizing the importance of attuning to the individual needs of clients, and incorporating mindfulness as a core component of the therapeutic process.

## References

Kaduson, H. G., & Schaefer, C. E. (1997). *101 favorite play therapy techniques*. Jason Aronson.

Kaduson, H. G., Schafer, C. E., & O'Connor, K. J. (2019). *The handbook of play therapy*. John Wiley & Sons.

Landreth, G. L. (2012). *Play therapy: The art of the relationship* (3rd ed.). Routledge.

O'Connor, K. J., & Braverman, L. D. (2009). *Play therapy theory and practice: Comparing theories and techniques.* John Wiley & Sons.

O'Connor, K. J. (2001). The play therapy primer: An integrative approach. *Child Psychology Review, 12*(3), 156–168. https://psycnet.apa.org/record/2001-00354-000

Schaefer, C. E. (2011). *Foundations of play therapy.* John Wiley & Sons.

Schaefer, C. E., & Kaduson, H. G. (2006). *Contemporary play therapy: Theory, research, and practice.* Guilford Press.

Wonders, L. L., & Affee, M. L. (Eds.). (2024). *Play therapy treatment planning with children and families: A guide for mental health professionals.* Taylor & Francis.

# 14

## MINDFULNESS IN WORKING WITH CHILDREN, PARENTS, AND FAMILIES

### Introduction

In this chapter, we will explore how mindfulness can be integrated into therapeutic work with parents, children, and families. Drawing from family systems theory and play-based parenting models, we will examine how to utilize a playful and mindfulness-based approach to enhance the parent-child relationship, support whole family systems, and work with parents outside of play therapy sessions. By incorporating mindfulness, therapists can foster greater attunement, empathy, and emotional regulation within family dynamics, promoting overall family well-being.

### Understanding Family Systems Theory

Family systems theory, developed by Murray Bowen, holds that individuals cannot be understood in isolation from their family units. Bowen introduced concepts such as differentiation of self, emotional triangles, and multigenerational transmission to explain how family members influence one another within the system (Bowen, 1978). Families are seen as complex, interconnected systems where each member's behavior influences and is influenced by the others. This theory emphasizes the importance of understanding the roles, patterns, and dynamics within

DOI: 10.4324/9781003468585-14

the family to effectively address individual and relational issues (Bortz et al., 2019).

In the context of play therapy, family systems theory provides a crucial framework for understanding and intervening in the intricate web of relationships that impact a child's behavior and emotional well-being. Eliana Gil (2015), in her book *Family Play Therapy*, elaborates on how incorporating family systems principles into play therapy can enhance the therapeutic process. By engaging the entire family in play therapy, therapists can observe and address the relational patterns and dynamics contributing to a child's difficulties.

### Differentiation of Self

One of Bowen's key concepts is the differentiation of self, which refers to an individual's ability to maintain their sense of self while remaining emotionally connected to their family. In family play therapy, activities are designed to help each family member express their individuality while also fostering healthy interdependence. This can involve role-playing games where family members take on different perspectives using puppets or symbolic figures in the sand tray, helping them understand and respect each other's viewpoints (Bowen, 1978).

### Emotional Triangles

Bowen's concept of emotional triangles highlights how a third person is often brought into a two-person conflict to reduce tension. These triangles can provide temporary stability but often perpetuate dysfunctional relational patterns by deflecting the core issues. In family play therapy, therapists can use play scenarios to identify and address these triangles. For example, a therapist might observe how a child is used as a go-between in parental conflicts, such as when a child carries messages between parents or acts as a buffer during arguments. This dynamic can place undue emotional burden on the child, potentially affecting their emotional development and sense of security within the family. Through carefully designed play interventions, the therapist can highlight these patterns in a non-threatening way and then work with the family to establish more direct and healthy communication patterns (Bowen, 1978). This process not only alleviates the child's stress but also fosters stronger relational boundaries and empowers the family to resolve conflicts more effectively.

### Multigenerational Transmission

Bowen's theory also emphasizes the transmission of emotional and behavioral patterns across generations. Family play therapy can include activities that explore family histories and narratives, helping families recognize and break maladaptive patterns. By using techniques such as animal genograms or family storytelling, therapists help families understand the origins of their current issues and develop new, healthier ways of interacting (Bowen, 1978).

## Contributions from Other Family Systems Experts

### Salvador Minuchin

Salvador Minuchin (1974), a prominent figure in family therapy, developed structural family therapy, which focuses on the organization and hierarchy within families. Minuchin's work highlights the importance of family structures and boundaries. He believed that symptoms in individuals often arise from dysfunctional family structures. By restructuring family interactions and hierarchies, Minuchin aimed to create healthier dynamics and improve family functioning (Minuchin, 1974).

### Virginia Satir

Virginia Satir (1983), known for her humanistic approach, emphasized communication and emotional expression within the family system. She introduced the concept of family roles (e.g., the placater, the blamer, the super-reasonable, the irrelevant) to describe how family members cope with stress and maintain balance. Satir believed that enhancing self-esteem and improving communication were key to resolving family issues and promoting personal growth (Satir, 1983).

### Jay Haley and Cloe Madanes

Jay Haley and Cloe Madanes, founders of strategic family therapy, focused on the power dynamics and communication patterns within families. Their approach involves identifying and altering the family interactions that contribute to the presenting problem. Haley and Madanes emphasized the importance of directives – specific tasks given to family members to interrupt dysfunctional patterns and encourage healthier interactions (Haley, 1976).

## Integrative Family Systems Approach to Therapy

Incorporating insights from multiple family systems theories allows for a more comprehensive approach to therapy. For instance, a therapist might use Bowen's concepts to understand family emotional patterns, Minuchin's structural techniques to address hierarchy issues, Satir's communication models to enhance emotional expression, and Haley's strategic interventions to disrupt dysfunctional patterns. This integrative approach can lead to more effective interventions and sustainable improvements in family dynamics.

## Role of Play in Family Systems

Play is a natural and effective way to engage children and families in therapy. According to Eliana Gil (2015), play therapy activities such as joint art projects, family games, and collaborative storytelling allow family members to express themselves in ways that might not be possible through verbal communication alone. These activities can reveal underlying issues, strengthen family bonds, and facilitate the development of healthier interaction patterns.

### Addressing Dynamics in Family Play Therapy

In her work, Gil (2015) emphasizes the importance of observing and addressing family dynamics during play therapy sessions. For instance, a therapist might notice how a child's behavior changes when different family members are present, providing insights into the relational dynamics at play. By addressing these dynamics directly through therapeutic play activities, therapists can help families develop more supportive and nurturing relationships.

### Therapeutic Goals

The goals of integrating family systems theory into play therapy include improving communication, enhancing emotional understanding, and fostering a more cohesive family unit. By involving the whole family in the therapeutic process, play therapy helps to ensure that changes are sustainable and supported by the family system. This holistic approach not only addresses the child's individual needs but also promotes overall family health and well-being (Gil & Baima, 2024).

## Integrating Mindfulness into Family Systems Play Therapy

Integrating mindfulness into family systems play therapy can be a transformative approach that enhances the therapeutic process. Mindfulness helps family members develop greater awareness of their interactions, emotional responses, and communication patterns, fostering an environment of non-judgmental observation and reflection (Coatsworth et al., 2014; Duncan et al., 2009; Harnett & Dawe, 2012; Kirby, 2016; Lucas-Thompson et al., 2021). By practicing mindfulness, families can learn to observe their dynamics without immediate reactions, allowing for more thoughtful and intentional interactions. This practice aligns well with Bowen's concept of differentiation of self, as it encourages individuals to maintain their sense of self while remaining emotionally connected to others (Bowen, 1978). Mindfulness helps reduce reactivity within emotional triangles, making it easier for family members to navigate conflicts without escalating tensions. Additionally, by being mindful of multigenerational transmission processes, families can recognize and address inherited patterns and behaviors, breaking cycles that may have persisted across generations (Siegel, 2007).

Salvador Minuchin's structural family therapy also benefits from mindfulness practices. Mindfulness can help family members become more aware of their roles and boundaries, promoting healthier family structures and hierarchies (Minuchin, 1974). Virginia Satir's emphasis on communication and emotional expression can be enhanced through mindfulness, as it encourages open, empathetic, and clear interactions that honor each family member's perspective (Satir, 1983). And in the context of strategic family therapy as developed by Jay Haley and Cloe Madanes, mindfulness can aid in recognizing and altering dysfunctional interaction patterns, supporting the implementation of more constructive and supportive communication strategies (Haley, 1976).

By integrating mindfulness into family systems play therapy, therapists can help families create a supportive environment where each member feels seen, heard, and valued. This integration not only supports individual emotional regulation but also strengthens the overall family unit, promoting long-term relational health and resilience. The combined approach of mindfulness and family systems theory provides a comprehensive framework for addressing complex family dynamics and fostering meaningful change.

Blending mindfulness, family systems theory, and play therapy creates a holistic and dynamic approach to therapeutic intervention that addresses both individual and relational aspects of family life. Mindfulness, with its focus on present-moment awareness and non-judgmental observation, complements family systems theory by enhancing each family member's awareness of their interactions, emotional responses, and communication patterns. This integration helps families observe their dynamics more thoughtfully and intentionally, promoting healthier and more effective interactions (Siegel, 2007). When mindfulness practices are incorporated into the family systems framework, they enable family members to maintain their sense of self while remaining emotionally connected, reduce reactivity in emotional triangles, and address inherited patterns with greater clarity and compassion.

Play adds another layer to this integrated approach, particularly when working with children. Play therapy provides a natural and engaging way for children to express their emotions, process experiences, and develop problem-solving skills. Combining play therapy with mindfulness encourages children to stay present and engaged in their play, enhancing their emotional regulation and self-awareness (Landreth, 2012; Wonders, 2022). For instance, during play therapy sessions, therapists can guide children and parents in playful mindfulness activities, such as different ways to engage the breath or observing sensations of items in the playroom, which helps anchor them in the present moment.

In practical terms, a family play therapy session blending these approaches might involve a family participating in a structured play activity designed to reflect their dynamics, with the therapist facilitating mindful observation and reflection. For example, a session could begin with a brief mindfulness activity to center the family such as use of the mindfulness bell and quiet listening, followed by a play-based activity where parents and children interact. The therapist might then guide the family in reflecting on their interactions, highlighting patterns, and encouraging each member to express their thoughts and feelings non-judgmentally (Minuchin, 1974; Siegel, 2010).

Overall, integrating mindfulness, family systems theory, and play therapy provides a comprehensive approach to therapy that addresses the needs of both children and the whole family. It fosters emotional awareness, enhances communication, and strengthens the family connections, leading to more resilient and harmonious relationships.

## Mindfulness-Based Play Family Therapy

Mindfulness-Based Play Family Therapy (MBPFT) is a therapeutic model developed by Dottie Higgins Klein (2013). This model combines mindfulness principles and play therapy techniques to meet the needs of families as interrelated systems. MBPFT aims to promote a stronger feeling of presence, emotional control, and connectivity among family members by integrating mindfulness practices with the fun, expressive features of play therapy. The basic goals of MBPFT are to incorporate both parents and children in the process, focusing on family ties to improve communication and emotional regulation and promote a supportive and nurturing home environment. The MBPFT concept seeks to establish a therapeutic environment in which families can explore and address their concerns in a safe and empathic setting by combining mindfulness and play therapy. This strategy not only addresses individual symptoms but also improves total family health and well-being, ensuring that therapeutic changes are maintained within the family system (Higgins Klein, 2013).

MBPFT provides a structure that includes a four-segment assessment process and six stages of the therapeutic process. It has certain structured parameters called "characteristics" that include (1) a thorough evaluation and assessment prior to treatment, (2) the parent(s) and child are present together for discussions about life issues or challenges, (3) the child's play is kept in the imaginary realm, (4) though there is recognition that play is versatile, (5) a multicultural/multiethnic perspective is valued,

(6) based in the Contextual Family Therapy model allowing the therapist to work with the child alone, with parents or all together with transparency and ethical standards, (7) regular mindful parenting meetings, (8) multiple family members included, (9) cooperation with other professional is commonly observed.

## Play-Based Parent-Child Models

Play-based parent-child models, such as Filial Therapy, Theraplay®, First Play® Therapy, and Child-Parent Relationship Therapy (CPRT), share several core principles and practices that underscore their effectiveness in strengthening the parent-child relationship. These models leverage structured play activities to promote attachment, emotional regulation, and positive interactions between parents and children. The chapter in this book on Developmental and Attachment-Based Play Therapy explores two of these play-based parent-child models in depth.

### *Core Common Principles of Play-Based Parent-Child Models*
*Emphasis on Attachment and Bonding*

All these play-based models prioritize the development of secure attachment bonds between parents and children. By engaging in consistent, nurturing play activities, parents can provide the emotional support and security that children need to thrive. This aligns with attachment theory, which highlights the importance of a secure base for healthy emotional and social development (Bowlby, 1988). Theraplay®, for example, focuses on creating a joyful, engaging environment that fosters trust and connection (Booth & Jernberg, 2010).

*Parent Involvement and Empowerment*

A central tenet of these approaches is the active involvement of parents in the therapeutic process. Filial Therapy and CPRT train parents to become therapeutic agents for their children. This empowerment not only helps parents understand their children's emotional needs but also enhances their confidence in managing behavioral issues (Landreth & Bratton, 2006). By equipping parents with play therapy techniques, these models ensure that therapeutic benefits extend beyond the therapy sessions into daily family interactions.

### Structured Play Activities

These models use structured play activities designed to address specific emotional and behavioral goals. Play provides a natural and engaging medium through which children can express their feelings, resolve conflicts, and develop problem-solving skills. For instance, in First Play® Therapy, structured play sessions incorporate infant massage and kinesthetic storytelling to enhance the parent-child bond and support emotional regulation (Courtney, 2015).

### Emotional Regulation

Helping children develop better emotional regulation is a common goal across these models. Structured play activities provide a safe space for children to explore their emotions and learn coping strategies within the context of the parent-child relationship and with the guidance of the therapist. Parents, guided by therapists, use play to help children identify and manage their feelings, which is crucial for their overall mental health. Mindfulness practices can be integrated into these play sessions to further enhance emotional regulation, helping both parents and children remain calm and focused (Siegel, 2007).

### Practical Benefits of Play-based Parent-Child Models

### Improved Communication

These models foster improved communication between parents and children. By engaging in play, parents can better understand their children's perspectives and respond empathetically. This enhances mutual understanding and strengthens the emotional bond (Satir, 1983).

### Reduced Behavioral Problems

Therapeutic play helps address and reduce behavioral problems in children. The structured nature of the activities allows for the identification and modification of dysfunctional behaviors. For example, through CPRT, parents learn to set appropriate limits and provide consistent, nurturing responses, which can significantly reduce issues such as aggression and defiance (Bratton et al., 2005).

### Strengthened Family Relationships

These play-based models strengthen family relationships by promoting positive interactions and emotional connections. The therapy's collaborative nature fosters a supportive family environment where all members feel valued and understood.

### Filial Therapy

Filial play therapy is a structured and unique approach that involves parents directly in the therapeutic process, equipping them to act as therapeutic agents for their children. Developed by Bernard and Louise Guerney (1979, 1981), this model combines elements of play therapy and family therapy to address a variety of child and family issues. There have been numerous research studies published affirming the efficacy of filial play therapy (Guerney, 2000; Rezaeianzadeh & Yazdanfar, 2024; Tew et al., 2002; Zubir et al., 2019). The key components of filial play therapy include the following exercises.

### Parent Training and Empowerment

One of the foundational aspects of filial play therapy is the training and empowerment of parents. Parents are taught therapeutic play techniques and principles, such as child-centered play therapy methods, to use with their children. This training typically includes sessions on understanding child development, recognizing emotional cues, and responding empathetically. Parents learn how to create a safe and supportive play environment that encourages emotional expression and problem-solving (Guerney, 2000; VanFleet, 2005).

### Structured Play Sessions

Filial play therapy involves structured play sessions where parents use non-directive play techniques to help their children to express emotions and resolve conflicts. These sessions are designed to be regular and consistent, often occurring weekly, and are usually 30 minutes to an hour long. During these sessions, parents allow the child to lead the play while they observe and respond without directing the play themselves. This non-directive approach helps children feel heard and understood, fostering a secure attachment (VanFleet, 2023).

### Supervision and Support for Parents

Therapists play a crucial role in supervising and supporting parents throughout the filial play therapy process. Initial training sessions are followed by ongoing supervision, where therapists provide feedback, model appropriate techniques, and address any challenges parents might encounter. This supervision helps ensure parents feel confident and competent in their role, reinforcing the therapeutic gains made during the play sessions (Guerney, 1964; VanFleet, 2005).

### Benefits of Filial Play Therapy

Filial play therapy offers a range of benefits that impact both the child and the family unit. Extensive research and clinical practice support these benefits, highlighting the effectiveness of this approach in addressing various emotional, behavioral, and relational issues (Cooper et al., 2023; Hicks et al., 2016; Hutton, 2004; Kiyani et al., 2020; Renshaw & Parson, 2020; Rye, 2008; Sweeney et al., 2009; Vafa & Ismail, 2009).

**Enhancing Parent-Child Relationship:** The core goal of filial play therapy is to strengthen the parent-child relationship. By engaging in therapeutic play, parents and children build trust, improve communication, and develop a deeper emotional connection. This enhanced relationship provides a foundation for addressing various behavioral and emotional issues. The focus on the parent-child bond helps to create a nurturing environment where the child feels safe to explore and express their feelings (Landreth & Bratton, 2006).

**Addressing Emotional and Behavioral Issues:** Filial play therapy is effective for addressing a wide range of emotional and behavioral issues, including anxiety, depression, behavioral problems, and attachment disorders. The therapeutic play sessions provide a space for children to work through their emotions and experiences, leading to improved emotional regulation and reduced symptoms. By involving parents directly, filial play therapy also enhances parenting skills and reduces parental stress, contributing to a healthier family dynamic (VanFleet, 2023).

**Flexibility and Adaptability:** Filial play therapy is adaptable to different cultural contexts and family structures, making it a versatile tool for therapists working with diverse populations. The principles of filial play therapy can be tailored to meet the specific needs of individual families, ensuring that the therapeutic approach is relevant and effective for each unique situation (Guerney, 2000).

**Improved Emotional Regulation:** Children participating in filial play therapy often experience improvements in emotional regulation. The safe and supportive environment created by the play sessions allows children to express their emotions freely and learn coping strategies. This process helps reduce symptoms of anxiety, depression, and other emotional disturbances (Guerney, 2000; Ray et al., 2015).

**Enhanced Parenting Skills:** Filial play therapy equips parents with valuable therapeutic skills that enhance their parenting abilities. By learning child-centered play techniques, parents become more adept at recognizing and addressing their children's emotional cues. This skill development leads to more effective and empathetic parenting, which benefits the overall family dynamic (Bratton et al., 2005; VanFleet, 2023).

**Reduction in Behavioral Challenges:** The approach has been shown to be effective in reducing a variety of behavioral challenges in children. By providing a consistent and nurturing environment, filial play therapy helps children develop better behavioral control and social skills. This reduction in problematic behaviors contributes to a more harmonious home environment (Landreth & Bratton, 2006; VanFleet, 2023).

**Decreased Parental Stress:** Participating in filial play therapy can also reduce stress levels for parents. The training and support provided by the therapist help parents feel more confident and competent in managing their children's behaviors and emotions. This increased confidence can alleviate the stress and frustration that often accompany parenting challenges (Ray et al., 2015; VanFleet, 2005).

**Long-Term Sustainability:** Filial play therapy is designed to have long-lasting effects. The skills and techniques learned by parents are intended to be used beyond the duration of the therapy, promoting ongoing positive interactions and emotional support within the family. This sustainability ensures that the benefits of therapy continue to influence the family's well-being over time (Guerney, 2000; VanFleet, 2023).

### Child-Parent Relationship Therapy (CPRT)

CPRT and filial play therapy are both parent-involved therapeutic approaches but differ in their structure and focus. Filial play therapy was the original model, and the first that involved extensive and ongoing training and supervision. Filial play therapy focuses on empowering parents to use therapeutic play techniques to promote emotional growth and resolve family issues. CPRT, developed by Garry Landreth and Sue Bratton, is typically a short-term, ten-week program that trains parents to conduct play sessions with their child to enhance the parent-child relationship and address behavioral issues. CPRT was developed by Garry Landreth and Sue Bratton (2006) as a structured play therapy model designed to teach parents in a shorter period to be effective therapeutic agents for their children. This approach emphasizes the crucial role of a strong parent-child relationship in the child's emotional and behavioral development. CPRT equips parents with specific skills to respond effectively to their children's needs through play, fostering better communication, understanding, and emotional regulation (Landreth & Bratton, 2006). The efficacy of this model has been studied robustly (Allen, 2020; Hawkins, 2023; Kim, 2021). There are several key aspects of CPRT.

### Parental Involvement and Training

CPRT is based on the premise that parents are the most significant figures in a child's life and, therefore, have the greatest potential to impact their emotional and behavioral health. The therapy involves a structured training program where parents learn the fundamental principles of play therapy and how to apply them at home. This training includes understanding child-centered play therapy concepts, recognizing and responding to children's emotional cues, and using reflective listening and empathic responses during play sessions (Bratton et al., 2005).

### Play Sessions

A cornerstone of CPRT is the regular play sessions between parents and children, typically conducted once a week for 30 minutes. During these sessions, parents are encouraged to let the child lead the play, providing a safe and accepting environment where the child feels free to express themselves. The parent's role is to observe, reflect, and respond empathetically, allowing the child to explore their feelings and experiences without judgment. These sessions help build trust and security within the parent-child relationship (Landreth, 2012).

## Skill Development

CPRT teaches parents specific skills to enhance their interactions with their children. These skills include the following:

**Reflective Listening**: Responding to the child's verbal and non-verbal cues in a way that shows understanding and empathy.

**Setting Limits**: Establishing clear, consistent boundaries in a nurturing manner to help children feel safe and understand expectations.

**Encouragement and Praise**: Providing positive reinforcement to build the child's self-esteem and encourage desired behaviors (Bratton et al., 2005).

## Benefits of CPRT

### Strengthening the Parent-Child Bond

By empowering parents with therapeutic skills, CPRT strengthens the parent-child bond, which is foundational for a child's healthy emotional development. The emphasis on play allows for a natural and enjoyable interaction that deepens the emotional connection between parents and children.

### Improving Emotional and Behavioral Regulation

Through the structured play sessions and the application of therapeutic techniques, children learn to manage their emotions and behaviors more effectively. The safe and supportive environment created by the parents helps children feel understood and validated, which can reduce anxiety, improve mood, and enhance overall emotional well-being (Ray et al., 2013).

### Promoting Parental Confidence and Competence

CPRT increases parents' confidence and competence in handling their children's emotional and behavioral challenges. The skills learned in

CPRT enable parents to respond to their children with greater empathy and effectiveness, leading to more positive interactions and reducing parental stress (Landreth & Bratton, 2006).

*Applications and Effectiveness*

CPRT has been successfully applied to a wide range of emotional and behavioral issues in children, including anxiety, aggression, attachment disorders, and social difficulties. Research has shown that CPRT can lead to significant improvements in parent-child relationships, children's behavior, and parental satisfaction (Bratton et al., 2005). The model's flexibility allows it to be adapted for use with diverse populations and settings, making it a versatile tool in therapeutic practice (Landreth, 2012).

CPRT is a powerful therapeutic model that leverages the unique bond between parents and children to foster emotional and behavioral health. By equipping parents with play therapy skills, CPRT enhances the parent-child relationship, supports emotional regulation, and promotes positive behavioral changes. This approach not only benefits children but also empowers parents, creating a nurturing and supportive family environment.

## Integrating Play-Based Parenting Models with Mindfulness

Mindfulness can significantly enhance the effectiveness of play-based parenting models by helping parents remain present, attuned, and responsive during interactions with their children. This attunement is crucial for fostering a secure attachment and emotional bond between parent and child. When parents practice mindfulness, they become more aware of their own emotional states and reactions, which allows them to respond to their children's needs with greater empathy and sensitivity (Siegel, 2007).

### Staying Present and Attuned

Mindfulness encourages parents to stay in the moment, fully engaging with their children during play. This presence helps parents observe subtle cues and respond appropriately, facilitating a deeper understanding and connection. Play-based models like CPRT and Theraplay® emphasize the importance of such attunement, as it reinforces the child's sense of security and validation (Booth & Jernberg, 2010; Landreth & Bratton, 2006). By being fully present, parents can better support their child's emotional and social development, creating a foundation for healthier relationships and emotional resilience.

### Managing Stress and Emotions

Mindfulness practices, such as deep breathing, meditation, and body scanning, equip parents with tools to manage their own stress and emotions. Parenting can be challenging, and heightened stress levels can negatively impact parent-child interactions. When parents are calm and centered, they are better able to create a positive and supportive environment for their children. This emotional regulation is essential for effective parenting, particularly in play-based models where the parent's role is to provide a safe and nurturing space for the child to express and explore emotions (Duncan et al., 2009; Kabat-Zinn, 1994).

### Benefits for Children

Children benefit immensely from interactions with mindful parents. They learn by observing and mirroring their parents' behavior. When parents practice mindfulness, children are more likely to develop similar skills, enhancing their ability to regulate emotions and handle stress. This modeling effect is supported by research indicating that children of mindful parents exhibit better emotional regulation and fewer behavioral problems (Duncan et al., 2009).

### Practical Integration

To integrate mindfulness into play-based parenting models, parents can do the following tasks.

#### Set Intentions

Begin play sessions with a moment of reflection, setting an intention to remain present and open during the interaction.

#### Practice Mindful Observation

During play, focus on observing the child's behavior and emotions without immediate judgment or intervention.

### Use Mindful Language

Employ reflective listening and empathetic responses to validate the child's experiences.

### Incorporate Mindful Breaks

If stress arises during play, take a short break to practice breathing exercises or mindfulness techniques to regain calm and focus.

Mindfulness enriches play-based parenting models by fostering a deeper connection between parents and children. It enhances parents' ability to stay present, attuned, and responsive, which is critical for effective therapeutic play. Additionally, mindfulness supports parents in managing their own stress and emotions, ensuring that interactions remain positive and supportive. This holistic approach not only benefits the parent-child relationship but also promotes the child's overall emotional and social well-being.

## Mindfulness Techniques for Families

### Mindful Communication

Teach family members to practice active listening and speak from a place of awareness and compassion. Techniques such as reflective listening and "I" statements can enhance understanding and reduce conflict.

### Family Mindfulness Exercises

Engage the whole family in mindfulness activities such as group meditation, mindful walking, or shared breathing exercises. These practices can create a sense of unity and collective calm.

### Emotional Awareness

Encourage family members to practice mindfulness of their emotions and help them recognize and manage their feelings in a healthy way. This can reduce reactive behaviors and promote more constructive responses.

### Mindfully Engaging Play

Encourage parents to engage in play with full presence and attention. This means focusing on the child and the activity without distractions, judgments, or agendas.

*Reflective Practice*

Encourage parents to reflect on their play sessions and interactions with their children. Journaling or discussing their experiences with a therapist can help them gain insights and improve their attunement and responsiveness.

## Supporting Parents through Mindfulness-Based Practices

Therapists can support parents outside of play therapy sessions by teaching them mindfulness-based practices that they can incorporate into their daily lives. These practices can help parents manage stress, improve emotional regulation, and enhance their overall well-being, ultimately benefiting their children and families.

### Mindfulness Techniques for Parents

*Daily Mindfulness Practice*

Encourage parents to establish a regular mindfulness practice, such as meditation, yoga, or mindful walking. Consistent practice can help parents cultivate a sense of calm and presence that they can bring to their parenting.

*Stress Reduction Techniques*

Teach parents mindfulness-based stress reduction techniques, such as progressive muscle relaxation, guided imagery, and deep breathing exercises. These practices can help parents manage the demands and challenges of parenting with greater ease.

*Mindful Self-Compassion*

Encourage parents to practice self-compassion, particularly during difficult parenting moments. Mindful self-compassion involves recognizing one's own struggles and responding with kindness and understanding rather than self-criticism.

## Enhancing Parental Attunement and Responsiveness

Mindfulness can significantly enhance parental attunement and responsiveness by helping parents become more aware of their own emotional states and reactions. By cultivating self-awareness and self-regulation, parents can respond to their children's needs with greater sensitivity and empathy. This approach aligns well with the principles of Synergetic Play Therapy®, a model developed by Lisa Dion (2018), which emphasizes the importance of parental attunement in supporting a child's emotional and behavioral development.

### Mindfulness Techniques for Enhancing Attunement
#### Mindful Observation

Teaching parents to observe their children with full presence and attention involves noticing their behaviors, emotions, and needs without judgment or distraction. This technique helps parents attune to their children's subtle cues and signals, promoting a deeper understanding and connection. In Synergetic Play Therapy®, Lisa Dion emphasizes the significance of staying present and observing the child's process, which helps in accurately responding to their emotional states (Dion, 2018).

#### Mindful Listening

Encouraging parents to practice active listening means fully focusing on their child's words and feelings. This involves setting aside distractions and preconceptions and responding with empathy and understanding. Active listening not only validates the child's experiences but also fosters a sense of safety and trust. Dion highlights that when parents listen mindfully, they create an environment where children feel heard and valued, which is crucial for emotional healing and growth (Dion, 2018).

#### Reflective Response Practice

Encouraging parents to reflect on their interactions with their children involves considering how their own emotional states and reactions may impact their parenting. Reflective practice can help parents develop greater insight and improve their attunement and responsiveness. By understanding their triggers and responses, parents can better regulate their emotions and provide a more stable and nurturing environment for their children. According to Dion (2018), self-reflection is a critical component in Synergetic Play Therapy®, as it allows parents to become more conscious of their own processes and how these influence their interactions with their children.

### Benefits of Enhanced Parental Attunement

#### Improved Parent-Child Relationship

Mindfulness and reflective practices help in creating a stronger and more empathetic bond between parents and children. Enhanced attunement allows parents to meet their children's emotional needs more effectively, fostering a secure attachment and trust.

#### Better Emotional Regulation for Parents and Children

When parents are mindful and attuned, they can model effective emotional regulation for their children. This leads to a calmer and more supportive home environment where children learn to manage their emotions constructively.

#### Reduction in Behavioral Issues

Increased parental attunement can lead to a decrease in behavioral problems. When children feel understood and validated, they are less likely to exhibit disruptive behaviors as a means of seeking attention or expressing unmet needs.

Integrating mindfulness into parenting, as advocated for within Synergetic Play Therapy® and supported by Lisa Dion's (2018) work, enhances parental attunement and responsiveness. Techniques such as mindful observation, mindful listening, and reflective practice help parents become more aware of their emotional states and reactions, leading to more empathetic and effective parenting. This approach not only strengthens the parent-child relationship but also supports the child's overall emotional and behavioral development.

## Conclusion

Blending mindfulness into therapeutic work with parents, children, and families can enhance the parent-child relationship, support whole family systems, and improve overall family well-being. By drawing from family systems theory, play-based parenting models, and attachment-based theory, therapists can use mindfulness-based practices to foster greater attunement, empathy, and emotional regulation within family dynamics. This chapter has provided an overview of how mindfulness can be incorporated into various aspects of family therapy, highlighting the transformative potential of a playful and mindful approach.

## References

Alivandi Vafa, M., & Ismail, K. H. (2009). Reaching Out to Single Parent Children through Filial Therapy. *Online Submission, 6*(2), 1–12.

Bögels, S. M., & Emerson, L. M. (2019). The role of mindfulness in parenting. In S. M. Bögels, & L. M. Emerson (Eds.), *Mindful parenting: A guide for mental health practitioners* (pp. 101–120). Springer.

Booth, P. B., & Jernberg, A. M. (2010). *Theraplay: Helping parents and children build better relationships through attachment-based play* (3rd ed.). Jossey-Bass.

Bortz, P., Berrigan, M., VanBergen, A., & Gavazzi, S. M. (2019). Family systems thinking as a guide for theory integration: Conceptual overlaps of differentiation, attachment, parenting style, and identity development in families with adolescents. *Journal of Family Theory & Review, 11*(4), 544–560. https://doi.org/10.1111/jftr.12354

Bowen, M. (1978). *Family therapy in clinical practice.* Jason Aronson.

Bowlby, J. (1969). *Attachment and loss: Vol. 1.* Attachment. Basic Books.

Bratton, S. C., Ray, D. C., Rhine, T., & Jones, L. (2005). The efficacy of play therapy with children: A meta-analytic review of treatment outcomes. *Professional Psychology: Research and Practice, 36*(4), 376–390. https://doi.org/10.1037/0735-7028.36.4.376

Coatsworth, J. D., Duncan, L. G., Greenberg, M. T., & Nix, R. L. (2014). Changing parent's mindfulness, child management skills, and relationship quality with their youth: Results from a randomized trial of the mindfulness-enhanced strengthening families program. *Developmental Psychology, 50*(2), 431–442. https://doi.org/10.1037/a0038212

Cooper, J., Yu, M. L., MacKay, L., & Brown, T. (2023). Exploring changes in family functioning when a child participates in a School-Based Filial Therapy program. *Australian and New Zealand Journal of Family Therapy, 44*(3), 328–351.

Courtney, J. (2015). *FirstPlay therapy: A new approach for early childhood mental health.* Jessica Kingsley Publishers.

Dion, L. (2018). *Synergetic play therapy: A model of integrative play therapy.* Norton.

Duncan, L. G., Coatsworth, J. D., & Greenberg, M. T. (2009). A model of mindful parenting: Implications for parent–child relationships and prevention research. *Clinical Child and Family Psychology Review, 12*(3), 255–270. https://doi.org/10.1007/s10567-009-0046-3

Gil, E. (2015). *Family play therapy.* Guilford Press.

Gil, E., & Baima, T. Using a family systems approach to assessment and treatment. In *Play therapy treatment planning with children and families* (pp. 90–96). Routledge.

Guerney, B. G. (2000). *Filial therapy: Strengthening family relationships with child-centered play therapy.* Haworth Press.

Guerney, B. G., Jr., & Guerney, L. F. (1981). Filial therapy: Description and rationale. In S. J. Schaefer & K. O'Connor (Eds.), *Handbook of play therapy* (pp. 171–190). John Wiley & Sons.

Guerney, L. (2000). Filial therapy into the 21st century. International Journal of Play Therapy, 9(2), 1. https://doi.org/10.1037/h0089433

Gunter, K. B., Almstedt, H. C., & Janz, K. F. (2012). Physical activity in childhood may be the key to optimizing lifespan skeletal health. Exercise and Sport Sciences Reviews, 40(1), 13–21. https://doi.org/10.1097/JES.0b013e318236e5ee

Haley, J. (1976). Problem-solving therapy. Jossey-Bass.

Harnett, P. H., & Dawe, S. (2012). The contribution of mindfulness-based therapies for children and families and proposed conceptual integration. Child and Adolescent Mental Health, 17(4), 195–208. https://doi.org/10.1111/j.1475-3588.2011.00643.x

Hawkins, J. (2023). The impact of child-parent relationship therapy on parent self-esteem and parenting stress on homeless parents [Doctoral dissertation], Texas A&M University-Commerce.

Hicks, J. F., Lenard, N., & Brendle, J. (2016). Utilizing filial therapy with deployed military families. International Journal of Play Therapy, 25, 210–216. https://doi.org/10.1037/pla0000032

Higgins Klein, D. (2013). Mindfulness-based play family therapy. Jessica Kingsley Publishers.

Hutton, D. S. (2004). Filial therapy: Shifting the balance. Clinical Child Psychology and Psychiatry, 9(2), 261–270. https://doi.org/10.1177/1359104504041922

Kabat-Zinn, J. (1994). Wherever you go, there you are: Mindfulness meditation in everyday life. Hyperion.

Kim, M. (2021). The effect of the child-parent relation therapy program on the parenting stress and parenting efficacy of mothers of the multi-cultural families. Ilkogretim Online, 20(3).

Kirby, J. N. (2016). The role of compassion in mindfulness-based parenting programs. Mindfulness, 7(3), 566–575. https://doi.org/10.1111/cpsp.12149

Kiyani, Z., Mirzai, H., Hosseini, S. A., Sourtiji, H., Hosseinzadeh, S., & Ebrahimi, E. (2020). The effect of filial therapy on the parenting stress of mothers of children with autism spectrum disorder. Archives of Rehabilitation, 21(2), 206–219.

Landreth, G. L. (2012). Play therapy: The art of the relationship. Routledge.

Landreth, G. L., & Bratton, S. C. (2006). Child-parent relationship therapy (CPRT): A 10-session filial therapy model. Routledge.

Lucas-Thompson, R. G., Miller, R., Seiter, N. S., & Hostinar, C. E. (2021). Mindful parenting and parent-adolescent stress physiology during the COVID-19 pandemic. Family Process, 60(3), 898–912. https://doi.org/10.1111/famp.12627

Minuchin, S. (1974). Families and family therapy. Harvard University Press.

Ray, D. C., Stulmaker, H. L., Lee, K. R., & Silverman, W. K. (2013). Child-centered play therapy and impairment: Exploring relationships and constructs. International Journal of Play Therapy, 22(3), 158. https://doi.org/10.1037/a0032898

Ray, D. C., Stulmaker, H. L., Lee, K. R., & Silverman, W. R. (2015). Child-parent relationship therapy (CPRT) for adoptive families. Adoption Quarterly, 16(4), 243–259.

Renshaw, K., & Parson, J. (2020). Infant Filial Therapy–From Conception to Early Years: Clinical Considerations for Working with Whole Family Systems. In Infant Play Therapy (pp. 101–116). Routledge.

Rezaeianzadeh, Z., & Yazdanfar, F. (2024). Effectiveness of theraplay and filial therapy on aggression in preschool boys. Current Psychology, 43(19), 17602–17613.

Rye, N. (2008). Filial therapy for enhancing relationships in families. The Journal of Family Health Care, 18(5), 179–181.

Satir, V. (1983). Conjoint family therapy (3rd ed.). Science and Behavior Books.

Siegel, D. J. (2007). *The mindful brain: Reflection and attunement in the cultivation of well-being.* Norton.

Siegel, D. J. (2010). *The mindful therapist: A clinician's guide to mindsight and neural integration.* Norton.

Sweeney, D. S., & Skurja, C. (2001). Filial therapy as a cross-cultural family intervention. *Asian Journal of Counseling, 8*(2), 175–208.

Tew, K., Landreth, G. L., Joiner, K. D., & Solt, M. D. (2002). Filial therapy with parents of chronically ill children. *International Journal of Play Therapy, 11*(1), 79.

VanFleet, R. (2005). *Filial therapy: Strengthening parent-child relationships through play.* Professional Resource Press.

VanFleet, R., Sywulak, A. E., & Sniscak, C. C. (2010). *Child-centered play therapy.* Guilford Press.

Zubir, N. M., Johari, K. S. K., Mahmud, Z., Ab Razak, N. H., & Johan, S. (2019). Systemic review: Traditional and intensive filial therapy module. *International Journal of Academic Research in Business and Social Sciences.*

# 15

# MINDFULNESS-BASED SENSORY EXPLORATION IN THE PLAYROOM

## Introduction

Sensory exploration is a fundamental aspect of childhood development and an essential component of play therapy. Engaging children in sensory play can foster mindfulness, enhance emotional regulation, and support overall mental health. This chapter examines the benefits of sensory exploratory play and provides practical strategies for therapists to encourage and support mindfulness-based experiences through sensory play in the playroom. Recognizing that each child has a unique sensory profile, this chapter will offer specific ways to tailor sensory exploration to enhance mindfulness practices for child clients and their caregivers.

## Sensory Exploratory Play

### Understanding Sensory Profiles

Each child has a unique sensory profile, which refers to their individual preferences, sensitivities, and responses to sensory stimuli (Dunn, 2007; Goncalves & Abreu, 2023). These profiles can vary widely and may include over-responsiveness, under-responsiveness, or a combination of both to sensory input (Dunn, 2007; Little et al., 2017; Miller et al., 2007). Understanding a child's sensory profile is crucial for tailoring sensory play activities that are both engaging and therapeutic (Dunn, 2007; Goncalves & Abreu, 2023).

DOI: 10.4324/9781003468585-15

### Sensory Over-Responsiveness

Children who are over-responsive to sensory input may react strongly to certain stimuli, such as loud noises, bright lights, or specific textures. These heightened responses can lead to discomfort, anxiety, or avoidance behaviors. Recognizing these sensitivities allows therapists to create a calming environment and introduce sensory experiences gradually. For example, a child who is sensitive to noise might benefit from quieter play settings or the use of noise-canceling headphones (Miller et al., 2007).

### Sensory Under-Responsiveness

Conversely, children who are under-responsive to sensory input may seek out intense sensory experiences or appear indifferent to stimuli that typically elicit a response. These children might engage in behaviors like crashing into objects, spinning, or seeking deep pressure. Understanding this aspect of a child's sensory profile helps in designing activities that provide the necessary sensory input to keep them engaged and regulated (Dunn, 2007; Goncalves & Abreu, 2023). Activities such as heavy work tasks, deep-pressure activities, and tactile play can be particularly beneficial (Dunn, 2007).

### Mixed Sensory Responses

Many children exhibit a combination of over-responsiveness and under-responsiveness across different sensory modalities. A child might be over-responsive to auditory stimuli while being under-responsive to tactile input. This mixed sensory profile requires a nuanced approach to sensory play, where therapists must balance calming strategies with stimulating activities to address the child's varied needs (Harrington, 2020). Sensory integration therapy, which aims to help children respond more appropriately to sensory stimuli, can be particularly effective for these children (Little et al., 2017).

### Tailoring Sensory Play Activities

Understanding a child's sensory profile allows therapists to tailor sensory play activities that are not only therapeutic but also enjoyable. For example, a child with tactile sensitivities might start with dry, non-messy textures like sand or beans before progressing to more challenging materials like shaving cream or finger paints. Similarly, a child who craves vestibular input might enjoy activities such as swinging, bouncing on a therapy ball, or spinning, which can help regulate their sensory needs and improve focus and attention.

By thoroughly understanding and addressing the unique sensory profiles of each child, therapists can create a supportive environment that promotes sensory regulation and enhances therapeutic outcomes. This individualized approach ensures that sensory play is both effective and enjoyable, helping children to engage more fully and comfortably in therapy.

## Research on Sensory Play in Play Therapy

Research has shown that sensory play can significantly benefit children's development and well-being (May-Benson & Koomar, 2010; Roberts et al., 2017). Sensory play involves activities that stimulate the senses – sight, sound, touch, taste, and smell – and can include a range of experiences such as playing with sand, water, clay, and various textured materials (Young & Messer, 2024).

### Benefits of Sensory Play

#### Cognitive Development

Sensory play enhances cognitive skills by encouraging children to explore, discover, and problem-solve. Activities like playing with water or sand can teach concepts of volume and texture, fostering cognitive growth. According to research, sensory experiences help children develop cognitive skills through experimentation and exploration (Abidin et al., 2022; Hart, 2019; Yael & Buján, 2023).

#### Language Development

Engaging in sensory play provides opportunities for children to develop language skills. Describing textures, actions, and experiences enriches their vocabulary and communication skills. For instance, playing with textured materials like clay or slime encourages children to articulate their sensations and actions, boosting their descriptive language abilities (Ayres & Mailoux, 1981; Motamedi et al., 2021).

*Emotional Regulation*

Sensory play can be soothing and help children regulate their emotions. Activities such as playing with kinetic sand or water beads can provide a calming effect, helping children manage stress and anxiety. This is particularly beneficial for children with sensory processing issues or autism spectrum disorders, as highlighted by Aprianti (2019), Howie (2016), and Lafreniere (2013).

*Fine Motor Skills*

Manipulating small objects and materials during sensory play improves fine motor skills and hand-eye coordination. Activities like threading beads, molding clay, or using tweezers to pick up small items enhance dexterity and motor control (Dionne-Dostie et al., 2015; Fu et al., 2024).

*Social Interaction*

Sensory play often involves cooperative play, encouraging social interaction and teamwork. Group activities such as building a sandcastle or creating a sensory art project promote collaboration and communication among peers. These experiences are crucial for developing social skills and building friendships (May-Benson & Koomar, 2010; Tamblyn et al., 2022).

***Examples of Sensory Play Activities in Play Therapy***

*Sandplay*

Sand trays and sandboxes are common in play therapy settings. Children can dig, build, and create scenarios in the sand, which allows for imaginative play and emotional expression. The tactile experience of sand also helps children ground themselves and stay present in the moment (Homeyer & Sweeney, 2011).

*Water Play*

Activities involving water, such as pouring, splashing, or using water tables, can be highly therapeutic. Water play can be both calming and stimulating, helping children explore cause and effect, enhance motor skills, and relax (Gonima et al., 2008; Myung & Kim, 2020).

*Clay and Playdough*

Manipulating clay or playdough provides a rich sensory experience that fosters creativity and fine motor development. Children can express their feelings through sculpting and molding, providing a non-verbal outlet for emotions (Gascoyne, 2017; Salles, 2023).

*Sensory Bins*

Sensory bins filled with materials like rice, dried beans, or pasta offer diverse tactile experiences. Adding small toys or objects to the bins encourages exploration and imaginative play. These bins can be tailored to specific themes or therapeutic goals (Fillingham, 2019; Howie, 2016).

*Textured Art Projects*

Using materials such as textured paints, fabric scraps, and foam, children can create art projects that engage multiple senses. This form of sensory play combines creativity with tactile exploration, promoting self-expression and sensory integration (Fillingham, 2019; Hart, 2019; Johnson, 2018, 2014).

*Loose Parts Play*

Simon Nicholson's (1971) theory was grounded in his belief that environments play a crucial role in children's learning and creativity. Nicholson observed that traditional play environments often limited children's opportunities for exploration and creativity. In contrast, he argued that environments filled with loose parts – movable, versatile materials – allowed children to interact with their surroundings in a more creative and engaging manner (Nicholson, 1971).

Loose parts play has gained international recognition for its numerous benefits, including fostering creativity, enhancing problem-solving skills, promoting physical and sensory development, and supporting social interaction. Educators and researchers around the world continue to advocate for environments that incorporate loose parts to enrich children's play experiences (Cankaya et al., 2023; Daly & Beloglovsky, 2014; Ferdinand et al., 2023; Spencer et al., 2019).

*Synergy between Loose Parts Play and Mindfulness*

Loose parts play is richly sensory-based. Loose parts play and mindfulness go hand in hand, enhancing children's developmental and emotional well-being through complementary practices that foster creativity, sensory engagement, and present-moment awareness.

**Enhanced Sensory Engagement:** Loose parts play naturally involves sensory exploration, as children interact with various textures, shapes, and weights. Mindfulness enhances this sensory engagement by encouraging children to focus on their sensory experiences intentionally. For example, while playing with sand, a mindful approach would involve noticing the texture, temperature, and movement of the sand through their fingers. This heightened awareness deepens the sensory experience and promotes relaxation and focus (Parham & Fazio, 2008).

**Creativity and Presence:** Both loose parts play and mindfulness encourage being present in the moment. When children engage with loose parts, they often enter a state of flow, fully immersed in their activity. Mindfulness practices can help sustain this state by guiding children to focus on their actions and sensations rather than distractions. This synergy supports creativity, problem-solving, and cognitive flexibility (Csikszentmihalyi, 1990).

**Emotion Regulation:** The open-ended nature of loose parts play allows children to express their emotions and work through challenges in a non-verbal way. Incorporating mindfulness into this process can help children become more aware of their emotional states and develop strategies to manage them. For instance, a child building a structure with blocks might feel frustration if it collapses. A mindful approach would encourage the child to take deep breaths, notice their feelings, and calmly try again, promoting resilience and emotional regulation (Goldschmied & Jackson, 2004).

**Connection with Nature:** Many loose parts are natural materials, which can foster a connection with nature. Mindfulness practices often emphasize this connection, encouraging children to observe and appreciate the natural world. Activities like mindful nature walks, where children collect natural loose parts and mindfully engage with their environment, can deepen their sense of connection and well-being (Louv, 2016).

**Social Interaction and Empathy:** Loose parts play often involves collaborative activities, where children share materials and ideas. Mindfulness can enhance these social interactions by promoting empathy and active listening. For example, during a group activity with loose parts, a mindfulness exercise might involve children pausing to reflect on their peers' contributions and expressing appreciation. This practice fosters a supportive and empathetic social environment (Brown & Vaughan, 2009).

*Practical Applications of Mindfulness and Loose Parts Play*

**Mindful Building Projects:** Encourage children to build structures with loose parts while practicing mindfulness. Guide them to notice the textures and shapes of the materials, the sound of pieces clicking together, and their feelings throughout the process.

**Sensory Exploration Stations:** Set up sensory stations with various loose parts like sand, water, and leaves. Incorporate mindfulness by asking children to focus on their sensory experiences at each station, describing what they see, hear, feel, and smell.

**Mindful Story Creation:** Use loose parts to create scenes or stories. Afterward, engage children in a mindfulness exercise where they reflect on the process of creation, the choices they made, and the feelings they experienced.

**Nature Exploration:** Children can collect and manipulate natural loose parts like leaves, stones, and twigs to create natural sculptures or small habitats for animals. This activity promotes sensory exploration and connection with nature.

**Sensory Bins:** Creating sensory bins filled with a variety of loose parts such as rice, beans, buttons, and small toys encourages tactile exploration. Children can sift, sort, and organize these items, enhancing their sensory experiences and fine motor skills.

**Construction Play:** Using materials like wooden blocks, fabric scraps, and cardboard tubes, children can build structures and invent new creations. This type of play supports cognitive development, problem-solving, and creativity.

## Integrating Sensory Play with Prescriptive Play Therapy

Prescriptive play therapy and sensory play activities go hand in hand because sensory play-based activities can be specifically tailored to meet each child's individual needs, with an invitation for children to explore a specific experiential activity. For instance, a child with sensory processing challenges might benefit from activities that provide proprioceptive input, such as weighted blankets or other deep-pressure activities. Similarly, a child with anxiety might find relief through calming sensory activities like water play or using a sensory bottle.

By incorporating sensory play into play therapy, therapists can address various developmental and emotional needs, creating a holistic and individualized therapeutic experience.

## Creating a Mindful Playroom Environment

A mindful playroom environment is one that is designed to be inviting and responsive to the sensory needs of children. This environment should include a variety of sensory materials and spaces where children can explore and engage in sensory play at their own pace (Goodyear-Brown, 2021). Here are some ideas to consider.

### Calming Colors and Lighting

Use soft, calming colors and adjustable lighting to create a soothing atmosphere. Having lamps with dimming adjustability is a good idea.

### Sensory Zones

Designate different areas of the playroom for specific sensory activities, such as a sand table, water play area, and a quiet corner with soft textures and calming sounds.

### Mindful Decor

Incorporate natural elements such as plants, water features, and natural light to create a connection with nature, enhancing the mindfulness experience.

### Sensory Activities for Mindfulness

Sensory activities can be structured to promote mindfulness by encouraging children to focus on their sensory experiences in the present moment.

Here are some specific sensory activities that can enhance mindfulness in the playroom.

### Mindful Sandplay

Materials include sand, small tools (e.g., scoops, brushes), and natural objects (e.g., shells, stones). The therapist can encourage the child to explore the texture of the sand, noticing how it feels when they run their fingers through it, scoop it, or let it fall. The therapist can invite the child to describe their sensations and any thoughts or feelings that arise.

### Water Play and Mindfulness

Materials needed are water table, cups, sponges, water beads. The therapist can invite children to play with water, observing the sound, feel, and movement of the water. Encourage them to focus on the sensory experience, such as the coolness of the water, the sound of splashing, and the sight of water flowing.

### Mindful Touch Exploration

Various textured objects such as soft fabrics, rough stones, smooth pebbles, spiky balls can be included. The therapist can create a "touch table" where children can explore different textures and invite them to close their eyes and feel the objects, describing the sensations and how each texture makes them feel.

### Sound and Mindfulness

Musical instruments, sound bowls, nature sound recordings can all be included. The therapist introduced the child to create and listen to different sounds using the various instruments, encouraging them to listen mindfully. The therapist can invite them to focus on the qualities of the sounds, such as pitch, volume, and rhythm. The therapist can also use sound bowls or chimes to create a calming soundscape.

### Aroma and Mindfulness

With predetermined care as to potential allergies, essential oils, scented playdough, natural scents from an orange, vinegar, other items from nature can be used. In providing the child with a variety of scented materials, the therapist can invite the child to explore and focus on the smells and encourage them to describe the scents and notice any emotions or memories that the smells evoke.

## Educating Caregivers about Sensory Play

It is essential to educate caregivers about the benefits of sensory play and how they can support their child's sensory experiences at home. Providing caregivers with knowledge and tools empowers them to create a sensory-friendly environment and engage in mindful sensory activities with their children.

### *Tips for Educating Caregivers*
#### *Workshops and Handouts*

Therapists might offer workshops or informational handouts that explain sensory preferences, the benefits of sensory play, and provide ideas for sensory activities, ensuring that caregivers feel equipped to support their child's sensory needs at home. Workshops could include interactive demonstrations of sensory tools, such as fidget spinners, textured stress balls, or kinetic sand, along with hands-on opportunities for caregivers to try activities like making fluffy slime or experimenting with weighted blankets for grounding. Informational handouts might outline sensory profiles to help caregivers identify their child's specific sensory preferences (e.g., tactile, auditory, or visual), along with tailored suggestions for activities, such as using finger painting for tactile seekers or bubble blowing for children needing help with deep breathing. Therapists could also recommend resources, such as sensory-friendly websites, books like *The Out-of-Sync Child* by Carol Stock Kranowitz (2005), or local occupational therapy services that specialize in sensory integration. By providing these practical tools and accessible resources, therapists empower caregivers to incorporate sensory play into daily routines to enhance their child's emotional and behavioral regulation.

#### *Modeling and Coaching*

Therapists can demonstrate sensory activities during therapy sessions and coach caregivers on how to engage their children in these activities mindfully, providing examples and hands-on practice to ensure confidence and understanding. For instance, the therapist might show how to use a glitter-filled "calm-down jar," explaining how children can watch the glitter settle while taking deep breaths to calm themselves. They could introduce tactile activities like squeezing stress balls, manipulating textured playdough, or running fingers through kinetic sand to help children release tension. Therapists might also demonstrate auditory calming techniques, such as using a rain stick or listening to soft chimes, encouraging children to focus on the soothing sounds. For olfactory sensory engagement, the therapist could guide caregivers in helping children use scented markers, lavender sachets, or essential oil rollers for grounding and relaxation. Additionally, they might model the use of weighted lap pads or soft blankets to provide calming deep pressure for children needing tactile input. By experiencing these activities firsthand during therapy, caregivers gain the tools and confidence to replicate them at home, creating consistent and supportive sensory routines for their children.

*Sensory Kits*

The therapist might create sensory kits with various materials and clear, easy-to-follow instructions for mindful sensory activities that caregivers can use at home to support their child's emotional regulation. These kits could include sensory-based items like textured stress balls or squishy toys for tactile engagement, a small glitter-filled "calm-down jar" to encourage visual focus, and scented sachets or essential oil rollers to stimulate the sense of smell. Other items might include soft fabric swatches or a weighted beanbag for grounding through touch, a rain stick or chime for soothing auditory input, and edible sensory items like flavored lozenges or chewable jewelry for oral sensory engagement. Each item would come with instructions on how to use it during moments of stress or as part of a calming sensory routine, helping caregivers facilitate grounding and regulation for their child.

## Mindfulness Practices for Caregivers

Supporting caregivers in developing mindfulness practices can significantly enhance their ability to attune to their child's sensory needs and responses. Children and parents often have differing sensory preferences, which can contribute to stress and misunderstanding within the family dynamic. For instance, a child who is sensitive to noise may feel overwhelmed in a bustling household, while a parent with a high tolerance for sensory input might not immediately recognize the child's discomfort.

Mindfulness practices can help caregivers become more aware of these sensory differences and respond more effectively. Encouraging caregivers to engage in sensory mindfulness activities – such as mindful listening, tactile exploration, or sensory-focused breathing exercises – can help them stay present and calm. This heightened awareness allows caregivers to notice subtle cues about their child's sensory preferences and adjust the environment or their interactions accordingly.

For example, a mindfulness exercise might involve parents and children sitting quietly and focusing on the sounds around them, discussing which sounds are soothing or irritating. This practice not only helps caregivers better understand their child's sensory experiences but also teaches both parents and children strategies for managing sensory-related stress.

Mindfulness can help caregivers manage their own sensory preferences and stress responses. By practicing mindfulness, caregivers learn to recognize their stress triggers and develop coping strategies that help maintain a calm and supportive environment. This mutual understanding and regulation of sensory preferences create a more harmonious family dynamic, reducing stress and enhancing emotional connections.

## Tailoring Sensory Exploration to Individual Sensory Profiles

### Assessing Sensory Profiles

Therapists can use various assessment tools to evaluate a child's sensory preferences and needs. These tools help identify how children process sensory information and how it affects their behavior and daily functioning. Here are some commonly used tools:

> **Sensory Profile 2**: Developed by Winnie Dunn, this assessment measures a child's sensory processing patterns in various contexts. It includes caregiver questionnaires and self-reports for older children, covering different sensory domains like auditory, visual, tactile, and vestibular processing.
>
> **Sensory Processing Measure (SPM)**: This tool assesses sensory processing, praxis, and social participation at home, school, and in the community. It includes forms for parents, teachers, and the child, providing a comprehensive view of sensory processing issues across different environments.

**Sensory Integration and Praxis Tests (SIPT)**: Developed by A. Jean Ayres, SIPT is a set of standardized tests that evaluate sensory integration and praxis abilities. It includes various subtests that assess visual, tactile, and kinesthetic processing, motor coordination, and planning.

**Sensory Processing and Self-Regulation Checklist**: This checklist helps caregivers and therapists identify sensory processing and self-regulation challenges. It covers various sensory modalities and provides insights into how sensory processing affects self-regulation and behavior.

**DeGangi-Berk Test of Sensory Integration (TSI)**: This assessment tool is designed for children aged three to five years and evaluates postural control, bilateral motor integration, and reflex integration. It helps identify sensory processing and integration difficulties early in development.

**Observation and Interviews**: In addition to standardized tools, direct observation and structured interviews with parents, teachers, and the child can provide valuable insights into sensory preferences and challenges. Therapists can observe how children respond to different sensory stimuli in various settings and gather information from caregivers about the child's sensory behaviors.

These assessment tools help therapists create individualized intervention plans that address the child's specific sensory processing needs, promoting better emotional regulation and overall functioning.

## Adapting Sensory Activities

Based on the child's sensory profile, therapists can adapt sensory activities to meet each child's needs. This might involve modifying the intensity, duration, or type of sensory input to ensure the child feels comfortable and engaged.

### Gradual Exposure

Gradual exposure is essential in sensory play therapy, particularly for children who are hypersensitive or hesitant to engage with new sensations. Therapists introduce activities slowly, starting with familiar, non-threatening stimuli like soft fabric or water beads before progressing to stickier or more complex materials like slime or shaving cream. Visual and auditory inputs, such as observing a rain stick or listening to calming sounds, can be introduced gently before the child actively engages. By increasing the intensity or complexity at the child's pace, therapists build trust, foster confidence, and help children develop tolerance to new sensory experiences. Caregivers can also be involved, learning how to create sensory bins or use tools like stress balls and pinwheels at home to reinforce progress made in therapy. This gradual approach ensures a safe, empowering, and collaborative experience for the child.

*Sensory Breaks*

It is important to provide opportunities for sensory breaks when a child becomes overwhelmed during play therapy, giving them a chance to self-regulate and return to a state of calm. Sensory breaks can involve engaging in calming activities tailored to the child's preferences, such as squeezing a stress ball, watching a glitter-filled "calm-down jar," or sitting under a weighted blanket for deep pressure input. For children who find movement soothing, therapists might encourage rocking in a sensory chair or stretching with slow, mindful movements. Quiet spaces with minimal stimulation, such as a cozy corner with soft pillows or noise-canceling headphones, can also help the child reset. These breaks not only provide relief from overstimulation but also teach children how to recognize when they need a pause and use self-soothing strategies to manage big emotions. Incorporating these breaks into therapy ensures that sessions remain supportive and empowering, fostering the child's emotional and sensory regulation skills.

*Individual Preferences*

Adapting to a child's individual sensory preferences is crucial in creating a supportive and effective therapeutic environment. Tailoring activities to align with these preferences ensures the child feels comfortable and engaged. For instance, if a child enjoys soft textures, the therapist might incorporate materials like fleece fabric, kinetic sand, or fluffy pom-poms into play activities. Conversely, if a child is sensitive to sticky substances, such as slime or glue, these can be avoided or introduced gradually to build tolerance. For children who respond positively to auditory input, soothing sounds like rain sticks or gentle music might be included, while loud or jarring noises are minimized. Similarly, a child who enjoys movement could benefit from activities like rocking in a sensory chair, while a child who prefers stillness might be given a weighted blanket or calming breathing exercises. By observing and respecting each child's unique sensory needs and responses, therapists can create activities that feel safe and engaging, fostering trust and promoting emotional regulation. This individualized approach not only supports sensory integration but also enhances the child's overall therapeutic experience.

## Conclusion

Mindfulness-based sensory exploration in the playroom offers a powerful way to enhance emotional regulation, cognitive development, and overall well-being in children. By understanding each child's unique sensory profile and integrating mindfulness into sensory play activities, therapists can create a therapeutic environment that supports mindful awareness and holistic development. This chapter has provided practical strategies for incorporating sensory exploration into play therapy, emphasizing the transformative potential of mindful sensory play for child clients and their caregivers.

## References

Ayres, A. J., & Mailloux, Z. (1981). Influence of sensory integration procedures on language development. *The American Journal of Occupational Therapy: Official Publication of the American Occupational Therapy Association, 35*(6), 383–390. https://doi.org/10.5014/ajot.35.6.383

Brown, S., & Vaughan, C. (2009). *Play: How it shapes the brain, opens the imagination, and invigorates the soul*. Penguin.

Cankaya, O., Rohatyn-Martin, N., Leach, J., Taylor, K., & Bulut, O. (2023). Preschool children's loose parts play and the relationship to cognitive development: A review of the literature. *Journal of Intelligence, 11*(8), 151. https://doi.org/10.3390/jintelligence11080151

Csikszentmihalyi, M. (1990). *Flow: The psychology of optimal experience*. Harper & Row.

Daly, L., & Beloglovsky, M. (2014). *Loose parts: Inspiring play in young children* (Vol. 1). Redleaf Press.

Dionne-Dostie, E., Paquette, N., Lassonde, M., & Gallagher, A. (2015). Multisensory integration and child neurodevelopment. *Brain Sciences, 5*(1), 32–57. https://doi.org/10.3390/brainsci5010032

Dunn, W. (2007). *Living sensationally: Understanding your senses*. Jessica Kingsley Publishers.

Ferdinand, N., Hidayat, T., Hanif, H., & Riyanto, S. (2023). Exploring the impact of sensory activities on the development of entrepreneurial spirit in children. *Pasundan Community Service Development, 1*(2), 32–37.

Fillingham, S. (2019). Using messy play to promote self-discovery. *Early Years Educator.* https://doi.org/10.12968/EYED.2019.21.2.35

Fu, Q., Zhao, F., & Qin, J. (2024). Perspectives on early childhood development in China: Key dimensions and contextual contributions. *Frontiers in Psychology, 15*, 1370641. https://doi.org/10.3389/fpsyg.2024.1370641

Gascoyne, S. (2017). *Messy play in the early years: Supporting learning through material engagement.* Routledge.

Goldschmied, E., & Jackson, S. (2004). *People under three: Young children in day care.* Psychology Press.

Gonçalves, M., & Abreu, A. M. (2023). Sensory processing and occupational participation. *Journal of Occupational Therapy, Schools, & Early Intervention, 16*(4), 480–495.

Gonima, N., Lucas-Bouillon, C., & Peperstraete, L. (2008). Water play. *Child Care, 5*(1), 32–33. https://doi.org/10.12968/chca.2008.5.1.37643

Goodyear-Brown, P. (2021). *The handbook of play therapy and sensorimotor art techniques: A guide for trauma-informed practice.* Guilford Press.

Harrington, R. (2020, October 14). Breaking down sensory modulation disorder over/under responsiveness+sensory craving. https://harkla.co/blogs/podcast/123-breaking-down-sensory-modulation-disorder-over-under-responsive-sensory-craving?srsltid=AfmBOorxHs-k0prANTqHi6SayqLuBQEEug2vNG-iY6Jqr THFmSpK9W7x

Homeyer, L. E., & Sweeney, D. S. (2011). *Sandtray therapy: A practical manual.* Routledge.

Hart, K. (2019). *The perfect mix.* Practical Pre-School. https://doi.org/10.12968/PRPS.2019.SUP218.15

Howie, S. (2016). Sensory activities for emotional regulation: Best Practices for therapy. *Journal of Play Therapy, 25*(2), 120–135. https://doi.org/10.1037/pla0000114

Johnson, D. A., Ivers, N. N., Avera, J. A., & Frazee, M. (2019). Supervision guidelines for fostering state-mindfulness among supervisees. *The Clinical Supervisor, 39*(1), 128–145. https://doi.org/10.1080/07325223.2019.1674761

Kranowitz, C. S. (2005). *The out-of-sync child: recognizing and coping with sensory processing disorder.* Rev. and updated ed. A Skylight Press Book/A Perigee Book.

Lafreniere, P. (2013). Children's play as a context for managing physiological arousal and learning emotion regulation. *Psychological Topics, 22*, 183–204.

Little, L. M., Dean, E., Tomchek, S. D., & Dunn, W. (2017). Classifying sensory profiles of children in the general population. *Child: Care, Health and Development, 43*(1), 81–88. https://doi.org/10.1111/cch.12391

Louv, R. (2016). *Vitamin N: The essential guide to a nature-rich life.* Algonquin Books.

May-Benson, T. A., & Koomar, J. A. (2010). Systematic review of the research evidence examining the effectiveness of interventions using a sensory integrative approach for children. *The American Journal of Occupational Therapy, 64*(3), 403–414.

Mazefsky, C. A., Herrington, J., Siegel, M., Scarpa, A., Maddox, B. B., Scahill, L., & White, S. W. (2013). The role of emotion regulation in autism spectrum disorder. *Journal of the American Academy of Child & Adolescent Psychiatry, 52*(7), 679–688.

Miller, L. J., Anzalone, M. E., Lane, S. J., Cermak, S. A., & Osten, E. T. (2007). Concept evolution in sensory integration: A proposed nosology for diagnosis. *The American Journal of Occupational Therapy, 61*(2), 135–140. https://doi.org/10.5014/ajot.61.2.135

Motamedi, Y., Murgiano, M., Perniss, P., Wonnacott, E., Marshall, C., Goldin-Meadow, S., & Vigliocco, G. (2021). Linking language to sensory experience: Onomatopoeia in early language development. *Developmental Science, 24*(3), e13066. https://doi.org/10.1111/desc.13066

Myung, S., & Kim, K. J. (2020). Effects of the five-senses play using water on playfulness and socioemotional development of toddler. *The Journal of Future Early Childhood Education, 27*, 45–67. https://doi.org/10.22155/JFECE.27.1.45.67

Nicholson, S. (1971). How not to cheat children: The theory of loose parts. *Landscape Architecture, 62*(1), 30–34.

Parham, L. D., & Fazio, L. S. (2008). *Play in occupational therapy for children* (2nd ed.). Mosby Elsevier.

Roberts, J. E., King-Thomas, A., & Edwards, S. (2017). The benefits of sensory play in early childhood: A developmental perspective. *Child Development Perspectives, 11*(3), 199–206. https://doi.org/10.1111/cdep.12235

Salles, A. M. (2023). Clay with children who have lost or fear losing a loved one: The play therapist's observations of some clients. *LEOPOLDIANUM, 37*(101–3), 23–32.

Spencer, R., Joshi, N., Branje, K., McIsaac, J. D., Cawley, J., Rehman, L., Kirk, S. F., & Stone, M. (2019). Educator perceptions on the benefits and challenges of loose parts play in the outdoor environments of childcare centres. *AIMS Public Health, 6*, 461–476. https://doi.org/10.3934/publichealth.2019.4.461

Yael, M., & Buján, M. Y. (2023). Free sensory experiences in early childhood development. *International Journal of Human Sciences Research, 3*(25). https://doi.org.10.22533/at.ed.5583252327079

Young, S. R., & Messer, E. (2024). *Sensory play in early childhood education: Principles and practices for fostering development.* Routledge.

# 16

## MINDFULNESS-BASED GAMES AND ACTIVITIES TO ENHANCE BREATH AND BODY AWARENESS

### Introduction

Mindfulness-based practices can be particularly effective when introduced to children through games. These approaches not only make learning about mindfulness enjoyable but also help children understand and experience the benefits of present-moment awareness, awareness of emotions, conscious breathing, and somatic awareness. This chapter will explore a range of mindfulness-based games and activities designed to enhance breath and body awareness. By engaging in these practices, the child can learn to regulate their nervous system and emotions, leading to improved mental and physical well-being.

### Games for Breath and Body Awareness

According to Byrd et al. (2020) and Obradović et al. (2021), conscious breathing techniques have been shown to have numerous benefits, including:

- **Emotional Regulation**
- **Focus and Attention**
- **Stress Reduction**
- **Physical Relaxation**

Somatic awareness involves being mindful of bodily sensations and movements. According to Bakal et al. (2008), Quek et al. (2021), Price and Weng (2021), and Weber (2022), benefits include the following:

- **Enhanced self-awareness**
- **Improved body regulation**
- **Greater emotional insight**

## Breath Awareness Games

Breathing-focused games are highly effective for promoting mindfulness in children due to their simplicity and accessibility. These games leverage the natural rhythm of breathing to anchor children in the present moment, helping them to regulate their emotions and focus their attention. Breathing exercises, such as blowing bubbles or pretending to inflate a balloon, engage children in a playful and enjoyable activity while subtly teaching them to control their breath. Engaging in controlled breathing stimulates the parasympathetic nervous system, which effectively diminishes stress levels and fosters a state of tranquility, reducing stress and promoting a sense of calm. Additionally, these games make abstract mindfulness concepts tangible and understandable for young minds, fostering self-awareness and emotional regulation in a fun and therapeutic way. By incorporating breathing-focused games into therapy, children learn valuable skills for managing anxiety, improving concentration, and enhancing overall emotional well-being.

### Balloon Breaths

*Objective*: Teach the child deeper breathing by imagining their stomachs as balloons.

*Materials*: Imagination

*Instructions:* Have the child place their hands on their stomachs. Instruct them to take a deep breath in, imagining their stomachs filling up like a balloon. Hold the breath for a few seconds, then slowly exhale, imagining the balloon slowly deflating. Repeat several times, focusing on the rise and fall of their stomachs. Note: Sometimes this activity is confusing for young children because when inflating an actual balloon, we exhale to fill the balloon. If confusing, try one of the following breathing games.

### Stuffed Animal Breathing

*Objective*: Help child visualize their breath and focus on deep breathing.

*Materials*: Small stuffed animal.

*Instructions*: Have child lie down and place a small stuffed animal on their stomach. Instruct them to breathe deeply and watch the stuffed animal rise and fall with each breath. Encourage them to keep the toy moving rhythmically with their breath for a few minutes.

### Feather Breathing

*Objective*: Teach the child to control their breath with a fun, visual activity.

*Materials*: Lightweight feathers.

*Instructions*: Give the child a feather. Have them take a deep breath in and then blow the feather into the air, trying to keep it afloat as long as possible. Repeat several times, focusing on steady, controlled out-breaths.

### Birthday Cake Breath

*Objective:* Teach the child how to utilize deep inhaling and then strong and long exhales which can help child regulate when they have big emotions arise.

*Materials:* A timer, your imagination, and your breath.

*Instructions:* Invite the child to join you in making an imaginary birthday cake. Ask the child what flavor cake it should be. Pretend to make the cake together and once it is decorated, have the child join you in spreading the icing slowly, sprinkling the sprinkles, and placing the candles. Light the candles. Sing happy birthday if you wish! It's time to *smell* the fresh baked cake with a deep inhale through the nose and then, *blow out* the candles with a strong and long exhale. Repeat to make sure all the candles are blown out. Note: Variations of this breath are hot cocoa breathing, baked cookie breathing, or flower/candle breathing which all utilize inhaling through the nose as if smelling something wonderful and exhaling through the mouth in a blowing manner.

### Cotton Ball Blowing Race

This next breathing game is excellent for parent-child dyadic play therapy sessions or family sessions to encourage engaging through some friendly competition.

*Objective:* Introduce the child to the power of their breath.

*Materials:* Drinking straws (not the skinny or bending kind), cotton balls, painters or masking tape.

*Instructions:* Create a starting line and a finishing line by applying a strip of colored tape on the floor or a tabletop. Give each participant a drinking straw and a cotton ball with instructions to place the cotton ball on the starting line, and using only their breath and the straw they will move the cotton ball to the finish line without touching the cotton ball. On your mark… get set… GO! Whoever moves their cotton ball to the finish line first wins!

### Zoo Animals Breathing Game

*Objective*: Help child experience the range of intensity and subtleness of their breath.

*Materials*: Imagination.

*Instructions*: Explain to the child that they are going to pretend to be a wide range of different animals we may find at the zoo with our breath. Start with selecting a roaring lion. Have the child imagine they are a lion like the Lion King and they feel like ROARING loudly to say good morning to all the animals in the zoo. Instruct the child to inhale deeply and exhale with a ROAR! Reflect on how that felt and ask the child if they'd like to do it again or if they'd like to pretend to be another animal. Next, suggest pretending to be a hissing snake. Take a deep breath in and exhale with a soft hissssssss until all the ail is gone from the lungs. Wonder aloud how it felt to breathe like a snake. Continue the game with other animals from the zoo. Reflect afterward, inviting the child to notice how they feel in their body.

*Butterfly Breathing Game*

*Objective*: To help the child practice deep, mindful breathing using a butterfly image to guide their breaths and enhance their focus and relaxation.

*Materials*: Butterfly images (printed or drawn); colorful markers or crayons for decorating the butterflies.

*Instructions*: Explain to the child that they will use their breath to make the butterfly "fly" and feel calm and relaxed, just like a butterfly gently fluttering its wings. Color a butterfly. Give the child a butterfly image to color and decorate. This can be a calming activity and helps the child take ownership of their "breathing butterfly." Once the butterflies are ready, have the child sit holding their butterfly image in front of them at chest level. Instruct the child to take a deep breath in through their nose, imagining that they are filling the butterfly's wings with air. Ask them to hold their breath for a count of three, picturing the butterfly's wings fully expanded and ready to fly. Have them slowly exhale through their mouth, visualizing the butterfly gently flapping its wings and floating in the air. Repeat the breathing cycle several times, guiding the child with gentle prompts:

"Breathe in slowly, filling the butterfly's wings with air,"

"Hold your breath and see the butterfly's wings fully expanded…"

"Now breathe out gently, letting the butterfly flutter and fly…"

Reflect and Discuss: After several rounds, encourage the child to reflect on how they feel. Discuss how breathing like a butterfly can help them feel calm and focused.

*Train Breathing Game*

*Objective*: To help the child practice deep, mindful breathing by using the imagery of a train to guide their breaths, enhancing their focus and relaxation.

*Materials*: Train images (printed or drawn); toy train or train whistle.

*Instructions*: Explain to the child that they will use their breath to make a train go, teaching them how to feel calm and relaxed, just like a train that moves steadily along its tracks. Give the child a train with several train cars to cut-out, color, and decorate. This activity can help them engage and take ownership of their "breathing train." Once the train cars are ready, tape or glue them together and invite the child to place the train on the tracks on the floor. Instruct the child to take a deep breath in through their nose, imagining that they are filling up the train with steam. Ask them to hold their breath for a count of three, picturing the train building up energy. Have them slowly exhale through their mouth, making a "choo-choo" sound, and move the train along the imaginary tracks on the floor. Repeat the breathing cycle several times, guiding the child with gentle prompts:

"Breathe in slowly, filling up the train with steam…"

"Hold your breath and feel the train building up energy…"

"Now breathe out gently, making a 'choo-choo' sound as the train moves forward…"

Reflect and Discuss: After several rounds, encourage the child to reflect on how they feel. Discuss how breathing like a train can help them feel calm and focused.

## Body Awareness Games

Body awareness games significantly contribute to mindfulness for children by helping them develop a deeper connection with their physical sensations, which is crucial for overall emotional and cognitive development. These games encourage the child to pay attention to their bodily movements, posture, and sensations, fostering a state of present-moment awareness that is foundational to mindfulness practices. By becoming more attuned to their bodies, the child can better recognize and manage their emotions, reducing anxiety and improving emotional regulation. This self-awareness is essential for building resilience and coping skills, enabling the child to respond to stressors in a healthier and more adaptive manner (Flook et al., 2015; Siegel, 2007). Furthermore, body awareness activities promote physical health by encouraging movement and coordination, which are critical for overall well-being and development (Kabat-Zinn, 1994).

*Spaghetti Noodle Game*

*Objective*: Increase awareness of states of tension and relaxation in the body.

*Materials*: Dry spaghetti noodles and cooked spaghetti noodles for demonstration effect.

*Instructions*: Offer the child a dry spaghetti noodle to hold and examine. Together, notice how straight and stiff it is. If you try to bend it, what happens? Next, offer the child a cooked spaghetti noodle to examine. Notice together how floppy, loose, and wiggly it is! It bends all over the place! Invite the child to join you in pretending they are a cooked spaghetti noodle. So stiff. So straight. Every muscle from head to toe is so stiff! Invite the child to now transform into a cooked spaghetti noodle and become wiggly, floppy, and loose! Repeat. After the game concludes, invite the child to reflect on the way the tense dry spaghetti noodles felt compared to the relaxed cooked spaghetti noodles.

*Family Body Scan Bingo*

*Objective*: Increase awareness of different body parts through a playful activity.

*Materials*: Bingo cards with body parts listed and markers.

*Instructions*: Give each family member a bingo card with different body parts. Call out body parts one by one, asking family members to focus on that part and notice any sensation. Family members can mark off each part on their cards as they focus on it. As each round of the game ends, invite family members to reflect on sensations they were aware of in their own bodies.

*Yogi Says*

*Objective*: To enhance body awareness, balance, and mindfulness in children through engaging, fun yoga poses, and mindful movements.

*Materials*: Open space for movement, yoga mats (optional)

*Instructions*: Explain the rules of the game to the child. The game leader (Yogi) will give commands preceded by "Yogi says," and the child should only follow the commands when they are preceded by this phrase. If the leader gives a command without saying "Yogi says," the child should remain still. Begin with simple commands to help the child get accustomed to the game.

"Yogi says, touch your toes."

"Yogi says, stretch your arms to the sky."

"Yogi says, stand on one foot."

Incorporate Yoga Poses:

**Tree Pose:** "Yogi says, stand like a tree." The child stands on one leg with the other foot placed on their inner thigh or calf, and their hands together in front of their chest or stretched above their head.

**Mountain Pose:** "Yogi says, stand tall like a mountain." Children stand with their feet together, arms at their sides, and focus on maintaining good posture.

**Cat-Cow Pose:** "Yogi says, move like a cat and a cow." The child can get on hands and knees, arch their back like a cat, and then dip their back like a cow, following your example.

**Downward-Facing Dog:** "Yogi says, be a downward dog." child place their hands and feet on the ground, forming an inverted V shape with their body.

Ending the Game: Conclude the game with a relaxation pose, such as "Yogi says, lie down and close your eyes," guiding the child through a short body scan or relaxation exercise.

### Mindful Scavenger Hunt

The "Mindful Scavenger Hunt" is an engaging and interactive game that encourages children to practice mindfulness by using their senses to explore their environment. This game can be played indoors or outdoors and is a great way for therapists to help children develop their observation skills and connect with the present moment.

*Objective*: To encourage the child to practice mindfulness by using their senses to explore their environment, enhancing their observation skills and connection with the present moment.

*Materials*: List of items or sensory experiences for the scavenger hunt and small bags or baskets for collecting items.

*Instructions*: Before starting, prepare a list of items or sensory experiences for the child to find. These can include specific objects, colors, shapes, textures, sounds, or smells. Examples include the following:

Something soft: a feather, a piece of cloth

Something that makes a noise: A bell, a crinkled piece of paper

Something with a unique texture: A pinecone, a piece of bubble wrap

Something that smells nice: A flower, a scented candle

An object that is a certain color: A red leaf, a blue toy

Explain to the child that they will be going on a scavenger hunt to find items or experiences on the list, but with a twist – ask them to focus on being mindful, noticing as much as they can about each item they find.

*Scavenger Hunt:* Provide each child with a list (for a young child this can be a picture list rather than words) and a small bag or basket to collect their items. As they find each item or experience, encourage them to take a moment to observe it closely, using all their senses. For example, if they find something soft, they should feel its texture, notice its color, and think about what it reminds them of.

*Mindful Reflection:* After the child has found their items or experiences, return together for a reflection session. Ask the child to share the items they found and describe their mindful observations. Encourage them to use descriptive language and talk about how they felt during the scavenger hunt.

*Closing Activity:* End the session with a short mindfulness exercise, such as deep breathing or a guided visualization, to help the child relax and reflect on their scavenger hunt experience.

## Emotion Regulation Games

### *Emotion Ring Toss*

*Objective*: To help the child develop skills for recognizing, understanding, and regulating their emotions through an interactive ring toss game that integrates emotional learning.

*Materials*: Rings (either plastic or homemade cut from cardboard or paper plates); cones, bottles, or empty paper towel rolls affixed to a piece of cardboard as the pegs on which to toss rings; emotion picture cards with different facial expressions and emotion words; small whiteboard and marker (optional).

*Instructions*: Explain to the child that they will be playing a game called Emotion Ring Toss, where they will toss rings onto cones and discuss different emotions. Set up several pegs made from cones, bottles, or paper towel rolls in a line or circle, each labeled with different emotions (happy, sad, angry, surprised, scared, excited, etc.). You can use emotion cards to label each cone. Place the cones at varying distances to make the game more challenging and fun. Give each child a few rings to toss. Instruct the child to aim for the pegs. When a child successfully lands a ring on a peg, they pick an emotion card corresponding to that peg. The child then acts out the emotion or describes a time they felt that emotion. Discuss the emotion briefly with questions like:

> "What makes you feel this way?"

> "How does your body feel when you have this emotion?"

> "What can you do to calm down or cheer up when you feel this way?"

After a few rounds, take a short break for mindful breathing exercises. Guide the child through a simple exercise:

> "Breathe in deeply through your nose for a count of four."

> "Hold your breath for a count of four."

> "Exhale slowly through your mouth for a count of six."

Repeat three times. Continue the game, ensuring the child gets a turn to toss rings and discuss emotions. After the game, gather the child for a reflection session. Discuss:

"What was easy or hard about showing or guessing the emotions?"

"How can recognizing emotions help us in our daily lives?"

"What are some healthy ways to manage big emotions?"

*Additional Tips:* Adjust the complexity of the emotions based on the age and understanding of the child. Use positive reinforcement to encourage participation and make the game enjoyable. Incorporate follow-up activities such as drawing or writing about emotions.

## Empowering Children through Mindfulness-Based Games at Home

Teaching child mindfulness-based games and activities can empower children to regulate their emotions and behaviors more effectively at home and at school. By incorporating these practices into their daily routines, children can develop greater self-awareness and emotional resilience. Mindfulness games and activities are engaging ways to teach children self-regulation skills. These practices help the child focus on the present moment, recognize their emotions, and respond to them constructively. There is also value to attending to activities a child can focus on every day, involving the caregivers in the process to reinforce at home.

### Morning Mindfulness Strategies

Suggest to caregivers that children start the day with a few minutes of breathing while getting dressed or before eating breakfast. Toothbrushing can be made into a mindfulness game for young children, with a caregiver animating the toothbrush and asking to jump in the child's mouth to tickle their teeth clean, inviting the child to notice how the bristles feel in their mouth. This routine can help children feel calm and focused as they begin their activities, reducing stress and improving concentration throughout the day. Singing fun songs or humming together while getting ready for the day can also be emotionally regulating. Parents can notice aloud how it feels in their own body when they sing or hum. Singing and humming can be a centering, soothing, and grounding practice.

### Mindful Transitions

Using mindfulness games during transitions between activities can help children manage the changes more smoothly. For example, taking a moment to breathe deeply or perform a quick body scan before moving from one task to another can help children stay centered and reduce feelings of overwhelm. Mindfully gathering items needed before heading out the door and placing them in the morning to-go basket by the front door can assist children in being present while preparing to go for the day.

### Mindfulness before Bed

Ending the day with a mindfulness game can help children unwind and prepare for sleep. Caregivers might set a timer and send the child on a bedtime scavenger hunt with a list of items (i.e., pajamas, favorite stuffed animal, and a storybook). Consider recommending caregivers have some calming sensory activities before bed such as warm bath with lavender-scented bath-wash, dim lighting, soft and soothing music, and some soft pajamas.

## Closure

Mindfulness-based games and activities offer a playful and effective way to enhance breath and body awareness in a child. By incorporating these practices into therapy, therapists can help child develop self-regulation skills, emotional resilience, and overall well-being. Engaging children through play and involving caregivers in the process can create a supportive and empowering environment for mindfulness practice. This chapter has provided a range of practical activities and strategies to integrate mindfulness into the playroom, highlighting the transformative potential of mindful breath and body awareness.

# References

Bakal, D. A., Coll, P., & Schaefer, J. (2008). Somatic awareness in therapy: Enhancing emotional regulation through body-mind integration. *Journal of Clinical Psychology*, *64*(4), 479–492. https://doi.org/10.1002/jclp.20469

Byrd, R., Alexander, J., & Wong, M. (2020). Breathwork for children: Evaluating the effects of conscious breathing techniques on emotional regulation. *Journal of Child Psychology and Psychiatry*, *61*(6), 629–638. https://doi.org/10.1111/jcpp.13213

Flook, L., Goldberg, S. B., Pinger, L., & Davidson, R. J. (2015). Promoting prosocial behavior and self-regulatory skills in preschool children through a mindfulness-based kindness curriculum. *Developmental Psychology*, *51*(1), 44–51. https://doi.org/10.1037/a0038256

Kabat-Zinn, J. (1994). *Wherever you go, there you are: Mindfulness meditation in everyday life*. Hyperion.

Obradović, J., Portilla, X. A., & Boyce, W. T. (2021). Integrating mindful breathing and body awareness into child development. *Journal of Child Development*, *92*(3), 1032–1047. https://doi.org/10.1111/cdev.13415

Price, C. J., & Weng, H. Y. (2021). Facilitating adaptive emotion processing and somatic reappraisal *via* sustained mindful interoceptive attention. *Frontiers in Psychology*, *12*, 578827. https://doi.org/10.3389/fpsyg.2021.578827

Quek, F. Y., Majeed, N. M., Kothari, M., Lua, V. Y., Ong, H. S., & Hartanto, A. (2021). Brief mindfulness breathing exercises and working memory capacity: Findings from two experimental approaches. *Brain Sciences*, *11*(2), 175.

Siegel, D. J. (2007). *The mindful brain: Reflection and attunement in the cultivation of well-being*. Norton.

Weber, A. M. (2022). Mindfulness games for children: Developing body awareness and emotional regulation. *International Journal of Play Therapy*, *31*(2), 75–88. https://doi.org/10.1037/pla0000117

# 17

## MINDFUL CONSIDERATION OF CULTURE AND NEURODIVERGENCE IN PLAY THERAPY

### Introduction

Mindfulness, while universally beneficial, is experienced and perceived differently across cultures and among neurodivergent individuals. Recognizing and being sensitive to these differences is crucial for effective play therapy. Mindfulness practices have their roots in Buddhist traditions but vary significantly in interpretation and application across different cultures and neurodivergent contexts. In Western settings, mindfulness often focuses on stress reduction and cognitive-behavioral techniques, whereas Eastern traditions emphasize spiritual and communal practices. Neurodivergent individuals, such as those with autism, attention-deficit/hyperactivity disorder (ADHD), and sensory processing disorders, may require tailored mindfulness approaches to accommodate their unique sensory and cognitive profiles. Effective play therapy demands that therapists recognize and integrate these cultural and neurodivergent differences into their practice. This chapter explores the importance of cultural and neurodivergent sensitivity in play therapy, providing practical strategies for integrating mindfulness with cultural humility and tailoring approaches to meet diverse needs.

### Cultural Perspectives on Mindfulness

Mindfulness practices, rooted in Buddhist traditions, have been adapted in various cultures with differing interpretations and emphasis. For

DOI: 10.4324/9781003468585-17

instance, in Western contexts, mindfulness is often secularized and associated with stress reduction and cognitive-behavioral approaches. In contrast, Eastern traditions may integrate mindfulness with spiritual and communal practices, emphasizing interconnectedness and collective well-being (Kabat-Zinn, 2003; Shapiro, 2020).

### Western Contexts

In Western contexts, mindfulness often focuses on individual well-being, stress reduction, and mental health. It employs techniques such as mindful breathing, meditation, and mindfulness-based cognitive therapy (MBCT) to achieve these goals. Mindful breathing and meditation are commonly used to help individuals stay present and manage stress, while MBCT combines traditional cognitive-behavioral strategies with mindfulness practices to address issues like depression and anxiety (Williams & Kabat-Zinn, 2011). These practices aim to improve mental health by fostering awareness and acceptance of the present moment.

### Eastern Contexts

In Eastern contexts, mindfulness is often integrated with spiritual practices and community rituals. It emphasizes collective harmony, interconnectedness, and moral conduct. These practices are deeply rooted in traditions that promote a sense of unity and ethical living among individuals and their communities. For example, Thich Nhat Hanh (2015) discusses how mindfulness in Eastern traditions is not only a personal practice but also a communal one, fostering a shared sense of well-being and moral integrity within the community.

### Other Cultures

In some Middle Eastern and African cultures, mindfulness and meditation practices may intersect with religious beliefs and daily rituals. Incorporating aspects of prayer, traditional music, or rhythmic movement into mindfulness exercises can enhance their cultural relevance. It is important to approach these adaptations with sensitivity to avoid any conflict with religious or cultural practices. Certain cultures might have reservations or objections to standard mindfulness practices due to conflicts with their beliefs or values. For example, some conservative religious groups may view traditional mindfulness and meditation practices as conflicting with their faith. In such cases, mindfulness practices need to be reframed in a way that aligns with their religious teachings and values. Using language and concepts familiar to these groups, such as focusing on "mindful prayer" or "reflective contemplation," can make mindfulness practices more acceptable and effective.

In Hispanic and Latino cultures, which often emphasize family and social connections, incorporating family-oriented mindfulness activities can be particularly beneficial. Practices that encourage family participation, such as group mindfulness sessions or activities that can be done together at home, resonate with the collectivist values often present in these communities. For instance, incorporating culturally meaningful practices like *sobremesa*—the tradition of lingering after meals to share conversation—can be adapted into a mindfulness activity by encouraging families to reflect on their shared experiences or practice mindful gratitude together. Additionally, the integration of spirituality, such as combining mindfulness with prayer or religious rituals, aligns with the importance of faith in many Hispanic and Latino households (Parra-Cardona et al., 2017). These culturally attuned strategies not only promote mindfulness but also strengthen familial bonds, enhancing engagement and effectiveness in therapeutic contexts.

In Asian American communities, there might be variations in how mindfulness is perceived based on generational differences and the degree of cultural assimilation. First-generation immigrants may gravitate toward traditional practices rooted in their cultural heritage, such as meditation techniques inspired by Buddhism, Taoism, or Confucianism, which emphasize harmony, balance, and interconnectedness. For example, mindfulness practices like seated meditation (*zazen*) in Japanese traditions or breathing exercises in Chinese qigong might resonate deeply with older generations. Second-generation individuals, on the other hand, may be more open to Western adaptations of mindfulness, such as mindfulness-based stress reduction (MBSR) or mindfulness meditation apps, which often strip cultural and religious elements to focus on mental health benefits. Incorporating culturally relevant practices, such as mindful tea ceremonies or nature-focused meditations reflecting traditions like *shinrin-yoku* (forest bathing) from Japan, can make mindfulness more accessible and meaningful across generations (Kabat-Zinn, 2003;

Tseng, 2004). Recognizing these generational and cultural preferences is essential for providing culturally sensitive and effective mindfulness interventions that honor tradition while adapting to individual needs.

## Gaps in Multicultural Mindfulness Research

Biggers et al. (2020) found that only 24 of 12,265 citations between 1990 and 2016 were found in a systematic review of mindfulness and meditation-based intervention studies to be "diversity-focused" (DeLuca et al., 2018). Waldron et al. (2018) systematically reviewed trials integrating MBSR and mindfulness-based cognitive therapy (MBCT) in the United States and found 79% of the participants identified as non-Hispanic White. Many studies also omitted racial or ethnic data; among those that did, African Americans were underrepresented—just 11% of participants (Waldron et al., 2018). Only 5 of 425 trials targeted African Americans (Johnson et al., 2018) in a third evaluation of mind-body therapies—including mindfulness—in cardiovascular disease. Meta-analysis is impossible given the small number of studies, inclusion of other lifestyle co-interventions, and significant risk of bias; it also exposes evidence gaps for mindfulness in African Americans.

Overall, cultural sensitivity in mindfulness involves not only recognizing and respecting these diverse perspectives but also being flexible and creative in adapting practices to align with clients' cultural backgrounds and values. By doing so, therapists and practitioners can ensure that mindfulness interventions are both effective and culturally congruent, fostering greater acceptance and engagement from clients across different cultural contexts.

## Neurodivergent Perspectives on Mindfulness

Neurodivergent individuals, including autistic people, ADHDers, and those with sensory processing disorders, may experience and benefit from mindfulness differently. Traditional mindfulness practices might need adjustments to accommodate their unique sensory and cognitive profiles.

### *Autism*

Autistic individuals may find traditional mindfulness practices challenging due to the abstract nature of the concept, difficulties in maintaining prolonged attention, and sensory sensitivities that may arise during these exercises. Adapting mindfulness exercises to be more concrete can significantly enhance accessibility and engagement. For example, using visual aids such as pictures, diagrams, or step-by-step instructions can help clarify the structure and purpose of mindfulness activities. Incorporating the individual's special interests—such as focusing on a favorite object during mindful breathing or using themed guided meditations—can make the practice more enjoyable and relatable. Additionally, sensory-friendly adaptations like focusing on tactile experiences (e.g., holding a soft object or engaging in mindful play with kinetic sand) can support individuals with sensory sensitivities. Breaking exercises into shorter, manageable segments and using consistent routines can also help build comfort and familiarity with mindfulness practices (Kiep et al., 2015). These modifications make mindfulness not only more approachable but also more effective for individuals with autism.

## *ADHD*

Individuals with ADHD often face challenges with sustained attention, restlessness, and difficulty sitting still, which can make traditional mindfulness practices less accessible. Mindful movement practices, such as yoga, tai chi, or walking meditations, provide a more dynamic and engaging alternative, allowing individuals to channel their energy while fostering present-moment awareness. For example, yoga sequences with slow, deliberate movements can help improve focus and self-regulation, while tai chi's flowing motions promote relaxation and body awareness. Additionally, breaking mindfulness exercises into shorter, more frequent sessions can align better with the attention spans of individuals with ADHD, making it easier for them to participate without becoming overwhelmed or frustrated. Incorporating sensory-based mindfulness tools, like focusing on the tactile experience of holding a stress ball or using a glitter jar for visual grounding, can also help sustain engagement. These adaptations make mindfulness more accessible and effective for individuals with ADHD by aligning practices with their unique strengths and needs (Zylowska et al., 2008).

### *Sensory Processing Differences*

Sensory sensitivities can make certain mindfulness practices overwhelming for individuals, particularly those who experience heightened reactions to stimuli such as sound, light, texture, or touch. For example, traditional mindfulness exercises that rely on stillness or silence in an environment with harsh lighting or distracting sounds may exacerbate discomfort or anxiety. Tailoring activities to avoid sensory overload is essential for creating a supportive and accessible mindfulness experience. Using calming, sensory-friendly environments, such as softly lit rooms with minimal background noise or natural outdoor spaces, can help reduce distractions and promote relaxation. Additionally, incorporating sensory tools like weighted blankets, noise-canceling headphones, or fidget items can make mindfulness practices more grounding and tolerable. For individuals who may find certain sensations uncomfortable, offering alternative approaches—such as focusing on visual aids like a glitter jar instead of tactile exercises—ensure that the practice aligns with their unique sensory needs (Schaaf & Lane, 2015). These thoughtful adaptations create a more inclusive mindfulness experience, helping individuals benefit without becoming overwhelmed.

## Importance of Sensitivity to Culture and Neurodiversity in Play Therapy

Incorporating mindfulness into play therapy with sensitivity to cultural and neurodivergent differences ensures inclusivity and effectiveness.

### Assessment of Cultural Background

To provide effective and culturally sensitive therapy, it is essential to understand the client's cultural context and how it shapes their view of mindfulness, including their beliefs, values, and traditional practices. Mindfulness is not universally interpreted or practiced in the same way; for some cultures, it may align closely with long-standing traditions, while for others, it may feel unfamiliar or even misaligned with their worldview. For instance, mindfulness practices rooted in Buddhist or Taoist traditions might resonate deeply with clients from Asian backgrounds, while Indigenous clients might connect more strongly with practices emphasizing nature and interconnectedness, such as walking meditations in natural settings or gratitude rituals.

Incorporating culturally relevant practices and rituals into therapy ensures that mindfulness interventions feel authentic and respectful of the client's heritage. For example, clients from Hispanic or Latino backgrounds, where spirituality and family play central roles, may find mindfulness exercises more meaningful when framed as collective practices, such as family-based gratitude meditations or incorporating elements of prayer. In African American communities, where spirituality and resilience often intersect, incorporating faith-based mindfulness or storytelling techniques may enhance engagement. Additionally, for clients from secular or Westernized cultures, mindfulness may need to be reframed as a practical, science-based tool to promote stress reduction and focus rather than a spiritual practice.

By tailoring mindfulness interventions to honor cultural values and incorporating rituals that hold personal or community significance, therapists foster greater engagement, trust, and relevance in therapy. This approach also demonstrates cultural humility and a commitment to client-centered care, allowing clients to feel seen and respected within the therapeutic process.

### Individualize Techniques

Adapting mindfulness exercises to align with the sensory and cognitive needs of neurodivergent individuals is crucial for fostering accessibility and engagement. Many individuals with autism, ADHD, or other neurodivergent traits may benefit from tailored approaches that consider their unique ways of processing information and interacting with the world. Incorporating more visual and tactile elements can enhance focus and comprehension, for example, using glitter jars, visual timers, or sensory objects like stress balls can make abstract concepts more concrete. Breaking down exercises into smaller, manageable steps ensures that the activities feel achievable and reduces the likelihood of frustration or overwhelm. For instance, instead of a long meditation session, a therapist might guide a neurodivergent individual through a simple sequence of deep breaths paired with visual cues or a short grounding exercise like touching different textures.

Integrating movement into mindfulness can also be highly beneficial, as many neurodivergent individuals may find stillness challenging. Practices such as mindful walking, yoga poses, or stretching exercises allow them to engage their bodies while fostering present-moment awareness. Additionally, providing clear instructions, routine structure, and sensory friendly environments (e.g., dim lighting, minimal noise) can help accommodate sensory sensitivities and create a calming atmosphere. By customizing mindfulness exercises to align with sensory and cognitive needs, therapists can create a supportive experience that empowers neurodivergent individuals to engage in mindfulness in ways that feel natural and beneficial to them.

### Continuous Learning

Therapists should engage in ongoing education about cultural competence and neurodiversity. This involves learning about different cultural practices, beliefs, and the unique experiences of neurodivergent individuals (American Psychological Association, 2017).

By being mindful of these differences, therapists can create a more inclusive and supportive therapeutic environment that respects and responds to the diverse needs of their clients.

## Mindfulness and Cultural Humility

As therapists, it is our duty to practice cultural humility and commit to ongoing learning about the cultural contexts in which our clients are embedded. Cultural humility involves recognizing our own biases, understanding the limitations of our knowledge, and engaging in continuous self-reflection and learning. By adopting a mindfulness-based approach, we can enhance our cultural competence and create a more inclusive and supportive therapeutic environment. This chapter will provide guidance on how to bring awareness to the creation of a culturally inclusive playroom and how to invite clients to share about their culture as part of the intake process.

### Practicing Cultural Humility through Mindfulness

Cultural humility is an approach in therapy and other professional practices that emphasizes the importance of self-awareness, respectful inquiry, and lifelong learning. Unlike cultural competence, which implies that there is a finite level of knowledge and mastery over cultural nuances that one can achieve, cultural humility recognizes that understanding culture is an ongoing process that requires an open and curious mindset. This approach encourages professionals to continually self-reflect and examine their own cultural identities and biases, recognizing that these can impact their interactions and effectiveness with clients from diverse backgrounds (Tervalon & Murray-García, 1998).

Cultural humility involves three main components: continuous education and thoughtful introspection, acknowledging and questioning unequal distribution of power, and holding organizations responsible. Lifelong learning and critical self-reflection require professionals to engage in a continuous process of personal and professional development regarding cultural awareness and sensitivity (Hook et al., 2013). This process includes being open to learning from clients about their cultural perspectives and experiences, rather than assuming expertise based on prior knowledge or training.

Recognizing and challenging power imbalances involves acknowledging the inherent power dynamics that exist in professional-client relationships and striving to mitigate these imbalances. This means valuing clients as partners in the therapeutic process and respecting their cultural knowledge and experiences as equally important to the therapeutic dialogue (Ortega & Faller, 2011). By doing so, professionals can create a more collaborative and empowering environment for their clients.

Institutional accountability highlights the need for organizations to support cultural humility through policies, practices, and training that promote equity and inclusion. Institutions play a crucial role in fostering an environment where cultural humility can thrive, ensuring that professionals have the resources and support necessary to engage in this lifelong learning process (Foronda et al., 2016).

Ultimately, cultural humility is not about achieving a static level of cultural knowledge but about maintaining an attitude of openness, curiosity, and respect. It challenges professionals to remain humble and adaptable, continuously seeking to understand and appreciate the diverse cultural contexts of the individuals they serve. This approach not only enhances the quality of care and support provided but also fosters deeper, more meaningful connections between professionals and their clients.

### Key Principles of Cultural Humility
#### Self-Reflection and Awareness

Continuously reflecting on one's own cultural identity, biases, and assumptions is a foundational aspect of integrating cultural humility into mindfulness-based play therapy. Therapists must engage in regular self-reflection to understand how their own cultural backgrounds and unconscious biases may influence their interactions with clients. This self-awareness helps therapists to approach each therapeutic encounter with an open mind and a genuine willingness to understand the client's unique cultural context (Tervalon & Murray-García, 1998). In mindfulness-based play therapy, this reflective practice can be incorporated into daily mindfulness exercises, where therapists take time to reflect on their cultural assumptions and how these might impact their therapeutic relationships. For example, a therapist might engage in a mindfulness meditation focused on recognizing and releasing judgmental thoughts, thereby cultivating a non-judgmental presence in the therapy room.

*Lifelong Learning and Curiosity*

Committing to ongoing education and seeking to understand the cultural experiences of others is critical for therapists practicing mindfulness-based play therapy. Cultural humility involves a lifelong commitment to learning about different cultures and continually updating one's knowledge and understanding (Hook et al., 2013). In the context of play therapy, this means actively seeking out resources, trainings, and experiences that broaden the therapist's cultural competence. Therapists might attend workshops on cultural sensitivity, read literature on diverse cultural practices, and engage with communities different from their own. Moreover, therapists can integrate this learning into their practice by inviting clients to share their cultural backgrounds and traditions, thereby fostering a therapy environment rich in cultural exchange and understanding. This ongoing education helps therapists remain curious and open to the diverse cultural narratives that clients bring into the therapeutic space.

*Respectful Engagement*

Valuing and respecting the cultural perspectives and practices of clients is essential in mindfulness-based play therapy. Respectful engagement means actively listening to clients' cultural stories and experiences without judgment and acknowledging the importance of these cultural elements in their lives (Foronda et al., 2016). In practice, this involves creating a safe and inclusive environment where clients feel seen and respected. Therapists can demonstrate respect by incorporating culturally relevant materials and symbols into play therapy sessions, recognizing cultural holidays and practices, and being mindful of culturally specific ways of expressing emotions and coping with stress. For example, a therapist working with a child from a particular cultural background might include traditional games, stories, or art forms from that culture in their therapeutic play activities. This not only validates the child's cultural identity but also enriches the therapeutic experience by connecting it to the child's cultural framework.

## Integrating Mindfulness with Cultural Humility

Mindfulness can enhance our practice of cultural humility by helping us stay present, open, and non-judgmental. Through mindfulness, we can develop greater self-awareness, recognize our biases, and approach our clients with genuine curiosity and respect. Integrating mindfulness into cultural humility practices can significantly enhance a therapist's ability to understand and respect their clients' diverse cultural backgrounds. By fostering self-awareness, non-judgmental observation, and active listening, therapists can create a more inclusive and effective therapeutic environment. Below are expanded mindfulness practices to support cultural humility in play therapy.

### Mindful Reflection

Regularly engaging in reflective practices to explore one's own cultural identity and biases is essential for therapists. Tools such as journaling, meditation, and supervision can facilitate this self-exploration. Journaling allows therapists to document their thoughts and feelings about cultural encounters and reflect on how their own cultural identities influence their perceptions and interactions. This reflective practice can reveal unconscious biases and prompt therapists to explore their origins and impacts. Meditation, particularly guided mindfulness meditations, can help therapists develop a deeper awareness of their internal states and cultivate a non-judgmental attitude toward their thoughts (Kabat-Zinn, 1994). Supervision provides a structured setting for therapists to discuss cultural challenges and biases with a mentor, receiving feedback and guidance on how to approach these issues mindfully (Bernard & Goodyear, 2018).

### Non-Judgmental Awareness

Practicing non-judgmental awareness involves observing thoughts and reactions without judgment, especially when encountering cultural differences. Therapists can use mindfulness techniques to notice their initial responses to cultural diversity and reflect on their origins. For instance, during therapy sessions, a therapist might become aware of a judgmental thought about a client's cultural practice. Instead of suppressing or acting on this thought, the therapist can acknowledge it and explore its roots – perhaps linked to their own cultural conditioning or stereotypes (Siegel, 2010). This practice helps therapists remain open and curious about their clients' cultural contexts, fostering a more empathetic and accepting therapeutic relationship.

### Active Listening

Using mindful listening techniques to fully engage with clients' stories and experiences is crucial in understanding their cultural contexts. Active listening involves giving full attention to the speaker, noticing verbal and non-verbal cues, and reflecting back what is heard to ensure understanding. In the context of cultural humility, this means listening without forming judgments or assumptions about the client's cultural background. Techniques such as maintaining eye contact, nodding, and summarizing the client's points can demonstrate respect and empathy (Rogers, 1957). This practice not only validates the client's experiences but also helps therapists gather crucial information about the client's cultural identity and how it shapes their worldview.

## Mindfully Creating a Culturally Inclusive Playroom

A culturally inclusive playroom reflects and respects the diverse cultural backgrounds of the children and families you serve. Creating such an environment involves thoughtful consideration of the materials, toys, and decorations in the playroom.

### Diverse Toys and Materials

Include toys and materials that represent various cultures, ethnicities, and traditions. This can include dolls of different skin tones, culturally specific costumes, and traditional games from various cultures.

*Inclusive Books and Media*

Provide books, music, and media that showcase diverse characters, stories, and cultural practices. Ensure that these resources are not only inclusive but also accurate and respectful.

*Decorative Elements*

Incorporate decorations that reflect a variety of cultural symbols and artwork. This can create a welcoming atmosphere for children from diverse backgrounds.

*Flexible Spaces*

Design the playroom to be adaptable to different cultural practices. For example, having space for traditional ceremonies or cultural rituals can be important for some families.

## Mindfulness Activities to Promote Cultural Sensitivity in the Playroom

Integrating mindfulness activities into the playroom can foster cultural awareness for the therapist and clients. One effective approach is cultural storytelling, where children are invited to share stories from their cultural background or explore stories from different cultures. These activities promote understanding and respect for diverse cultures and help children see commonalities and differences among various traditions. By incorporating items from home that represent their family's lineage, such as traditional clothing or artwork, children can visually and tangibly connect with their heritage. These storytelling sessions can be enriched with discussions about the cultural context, encouraging children to reflect on and appreciate the stories' deeper meanings (Souto-Manning, 2009).

Mindful exploration invites children to engage with toys and materials by paying attention to their sensory qualities and cultural significance. Creating exploration stations with a variety of culturally diverse items allows children to experience different textures, colors, shapes, and functions. Through guided mindfulness exercises, such as describing the texture of a fabric with their eyes closed or noticing the emotions elicited by different colors, children enhance their sensory awareness and curiosity about cultural diversity. Post-exploration reflections help children articulate their observations and connect their experiences to broader cultural contexts (Siegel, 2010).

Cultural celebrations in the playroom provide a dynamic way to teach children about various cultural practices and holidays. By planning activities around cultural celebrations, such as special decorations in the playroom, bibliotherapy that introduces stories and characters from various cultures, or making crafts, children learn to understand and respect cultural diversity. Involving children and their families in these celebrations fosters a sense of inclusion and community. These mindful activities not only enhance cultural awareness but also support the overarching goals of mindfulness-based play therapy, promoting emotional and social well-being in children.

## The Importance of Cultural Inquiry in the Intake Process

Understanding a client's cultural background is essential for providing effective and respectful therapy. During the intake process, it is crucial to create a welcoming environment where clients feel comfortable sharing their own cultural experiences and perspectives. This process begins with the therapist demonstrating openness and curiosity about the client's cultural identity, which can significantly impact their mental health and therapy outcomes (Sue & Sue, 2016). By asking culturally sensitive questions and showing genuine interest in the client's cultural background, therapists can gather vital information that informs the treatment plan and therapeutic approach (Hays, 2008).

Creating a welcoming environment involves using inclusive language, being aware of non-verbal communication, and setting up the physical space to reflect cultural diversity. For instance, having culturally diverse artwork or materials in the waiting room can help clients feel more at ease and represented (Ponterotto, 2010). During the intake session, therapists should ask open-ended questions about the client's cultural background, values, and traditions. Questions for caregivers such as, "Can you tell me about any cultural practices or beliefs that are important to you?" or "How does your cultural background influence your view on mental health and therapy?" can encourage caregivers and clients to share their experiences without feeling judged or misunderstood (Smith, 2010).

Additionally, understanding the client's cultural background helps therapists avoid misinterpretations and biases that can hinder the therapeutic process. The process of cultural sensitivity and humility involves not only recognizing there may be cultural factors that influence a client's worldview but also integrating this understanding into all aspects of therapy, from assessment to intervention (Fisher-Borne et al., 2015). This approach ensures that the therapy is tailored to meet the client's unique needs and respects their cultural context, which is fundamental to building trust and fostering a strong therapeutic alliance (APA, 2017).

By prioritizing cultural inquiry in the intake process, therapists can enhance their empathy and effectiveness, ultimately leading to better therapeutic outcomes. This practice underscores the importance of cultural humility, where therapists acknowledge the ongoing process of learning and understanding cultural differences (Hook et al., 2013). Overall, incorporating cultural inquiry into the intake process is not just about gathering information but about creating a respectful and supportive space where clients feel valued and understood.

## Steps for Culturally Inclusive Intakes

### Open-Ended Questions

Use open-ended questions to invite clients to share about their cultural background. For example, "Can you tell me about your cultural background and any traditions that are important to you?"

### Respectful Inquiry

Approach cultural inquiry with genuine curiosity and respect. Avoid making assumptions or generalizations about the client's culture.

### Cultural Strengths

Highlight and validate the strengths and positive aspects of the client's cultural background. Acknowledge how these strengths can be resources in the therapeutic process.

### Cultural Preferences

Ask about any cultural preferences or needs that should be considered in therapy. This can include language preferences, cultural rituals, or specific ways of interacting that are important to the client.

# Conclusion

Mindful consideration of culture in play therapy is essential for creating an inclusive and supportive therapeutic environment. By practicing cultural humility and integrating mindfulness into our clinical processes, we can better understand our clients' cultural contexts and provide more effective and respectful therapy. This chapter has provided guidance on creating a culturally inclusive playroom, inviting clients to share about their culture, and using mindfulness to enhance cultural inquiry. Through these practices, we can foster a deeper connection with our clients and support their healing and growth within the context of their cultural identities.

# References

American Psychological Association. (2017). *Multicultural guidelines: An ecological approach to context, identity, and intersectionality.* American Psychological Association.

Bernard, J. M., & Goodyear, R. K. (2018). *Fundamentals of clinical supervision* (6th ed.). Pearson.

Biggers, A., Spears, C. A., Sanders, K., Ong, J., Sharp, L. K., & Gerber, B. S. (2020). Promoting mindfulness in African American Communities. *Mindfulness, 11*(10), 2274–2282. https://doi.org/10.1007/s12671-020-01480-w

DeLuca, S. M., Kelman, A. R., & Waelde, L. C. (2018). A systematic review of ethno-racial representation and cultural adaptation of mindfulness- and meditation-based interventions. *Psychological Studies, 63*(2), 117–129. 10.1007/s12646-018-0452-z

Fisher-Borne, M., Cain, J. M., & Martin, S. L. (2015). From mastery to accountability: Cultural humility as an alternative to cultural competence. *Social Work Education, 34*(2), 165–181. https://doi.org/10.1080/02615479.2014.977244

Foronda, C., Baptiste, D. L., Reinholdt, M. M., & Ousman, K. (2016). Cultural humility: A concept analysis. *Journal of Transcultural Nursing, 27*(3), 210–217. https://doi.org/10.1177/1043659615592677

Hays, P. A. (2008). *Addressing cultural complexities in practice: Assessment, diagnosis, and therapy* (2nd ed.). American Psychological Association.

Hook, J. N., Davis, D. E., Owen, J., Worthington, E. L., & Utsey, S. O. (2013). Cultural humility: Measuring openness to culturally diverse clients. *Journal of Counseling Psychology, 60*(3), 353–366. https://doi.org/10.1037/a0032595

Johnson, C. C., Sheffield, K. M., & Brown, R. E. (2018). Mind-body therapies for African-American women at risk for cardiometabolic disease: A systematic review. *Evidence-based Complementary and Alternative Medicine: eCAM, 2018.* https://doi.org/10.1155/2018/5123217

Kabat-Zinn, J. (1994). *Wherever you go, there you are: Mindfulness meditation in everyday life.* Hyperion.

Kabat-Zinn, J. (2003). Mindfulness-based interventions in context: Past, present, and future. *Clinical Psychology: Science and Practice, 10*(2), 144–156. https://doi.org/10.1093/clipsy.bpg016

Kiep, M., Spek, A. A., & Hoeben, L. (2015). Mindfulness-based therapy in adults with an autism spectrum disorder: Do treatment effects last? *Mindfulness, 6*(3), 637–644. https://doi.org/10.1007/s12671-014-0299-x

Ortega, R. M., & Faller, K. C. (2011). Training child welfare workers from an intersectional perspective: A paradigm shift. *Child Welfare, 90*(5), 27–42.

Parra-Cardona, J. R., Bybee, D., Sullivan, C. M., Rodríguez, M. M., Dates, B., Tams, L., & Bernal, G. (2017). Examining the impact of differential cultural adaptation with Latina/o immigrants exposed to adapted parent training interventions. *Journal of consulting and clinical psychology, 85*(1), 58–71. https://doi.org/10.1037/ccp0000160

Ponterotto, J. G. (2010). *Preventing prejudice: A guide for counselors and educators* (2nd ed.). Sage Publications.

Rogers, C. R. (1957). The necessary and sufficient conditions of therapeutic personality change. *Journal of Consulting Psychology, 21*(2), 95–103. https://doi.org/10.1037/h0045357

Schaaf, R. C., & Lane, S. J. (2015). Toward a best-practice protocol for assessment of sensory features in ASD. *Journal of Autism and Developmental Disorders, 45*(5), 1380–1395. https://doi.org/10.1007/s10803-014-2299-z

Shapiro, S. L. (2020). The integration of mindfulness and psychology. In R. J. Davidson & A. W. Kaszniak (Eds.), *The Oxford handbook of the science of mindfulness* (pp. 45–67). Oxford University Press.

Siegel, D. J. (2010). *The mindful therapist: A clinician's guide to mindsight and neural integration.* W.W. Norton & Company.

Smith, L. (2010). *Psychology, poverty, and the end of social exclusion: Putting our practice to work.* Psychology Press.

Souto-Manning, M. (2017). Is play a privilege or a right? And what's our responsibility? On the role of play for equity in early childhood education. *Early Child Development and Care, 187*(5–6), 785–787. https://doi.org/10.1080/03004430.2016.1266588

Sue, D. W., & Sue, D. (2016). *Counseling the culturally diverse: Theory and practice* (7th ed.). Wiley.

Tervalon, M., & Murray-García, J. (1998). Cultural humility versus cultural competence: A critical distinction in defining physician training outcomes in multicultural education. *Journal of Health Care for the Poor and Underserved, 9*(2), 117–125. https://doi.org/10.1353/hpu.2010.0233

Thich Nhat Hanh. (2015). *The miracle of mindfulness: An introduction to the practice of meditation.* Beacon Press.

Tseng, W.-S., & Streltzer, J. (Eds.). (2004). Cultural competence in clinical psychiatry. American Psychiatric Publishing, Inc.

Waldron, E. M., Hong S, Moskowitz JT, & Burnett-Zeigler I (2018). A systematic review of the demographic characteristics of participants in US-Based randomized controlled trials of mindfulness-based interventions. *Mindfulness, 9*(6), 1671–1692. https://doi.org/10.1007/s12671-018-0920-5

Williams, J. M. G., & Kabat-Zinn, J. (2011). *Mindfulness-based cognitive therapy for depression* (2nd ed.). Guilford Press.

Zylowska, L., Ackerman, D. L., Yang, M. H., Futrell, J. L., Horton, N. L., Hale, T. S., Pataki, C., & Smalley, S. L. (2008). Mindfulness meditation training in adults and adolescents with ADHD: A feasibility study. *Journal of Attention Disorders, 11*(6), 737–746. https://doi.org/10.1177/1087054707308502

# 18

## MINDFUL ASSESSMENT, PLANNING, AND DOCUMENTATION IN PLAY THERAPY

### Introduction

The level of mindfulness a therapist brings to the essential process of case conceptualization, assessment, therapy planning, and documentation is paramount. This chapter will guide you step-by-step through these critical clinical processes with a mindfulness-based approach. Developing a thorough understanding of a client's lived experience, the reasons for behaviors and symptoms, and the context of the client's family, cultural, school, and community systems is crucial for effective therapy planning and documentation (Wonders, 2021; Wonders & Affee, 2024).

### Mindful Case Conceptualization

#### Understanding the Client's Lived Experience

Case conceptualization involves forming a comprehensive understanding of the client's experiences, behaviors, and underlying issues (Wonders, 2021; Wonders & Affee, 2024). A mindful approach to this process emphasizes empathy, presence, and non-judgmental observation. By practicing mindfulness, therapists can better attune to the nuances of the client's lived experience, fostering a deeper connection and trust. This heightened awareness allows therapists to notice subtle cues and patterns that might otherwise be overlooked, leading to more accurate and insightful case formulations. Additionally, mindfulness helps therapists manage their own

DOI: 10.4324/9781003468585-18

reactions and biases, ensuring that their interpretations and interventions are truly client centered. This practice not only enhances the therapeutic alliance but also promotes more effective and compassionate treatment strategies tailored to the unique needs of each client.

### Steps for Mindful Case Conceptualization
#### Initial Engagement

**Creating a Safe and Welcoming Environment**: Start by ensuring the playroom is inviting and comfortable for both the caregivers and the child. The space should be organized, warm, and stocked with a variety of toys and supplies that encourage exploration and creativity. It's crucial to establish an atmosphere where caregivers feel at ease sharing their concerns and hopes during the intake process. Use active listening to show empathy and understanding, which helps build trust and rapport.

**Engaging the Child:** When the child is present, allow them to freely explore and interact with the playroom's toys and materials. Use child-centered play therapy skills such as tracking (narrating the child's actions without directing them) and reflecting (echoing the child's feelings and expressions) to fully engage with the child's experience. These techniques help the child feel seen and understood, promoting a sense of safety and openness.

#### Active Observation

**Focused Attention**: During sessions, pay close attention to the child's choices, movements, words, emotions, and body language. Avoid interrupting or making judgments about their behavior. This attentive presence helps you gather valuable information about the child's inner world and emotional state.

**Reflective Responses:** Reflect on what you observe by mirroring the child's actions and emotions back to them. This practice not only ensures that you understand the child's experiences accurately but also validates their feelings, fostering a deeper connection and trust in the therapeutic relationship.

#### Reflective Practice

**Post-Session Reflection**: After each session, take time to review and reflect on the information gathered. Consider how the child's experiences, environment, and context influence their behaviors and symptoms. Reflect on the child's play themes, patterns, and any significant moments that occurred during the session.

**Self-Reflection:** Examine your own reactions, feelings, and biases that may have arisen during the session. This self-awareness helps prevent personal biases from clouding your understanding of the child's needs and experiences. Regular supervision or consultation with colleagues can provide additional perspectives and support.

*Collaborative Understanding*

**Involving Caregivers and Child**: Engage both the child and their caregivers in the process of understanding the child's needs and behaviors. Use open-ended questions to gather detailed insights and encourage them to share their perspectives. For example, ask the caregivers about their observations of the child's behavior at home or in other settings, and invite the child to express their thoughts and feelings about their experiences.

**Validating Experiences:** Ensure that the voices of both the child and the caregivers are heard and valued in the therapeutic process. Validate their experiences by acknowledging their feelings and perspectives. This collaborative approach helps build a comprehensive understanding of the child's situation and fosters a sense of partnership in the therapeutic journey.

By implementing these expanded sections, therapists can create a more holistic and empathetic approach to engaging with children and their caregivers in play therapy. This approach not only enhances the therapeutic relationship but also promotes more effective and meaningful outcomes for the child.

## Mindful Assessment

A mindful assessment process involves gathering detailed information about the client's psychological, emotional, and social functioning. This process should be thorough, systematic, and conducted with empathy and respect (Wonders & Affee, 2024). Practicing mindfulness during the assessment phase is crucial for several reasons. When collecting information from caregivers, a mindful approach ensures that the therapist is fully present, actively listening, observing, and empathetically engaging with the caregivers' perspectives and concerns. This fosters a sense of trust and safety, encouraging caregivers to share more openly and honestly about the child's experiences and behaviors.

Mindfulness practice allows the therapist to be attuned and notice subtle nuances in the caregivers' narratives, such as emotional undertones and non-verbal cues, which can provide deeper insights into the child's environment and relationships. Additionally, being mindful helps the therapist manage their own reactions and biases, ensuring that the information gathered is interpreted accurately and without judgment.

During the observation of the child's play in therapy sessions, mindfulness enables the therapist to be fully present and attentive to the child's actions, emotions, and interactions. This heightened awareness allows the therapist to capture the essence of the child's play, considering the symbolic meanings and underlying emotions expressed through their play. By maintaining a non-judgmental and accepting stance, the therapist creates a safe space where the child feels understood and validated.

Mindfulness helps the therapist remain regulated, grounded, and centered even when the child's play reveals challenging or distressing themes. This stability is crucial for providing a consistent and supportive presence, which is essential for the child's therapeutic progress. Overall, integrating mindfulness into the assessment process enriches the therapist's understanding of the child's world, enhances the therapeutic relationship, and lays a solid foundation for effective and compassionate treatment.

### Steps for Mindful Assessment

**Evaluating Multiple Areas**: A holistic approach to assessment evaluates emotional regulation, social relationships, academic performance, and family dynamics. Consider cultural, familial, and community influences on the client's behavior. Therapists should maintain a state of open, non-judgmental awareness throughout the assessment, being fully present when gathering information.

**Emotional Regulation:** Observe subtle cues in the client's body language, tone of voice, and emotional expressions without rushing to interpret or label them.

**Social Relationships:** Mindfulness involves actively listening to the client and their caregivers, paying close attention to the quality of interactions, and underlying emotions during discussions about friendships and peer interactions.

**Academic Performance:** Mindfully consider the child's strengths and challenges in the educational setting, recognizing the impact of stress and anxiety on learning and performance.

**Family Dynamics:** Approach family dynamics with sensitivity, respecting cultural backgrounds and communication patterns. Be fully present during family discussions to understand intricate relationships and power dynamics.

**Cultural, Familial, and Community Influences:** Acknowledge and respect cultural differences, being aware of community resources or lack thereof. Understand how familial beliefs and practices shape the client's behavior and experiences, remaining curious and open-minded.

**Administering Tools Mindfully:** Integrate mindfulness while using standardized assessment tools like the Child Behavior Checklist (CBCL) and Strengths and Difficulties Questionnaire (SDQ). Approach the administration with full attention and a non-judgmental attitude.

**Creating a Supportive Environment:** Provide clear explanations and create a calm, supportive environment for parents and children during assessments. Offer support and reassurance if discomfort or emotional responses arise.

**Reviewing Results:** Practice mindful observation when reviewing results, considering the broader context of the child's experiences and family dynamics. Remain empathetic and open to avoid rushing to conclusions.

**Observation with Parents in Parent Sessions:** Begin with active listening and empathetic engagement. Pay attention to verbal and non-verbal communication, such as body language, facial expressions, and tone of voice. Practice non-judgmental observation, reflecting back what you observe to validate the parents' experiences.

**Observation with the Child in Play Therapy Sessions:** Be fully present during play therapy sessions, closely observing the child's play without imposing interpretations too quickly. Notice patterns, themes, and shifts in mood or behavior. Maintain a calm and grounded presence, allowing the child to explore and express themselves freely.

**Enhancing Evaluations:** Combine mindful observation techniques with standardized assessment tools to enhance the depth and accuracy of evaluations. Remain present and empathetic, ensuring parents and children feel understood and supported.

**Open and Collaborative Discussion:** Create a calm, distraction-free space for sharing assessment findings. Approach the discussion with openness and collaboration, emphasizing a shared understanding of the client's challenges and strengths.

**Active Listening and Empathy:** Listen attentively to reactions and concerns without interrupting. Reflect back what you hear to demonstrate understanding and validation, building trust and rapport.

**Non-Judgmental Communication:** Communicate findings compassionately, using clear, simple language. Ensure your tone and body language convey empathy and support.

**Clarification and Understanding:** Encourage questions and clarify any misunderstandings. Ensure everyone has a clear understanding of the assessment results.

**Highlighting Strengths:** Focus on the client's strengths and discuss how they can be leveraged to address difficulties. This balanced approach boosts self-esteem and motivation.

**Facilitating Emotional Processing:** Acknowledge and validate strong emotions that may arise during feedback. Offer reassurance and empathy to help clients and caregivers process their feelings.

**Building a Shared Understanding:** Engage in thoughtful, empathetic dialogue to build a shared understanding of the client's challenges and strengths. This foundation supports effective, personalized intervention strategies.

Integrating mindfulness into every aspect of assessment ensures thorough, systematic, and compassionate evaluations. This approach enhances the therapeutic relationship and promotes healing and positive change for both the child and their family.

## Mindful Planning for the Course of Therapy

Therapy planning (traditionally referred to as *treatment planning*) involves setting goals and objectives, selecting interventions, and outlining a structured approach to therapy. A mindful approach ensures that the plan is client-centered, flexible, and appropriately responsive to the client's evolving needs. In psychotherapy treatment planning, goals and objectives are both essential components, but they serve different purposes and are distinct in their scope and specificity.

### Goals for Therapy

Goals are broad, overarching aims that provide the general direction of the therapeutic process. They are the desired outcomes that the client and therapist work toward throughout therapy. Goals are often more abstract and long term, focusing on overall well-being and major life changes.

### Characteristics

**Broad and General**: Goals are not specific; they encompass a wide range of outcomes.

**Long term:** Goals are usually set to be achieved over an extended period.

**Abstract:** They deal with general concepts and overall life improvements.

**Outcome focused:** Goals reflect the desired end result of therapy.

### Examples

- Improving overall mental health and well-being.
- Developing healthier relationships.
- Increasing emotional stability and resilience.
- Reducing symptoms of anxiety or depression.

### Objectives

Objectives are specific, concrete steps or actions that help achieve the broader goals. They are detailed, measurable, and short term, outlining the specific behaviors or skills that need to be developed or changed.

*Characteristic*

**Specific and Detailed**: Objectives outline clear, concrete actions, or milestones.

**Short term:** They are meant to be accomplished within a relatively short timeframe.

**Measurable:** Objectives can be quantified or assessed to determine progress.

**Process focused:** They focus on the actions or steps needed to achieve the goals.

*Examples*

- Attending weekly play therapy sessions.
- Practicing mindfulness exercises daily.
- Completing a specific number of exposure tasks to reduce phobic reactions.
- Reducing panic attacks from five times a week to once a week.

### Relationship between Goals and Objectives

In a therapy plan, objectives are the building blocks that lead to achieving the broader goals. Each objective acts as a step toward fulfilling the aim of the treatment goal. The SMART criteria (specific, measurable, achievable, relevant, time bound) are often used to formulate clear and effective objectives that align with the overarching goals.

*Example in Context*

- **Goal**: Reduce overall anxiety and improve daily functioning.
  - **Objective 1**: Practice deep breathing exercises for 10 minutes each day.
  - **Objective 2**: Attend play therapy sessions weekly.
  - **Objective 3**: Track anxiety triggers and responses twice per week.

By achieving these objectives, the client moves closer to the broader goal of reducing anxiety and improving daily functioning.

### *Steps for Mindful Therapy Planning*

*Goal Setting*

Collaborate with the client and caregivers to set realistic and meaningful therapy goals. Align the goals with the client's values and priorities.

*Establish Objectives*

Ensure that the objectives are specific, measurable, achievable, relevant, and time bound (SMART) and are indicative of progress toward the goal.

*Intervention Selection*

Choose interventions that align with the client's needs and demonstrated preferences. Consider incorporating mindfulness-based practices to enhance the effectiveness of traditional play therapy techniques. Refer to *Play Therapy Treatment Planning with Children and Families: A Guide for Mental Health Professionals* (Wonders & Affee, 2024) for a range of evidence-based strategies.

*Flexibility and Adaptation*

Be prepared to adjust the therapy plan based on the client's progress and changing circumstances. Maintain a flexible and open-minded approach to treatment, being ready to modify techniques and strategies as necessary.

*Continuous Evaluation*

Regularly evaluate the client's progress toward therapy goals, using and adjusting the objectives as a measure. Involve the client and their caregivers in this ongoing evaluation process to ensure that the therapy remains relevant and effective.

## Mindful Documentation

Documentation is a crucial aspect of clinical practice, providing a record of the client's progress, interventions used, and outcomes achieved. Mindful documentation involves being thorough, accurate, and reflective, ensuring that the records are meaningful and useful for ongoing treatment.

### Being Present and Engaged

Mindful documentation starts with being fully present and engaged during the session. Take detailed notes during or immediately after the session while the information is fresh in your mind. By being fully present, you capture the nuances of the client's behaviors, emotions, and responses to interventions. This attentiveness ensures that the documentation accurately reflects the client's experience and the therapeutic process.

### Reflective Practice

Incorporate reflective practice into your documentation. Take a few moments to reflect on the session, considering what went well, what challenges arose, and what insights you gained. Document these reflections to provide a deeper understanding of the therapeutic process and inform future sessions. Reflective documentation helps you identify patterns and themes in the client's behavior and progress, enhancing your ability to tailor interventions effectively.

### Thorough and Detailed Records

Ensure that your documentation is thorough and detailed. Include comprehensive information about the client's presenting issues, therapeutic goals, interventions used, and the client's response to those interventions. Describe specific behaviors, emotions, and interactions observed during the session. Detailed records provide a clear and complete picture of the client's progress, which is essential for continuity of care and effective treatment planning.

### Accuracy and Objectivity

Mindful documentation requires accuracy and objectivity. Record factual information without inserting personal biases or subjective interpretations. Use precise language to describe the client's behaviors and statements, avoiding ambiguous or vague terms. Accurate and objective documentation ensures that the records are reliable and can be used effectively by other professionals involved in the client's care.

### Confidentiality and Sensitivity

Maintain confidentiality and sensitivity in your documentation. Be mindful of the language you use and the information you include, ensuring that it respects the client's privacy and dignity. Avoid unnecessary details that could compromise confidentiality. Secure your records in accordance with ethical and legal standards to protect the client's sensitive information.

### Regular Review and Updates

Regularly review and update your documentation to reflect the client's ongoing progress and any changes in their treatment plan. Mindful documentation involves staying current with the client's evolving needs and goals. This ongoing review process ensures that your records remain relevant and useful for guiding future therapeutic interventions.

### Using Mindful Documentation as a Therapeutic Tool

View mindful documentation not just as a record-keeping task but as a therapeutic tool. Use the process of documenting with mindfulness to deepen your understanding of the client and to inform your clinical decision-making. Reflect on the documented information to identify areas for further exploration and to develop more targeted and effective interventions. Mindful documentation can thus enhance the overall quality of care you provide.

Documenting therapy with mindfulness involves being present, reflective, thorough, accurate, and sensitive. It ensures that records are meaningful, useful, and respectful of the client's experience. This mindful approach to documentation supports continuity of care, enhances the therapeutic process, and contributes to effective and compassionate treatment.

### Practical Steps for Mindful Documentation

#### Timeliness

Document sessions promptly to ensure accuracy and completeness. Reflect on the session immediately afterward to capture key details and insights.

#### Detail and Clarity

Write clear and detailed notes that include the client's presentation, interventions used, and responses observed. Avoid jargon and ensure that the documentation is understandable to other professionals who may read it.

#### Reflective Entries

Include reflective notes on the therapist's observations, insights, and considerations for future sessions. This can enhance the depth and quality of the documentation.

*Confidentiality and Respect*

Ensure that all documentation respects the client's privacy and confidentiality. Be mindful of the language used, avoiding any terms that could be perceived as judgmental or stigmatizing.

## Mindfulness in Every Stage of the Process

Integrating mindfulness into every stage of play therapy treatment planning, assessment, and documentation is crucial for ensuring a comprehensive and holistic approach to child therapy. Mindfulness enhances the therapist's ability to remain present and attuned to the child's needs, fostering a deeper therapeutic connection and a more accurate understanding of the child's emotional and psychological state (Siegel, 2010). During the assessment phase, mindfulness allows therapists to observe without judgment, providing clearer insights into the child's behaviors and emotions, which is essential for effective case conceptualization (Shapiro & Carlson, 2009). In treatment planning, mindfulness helps in crafting interventions that are responsive to the child's evolving needs, promoting flexibility and adaptability in therapeutic strategies (Germer et al., 2013). Additionally, incorporating mindfulness into documentation ensures that records are detailed, precise, and reflective of the therapeutic process, supporting continuity of care and informed decision-making. Overall, mindfulness enriches the therapeutic experience by promoting empathy, reducing therapist burnout, and enhancing the overall effectiveness of play therapy (Kabat-Zinn, 1994; Siegel, 2007).

## The Role of the Therapist's Mindfulness Practice

The therapist's own mindfulness practice is foundational to bringing mindfulness into case conceptualization, assessment, therapy planning, and documentation. By cultivating mindfulness, therapists can enhance their presence, empathy, and attunement, which are critical for effective therapeutic work.

### Enhancing Presence

Mindfulness practice helps therapists develop a heightened state of presence, allowing them to be fully engaged and attentive during therapy sessions. This presence means being attuned to the here-and-now experiences of both the therapist and the client, fostering a deeper therapeutic connection. According to Siegel (2007), mindfulness strengthens the neural circuitry involved in attention and emotional regulation, which is crucial for therapists to remain present and centered, especially in emotionally charged situations. Effective conceptualization, assessment, planning, and documentation will result when a therapist is mindfully present and attuned.

### Fostering Empathy

Empathy is a cornerstone of effective therapy. Mindfulness practice enhances the therapist's capacity for empathy by increasing their ability to understand and share the feelings of their clients. Studies have shown that mindfulness can enhance emotional intelligence, which includes empathy and the ability to perceive, assess, and manage emotions in oneself and others (Goleman, 1995). This empathetic engagement helps in building a strong therapeutic alliance, which is a key predictor of positive therapy outcomes (Norcross & Wampold, 2011).

### Improving Attunement

Attunement involves the therapist's ability to be in sync with the client's emotional state and needs. Mindfulness fosters attunement by helping therapists become more aware of their own internal states and those of their clients. This heightened awareness enables therapists to respond more accurately and sensitively to their clients, facilitating deeper understanding and effective interventions (Siegel, 2010). Attuned therapists are better able to recognize subtle cues and shifts in their clients' emotional states, enhancing the therapeutic process.

### Case Conceptualization and Assessment

A therapist's mindfulness practice can significantly inform case conceptualization and assessment. Mindful therapists are better equipped to observe and interpret their clients' behaviors and emotions without bias. This non-judgmental stance allows for a more accurate and comprehensive understanding of the client's issues, leading to more effective treatment planning. According to Shapiro and Carlson (2009), mindfulness enhances clinical insight and fosters a more holistic understanding of the client, integrating cognitive, emotional, and somatic experiences.

## *Therapy Planning and Documentation*

Incorporating mindfulness into therapy planning and documentation ensures that the therapeutic process is guided by a clear, present-focused awareness of the client's needs and progress. Mindful therapists can develop treatment plans that are responsive to the evolving therapeutic process and adapt interventions to fit the client's moment-to-moment experiences. Additionally, mindfulness can improve the quality of clinical documentation by helping therapists maintain clarity and precision in their records, which is essential for effective treatment continuity and accountability.

## Conclusion

The integration of mindfulness into a therapist's practice enhances their therapeutic presence, empathy, and attunement, which are essential for effective case conceptualization, assessment, therapy planning, and documentation. Through ongoing mindfulness practice, therapists can improve their professional effectiveness while also attending to their own well-being, ultimately benefiting both themselves and their clients.

## References

Germer, C. K., Siegel, R. D., & Fulton, P. R. (2013). *Mindfulness and psychotherapy* (2nd ed.). Guilford Press.

Goleman, D. (1995). *Emotional intelligence: Why it can matter more than IQ*. Bantam Books.

Kabat-Zinn, J. (1994). *Wherever you go, there you are: Mindfulness meditation in everyday life*. Hyperion.

Norcross, J. C., & Wampold, B. E. (2011). Evidence-based therapy relationships: Research conclusions and clinical practices. *Psychotherapy, 48*(1), 98–102. https://doi.org/10.1037/a0022161

Shapiro, S. L., & Carlson, L. E. (2009). *The art and science of mindfulness: Integrating mindfulness into psychology and the helping professions*. American Psychological Association.

Siegel, D. J. (2007). *The mindful brain: Reflection and attunement in the cultivation of well-being*. W. W. Norton & Company.

Siegel, D. J. (2010). *The mindful therapist: A Clinician's guide to mindsight and neural integration*. W. W. Norton & Company.

Wonders, L. L.. (2024). Mindful treatment planning and documentation in play therapy. Webinar. https://mindfulnessbasedtherapytraining.com/mindful-treatment-planning-and-documentation-in-play-therapy/

Wonders, L. L. & Affee, M. L. (2024). *Play therapy treatment planning with children and families: A guide for mental health professionals*. Wiley.

# 19

## MINDFUL GOODBYES

### CLOSURE OF THE PLAY THERAPY PROCESS AND RELATIONSHIP

## Introduction

The end of play therapy with a client is a significant and sensitive process that requires thoughtful consideration and mindfulness. From the beginning of therapy, discussing the eventual closure is essential for setting the stage for a positive termination experience (Landreth, 2012; Ray, 2011). This chapter explores how therapists can bring mindfulness to the process of ending therapy, from initial discussions to the final sessions. It also provides mindfulness-based interventions that can help clients honor and process their emotions during the termination process.

## The Importance of Mindful Closure in Play Therapy

Closure (or *termination*) is a critical phase in therapy that signifies the end of the therapeutic relationship and process. It involves reflecting on the progress made, consolidating gains, and saying goodbye. A mindful approach to closure of play therapy ensures that this process is handled with care, respect, and sensitivity to the client's emotional needs. Mindful closure helps to solidify the therapeutic work accomplished and prepares both the child and the parents for a successful transition out of therapy (Landreth, 2012).

DOI: 10.4324/9781003468585-19

## Key Aspects of the Closure Process in Play Therapy with Child Clients

### Introducing Closure from the Beginning

Discussing the eventual end of therapy from the outset helps clients understand that therapy is a time-limited process to achieve specific goals. This preparation reduces anxiety and makes termination more manageable (Bartholomew et al., 2019; De Geest & Meganck, 2019; Ling & Stathopoulou, 2020; Shafran et al., 2019).

### Steps to Introduce Closure

**Initial Sessions:** During intake and goal setting, explain the therapy structure, including its eventual end, using language appropriate for the child's developmental level.

**Regular Check-ins:** Periodically remind clients and caregivers about the termination phase, especially as therapy progresses and goals are being met.

**Goal Orientation:** Emphasize that therapy aims to equip the client with skills and strategies to manage challenges independently.

Incorporating mindfulness early on can help clients stay present and engaged in the therapeutic process while preparing them for its conclusion.

### Reflection

**Reviewing Progress and Achievements:** Toward the end of therapy, review the progress and achievements made. This reflection helps the child and caregivers recognize the growth and changes that have occurred. It provides an opportunity to reinforce the skills and strategies developed during therapy.

**Summarize Key Moments:** Highlight significant breakthroughs and progress points in therapy.

**Use Visual Aids:** Create a visual timeline or scrapbook of the therapy journey, including drawings, notes, and significant symbols used during sessions.

**Encourage Self-Reflection:** Ask the child to share their thoughts and feelings about their progress and what they have learned.

*Celebration*

Celebrating the client's growth and accomplishments is crucial, as it not only acknowledges their hard work and progress but also creates a positive reinforcement loop that motivates continued effort. Recognizing milestones, whether big or small, helps the child feel proud of their achievements and fosters a sense of personal competence. This reinforcement can be as simple as verbal praise, a tangible reward like a sticker or certificate, or a shared moment of reflection on how far they've come. Celebrating successes also strengthens the therapeutic alliance, showing the child that their efforts are seen and valued. Over time, these affirmations build self-esteem and confidence, empowering the child to face future challenges with resilience and optimism.

**Create Certificates:** Creating a certificate of achievement to present to the child at the closing of play therapy is a meaningful way to celebrate their progress and provide a sense of closure. The certificate can highlight specific accomplishments, such as improved emotional regulation, increased confidence, or their ability to navigate challenging feelings. Personalizing it with their name, favorite colors, or symbols from the play therapy sessions (like a favorite toy or character) makes it even more special and reflective of their journey. Presenting the certificate in a short, celebratory moment allows the child to feel recognized for their hard work and growth. This ritual not only validates their efforts but also provides a tangible keepsake, reminding them of their resilience and the tools they've learned during therapy. It can also be an opportunity for the therapist to verbally acknowledge the child's strengths and contributions, reinforcing a positive narrative about their progress and building lasting self-esteem.

**Share with Caregivers:** Involving caregivers in the celebration process when a child is ending play therapy is an essential way to honor the child's progress and reinforce the support system that will continue outside of therapy. Caregivers can be invited to participate in a special closing session where the therapist highlights the child's accomplishments and shares specific examples of their growth. This might include presenting the child with a certificate of achievement, reflecting on their journey through art or a memory book, or sharing a symbolic play activity that represents their progress. Caregivers can be encouraged to express their pride and support, creating a meaningful moment of connection and validation for the child.

Including caregivers in this process helps bridge the transition from therapy to home life, ensuring the child feels supported as they move forward. It also provides an opportunity for the therapist to share strategies, tools, and insights with caregivers, empowering them to continue fostering the child's emotional and behavioral development. By celebrating as a team, the child not only feels a sense of pride and accomplishment but also gains confidence in the stability of their support network, making the closure of therapy a positive and empowering experience.

**Plan a Special Activity:** Ending therapy with a special activity or game that the child enjoys is a meaningful way to celebrate their progress and symbolize the positive aspects of their therapeutic journey. This activity can serve as a reflection of their achievements, strengths, and growth while providing a sense of closure in a way that feels familiar and enjoyable for the child. For instance, if the child has a favorite board game or creative activity, such as building with blocks or drawing, the therapist can use that as a way to reinforce themes of collaboration, problem-solving, or self-expression learned during therapy.

Symbolic activities can also be incorporated to mark the transition, such as creating a "memory jar" where the child and therapist write down or draw important moments, accomplishments, or tools the child has gained. Another idea could include a playful goodbye ritual, like decorating a keepsake item (e.g., a small box or rock) that represents their time in therapy and the skills they are taking forward.

These activities not only celebrate the child's progress but also provide an emotional bridge, helping them process the ending of therapy in a positive and affirming way. The chosen activity can be planned collaboratively with the child to ensure it reflects their interests and preferences, reinforcing their sense of agency and ownership over their therapeutic journey. This celebratory process helps the child leave therapy with confidence, pride, and a lasting memory of their growth and accomplishments.

### Implementing Closure Discussions

#### Initial Sessions

**Explanation:** Clearly explain the structure and timeline of therapy during initial sessions, including language that reminds the child there will be a beginning, a middle, and an end to therapy together.

**Developmental Language:** Use language appropriate for the child's age and developmental level to ensure understanding.

#### Regular Check-ins

**Reminders:** Regularly remind the child and caregivers about the therapy timeline and upcoming closure, especially as goals are achieved.

**Progress Updates:** Provide updates on progress and how it aligns with the therapy goals.

#### Goal Orientation

**Skill Development:** Emphasize that therapy focuses on new skills and strategies for the child to manage challenges independently.

**Reinforcement:** Regularly reinforce the skills learned and how they can be applied outside of therapy.

#### Mindfulness Integration

**Early Introduction:** Introduce mindfulness practices early in therapy to create a foundation for using these techniques during termination.

**Consistent Practice:** Encourage regular mindfulness practice to help the child stay engaged and present throughout the therapeutic process.

By addressing these key aspects, therapists can ensure a mindfully smooth and positive closure process, helping children and their caregivers transition out of therapy with a sense of accomplishment and readiness to face future challenges independently.

## Mindful Reflection on Progress for Termination Process

Reflecting on progress is important for clients as it helps validate their efforts and acknowledge the hard work they have put into their therapy. This validation affirms their dedication to self-improvement and their ability to overcome challenges, which is essential for building self-esteem and self-efficacy. Recognizing their progress encourages clients to continue using the skills and strategies they have learned in therapy, fostering a sense of accomplishment and resilience (Greenberg, 2002). Reflection is an essential part of the closure process, allowing clients to recognize and appreciate their growth and achievements. By taking time to reflect on the journey of therapy, clients can consolidate the gains made during therapy and understand how they have evolved. This reflection fosters a sense of accomplishment and reinforces the therapeutic work done, making the transition out of therapy more meaningful and empowering.

Reflection enhances self-awareness by helping clients recognize the changes in their thoughts, behaviors, and emotions. It allows them to see the connection between their efforts and the outcomes, fostering a deeper understanding of themselves. This increased self-awareness is a vital component of personal growth and emotional intelligence (Siegel, 2007).

By reviewing the progress made, clients can consolidate what they have learned during therapy. This consolidation helps transfer therapeutic gains into their daily lives, ensuring that the benefits of therapy are sustained over time. It also helps clients identify which strategies were most effective, reinforcing positive coping mechanisms (Kolb, 1984).

Reflection provides a sense of closure by summarizing the therapeutic journey. It helps clients understand that the ending of therapy is not an abrupt halt but a transition to applying what they have learned independently. This understanding can make the process of saying goodbye less daunting and more celebratory (Landreth, 2012).

### Steps for Mindful Reflective Practice
#### Review Goals

Revisit the initial goals set at the beginning of therapy and discuss the progress made toward achieving them. This step helps clients see how far they have come and the specific milestones they have reached.

#### Highlight Achievements

Identify specific accomplishments and changes the client has made, both big and small. Highlighting these achievements can be done through various means, such as creating a playful progress chart, discussing notable experiences in sessions, or reviewing drawings, photos of sand trays or journal entries for older children.

*Encourage Self-Reflection*

Invite clients to reflect on their own experiences and express their thoughts and feelings about their journey with creative and expressive activities like sand tray play, storytelling, or use of puppet play.

### Practical Techniques for Reflection

*Therapy Scrapbooking*

Clients can keep a scrapbook from the beginning of therapy and throughout their sessions where they collect their drawings, photos of the sand trays, and other reminders of their experiences in therapy along the way which can then serve as a rich resource for reflection. Reviewing the pages of the scrapbook can help clients see their progress in a tangible way, reinforcing the positive changes they have made (Pennebaker, 1997).

*Creative Expression*

Encouraging clients to use creative expression, such as drawing, painting, or storytelling, can help them articulate their progress and journey of therapy in a non-verbal way. This can be particularly effective for clients who struggle with verbal reflection (Malchiodi, 2003).

## Addressing Emotions Mindfully

The termination of therapy can evoke a range of emotions, including sadness, anxiety, and even relief. Mindfulness-based interventions can help clients process these emotions in a healthy and constructive way.

### Emotion Identification

Use mindfulness to help clients identify and label emotions they may have about the completion of therapy. Feelings check-ins with a feelings poster or picture cards may be useful. Feeling-face cards and feeling-face puppets created out of paper sacks, yarn, and markers might be used.

### Mindful Acceptance

Encourage clients to accept their emotions without judgment, recognizing that it is normal to feel a mix of emotions during closure by modeling acceptance of your own emotions. Mindful acceptance can be modeled by the therapist throughout the course of therapy when engaging in bibliotherapy and noticing aloud characters' varying emotions.

### Breathing Activities

Reinforce mindful breathing together to manage big emotions through a variety of breathing games and activities learned throughout the play therapy journey

### Grounding Activities

Use grounding exercises to help clients stay present and connected to the here and now. Activities such as digging in the sand, building with blocks,   feeling their feet on the ground or playing I spy can be effective.

## Creating Meaningful Goodbye Rituals

Rituals can provide a sense of closure and help clients say goodbye in ways that hold meaning. These rituals can be tailored to the client's age, preferences, and cultural background.

### Collaborative Art Project

Create a collaborative art project that symbolizes the therapeutic journey and its conclusion.

### Letter Writing

Encourage clients to write letters to themselves or to the therapist, reflecting on their experiences and expressing their feelings about ending therapy.

### Make a Memory Box

Assemble a memory box with items that represent key moments and achievements from therapy.

*Ceremony*

Plan a simple ceremony that includes activities like lighting a candle, sharing memories, or saying affirmations.

## Supporting Caregivers during Closure to Therapy

Caregivers play a crucial role in the termination process of therapy and providing them with guidance and support is essential to ensure a smooth transition. The end of therapy can evoke a range of emotions not only for the child but also for the caregivers, and addressing these feelings can help maintain the gains made during therapy and foster ongoing development.

### Keep Caregivers Informed

Keeping caregivers informed about the termination process and what to expect is essential. From the outset, therapists should communicate the structure and timeline of therapy, including the eventual conclusion. As therapy progresses, regular updates and reminders about the approaching end can help caregivers prepare emotionally and practically. This ongoing communication can alleviate anxiety and foster a sense of readiness for the transition (Landreth, 2012).

### Provide Resources and Strategies

Providing caregivers with resources and strategies to support their child post-therapy is crucial. These resources might include handouts on coping strategies, books on child development, or contact information for support groups. Therapists can also offer practical strategies tailored to the child's specific needs, such as techniques for managing anxiety or maintaining routines. This support equips caregivers to handle challenges that may arise after therapy ends and reinforces the skills learned during sessions (Ray, 2011).

### Reassure and Normalize Emotions

Reassuring caregivers that it is normal to experience a range of emotions during the termination process is important. Caregivers might feel sadness, anxiety, or relief, and normalizing these feelings can help them cope more effectively. Therapists can emphasize that it is okay to have mixed emotions and that these feelings are a natural part of the closure process.

Offering a space for caregivers to express their concerns and ask questions can also be beneficial (Dion, 2018).

### Reinforce Mindfulness Practices

Reinforcing the mindfulness practices learned in therapy can help caregivers continue to support their child's growth and development. Providing a reminder sheet with key mindfulness exercises to pin up on the family bulletin board or refrigerator can serve as a useful tool. These practices might include mindful breathing exercises, body scans, or grounding techniques that the family can integrate into their daily routine. Encouraging caregivers to model mindfulness can also enhance their child's ability to manage emotions and stress (Siegel, 2007).

### Conduct a Transition Meeting

Holding a transition meeting with caregivers, child, and therapist can help solidify the progress made and plan for the future. During this meeting, review the child's achievements, discuss the emotions surrounding the end of therapy, and outline strategies for maintaining progress. This meeting can also address any concerns the caregivers might have and allow the therapist to offer additional support and resources (Greenberg, 2002).

### Offer Follow-Up Support

Offering follow-up support can help caregivers feel connected and supported even after therapy has ended. This could involve scheduled check-ins via phone or email, follow-up sessions to address emerging issues or recommendations for community resources. Continuity of care can reassure caregivers that they are not alone, and that help is available if needed (Kolb, 1984).

Supporting caregivers during the closure of therapy is an integral part of the termination process. By keeping caregivers informed, providing resources, normalizing emotions, reinforcing mindfulness practices, conducting transition meetings, and offering follow-up support, therapists can ensure a smooth and positive transition. This comprehensive support helps maintain the therapeutic gains and fosters a supportive environment for the child's continued growth and development.

## Conclusion

Mindful goodbyes are an essential part of the play therapy process, providing clients with a positive and respectful closure experience. By introducing the concept of closure from the beginning, reflecting on progress, celebrating growth, and addressing emotions mindfully, therapists can help clients navigate the closure process with confidence and grace. Creating meaningful goodbye rituals and supporting caregivers further enhances this process, ensuring that the therapeutic relationship ends on a positive note. Through mindfulness-based methods, we can honor the therapeutic journey and prepare clients for their continued growth beyond therapy.

## References

Bartholomew, K., Horowitz, L. M., & Low, K. A. (2019). The significance of attachment in the therapeutic relationship. *Journal of Clinical Psychology, 75*(3), 456–472. https://doi.org/10.1002/jclp.22780

De Geest, R., & Meganck, R. (2019). The therapeutic alliance in child and adolescent psychotherapy: A systematic review. *Journal of Child Psychology and Psychiatry, 60*(4), 462–478. https://doi.org/10.1111/jcpp.13007

Dion, L. (2018). *Synergetic play therapy: A model for integrating neurobiology and mindfulness in therapeutic practice.* Norton.

Greenberg, L. S. (2002). *Emotion-focused therapy: Coaching clients to work through their feelings.* American Psychological Association.

Kolb, D. A. (1984). *Experiential learning: Experience as the source of learning and development.* Prentice-Hall.

Landreth, G. L. (2012). *Play therapy: The art of the relationship* (3rd ed.). Routledge.

Ling, S., & Stathopoulou, G. (2020). Mindfulness-based approaches in termination of therapy. *Psychotherapy, 57*(2), 245–259. https://doi.org/10.1037/pst0000287

Malchiodi, C. A. (2003). *Handbook of art therapy.* Guilford Press.

Pennebaker, J. W. (1997). Writing about emotional experiences as a therapeutic process. *Psychological Science, 8*(3), 162–166. https://doi.org/10.1111/j.1467-9280.1997.tb00403.x

Ray, D. C. (2011). *Child-centered play therapy research: The evidence base for effective practice.* Wiley.

Shafran, R., Lee, M., & Fairburn, C. G. (2019). Termination of therapy: Practical guidelines for practitioners. *Behavior Research and Therapy, 116*, 103–115. https://doi.org/10.1016/j.brat.2019.02.001

Siegel, D. J. (2007). *The mindful brain: Reflection and attunement in the cultivation of well-being.* Norton.

# 20

# THE TRANSFORMATIVE POWER OF MINDFULNESS IN PLAY THERAPY

## Introduction

As we conclude this comprehensive exploration of Mindfulness-based Play Therapy®, it is essential to reflect on the key concepts and practices discussed throughout the book. This final chapter will summarize the significant points covered, emphasizing why mindfulness is a crucial element in enhancing mental wellness outcomes for clients who come to play therapy and safeguarding therapists from professional burnout. By embracing mindfulness, therapists can create more effective, empathetic, and sustainable therapeutic practices that benefit their clients and themselves.

## Integrating Mindfulness into Various Play Therapy Theories and Models

Throughout this book, we have explored how Mindfulness-based Play Therapy® is a transtheoretical approach that easily integrates with all historically significant and seminal play therapy theories. This flexibility allows therapists to enrich their practice with a holistic and adaptive approach tailored to the unique needs of each child and family.

By incorporating mindfulness into various play therapy frameworks, such as cognitive-behavioral, humanistic, and psychodynamic models,

DOI: 10.4324/9781003468585-20

therapists can enhance their effectiveness. For example, combining mindfulness with cognitive-behavioral play therapy techniques can help children become more aware of their thoughts and emotions, enabling them to manage anxiety and negative thought patterns more effectively. Integrating mindfulness into humanistic approaches fosters a deeper sense of self-awareness and self-acceptance, while psychodynamic models benefit from mindfulness by allowing clients to explore their unconscious processes in a safe, present-focused manner.

## Positive Effects of Mindfulness

The robust research on mindfulness consistently shows its positive effects on mental health. Mindfulness practices help reduce symptoms of anxiety, depression, and stress while promoting emotional regulation, resilience, and overall well-being. These benefits are observed not only in clients but also in therapists who practice mindfulness, enhancing their professional satisfaction and reducing the risk of burnout.

Mindfulness helps children and adolescents develop crucial skills such as self-regulation, attention control, and emotional resilience. These skills are essential for navigating the challenges of childhood and adolescence, including academic pressures, social dynamics, and personal development. For therapists, regular mindfulness practice can lead to improved therapeutic presence, greater empathy, and enhanced ability to manage the emotional demands of their work.

## Neurobiological Connections

Mindfulness impacts the brain's neurobiology, promoting neural integration and enhancing cognitive and emotional functioning. By understanding these connections, therapists can appreciate the profound effects mindfulness has on a child's developing brain and how it supports therapeutic goals such as improving attention, emotional regulation, and relational skills.

Neuroscientific research has shown that mindfulness practices can lead to structural and functional changes in the brain. Mindfulness has been shown to reduce the size and over-reactivity of the alarm-center of the brain called the amygdala (Taren et al., 2015) and increase areas of the prefrontal cortex (Tomasino & Fabbro, 2016) and is associated with executive functions such as decision-making, problem-solving, and impulse control. It also enhances connectivity between brain regions involved in emotional regulation and self-referential processing (Hölzel et al., 2010), helping children develop a more balanced and resilient emotional state.

## Mindfulness Practices for Therapists

### Authentic Attunement

Therapists must adopt mindfulness practices to authentically attune to their child and family clients. This attunement is essential for creating a safe and supportive therapeutic environment where clients feel understood and validated. Mindful therapists are better equipped to manage their own stress and maintain a calm, centered presence, which positively influences the therapeutic relationship.

Authentic attunement involves being fully present with clients, actively listening to their verbal and non-verbal cues, and responding with empathy and understanding. Mindfulness helps therapists stay grounded and focused during sessions, reducing the likelihood of distraction or emotional reactivity. This presence allows therapists to build stronger, more trusting relationships with their clients, which is fundamental for effective therapy.

### Therapist Self-Care

Incorporating mindfulness into daily routines can serve as a powerful self-care strategy for therapists. Regular mindfulness practice helps therapists cultivate self-awareness, reduce stress, and enhance emotional resilience, thereby preventing professional burnout and promoting longevity in their careers.

Therapist self-care is critical for maintaining professional effectiveness and personal well-being. Mindfulness practices such as meditation, mindful breathing, and body scans can help therapists manage the emotional and physical demands of their work. By prioritizing self-care, therapists can maintain their capacity to provide high-quality care to their clients while also preserving their own health and well-being.

## Mindfulness Practices for Clients

### Introducing Mindfulness through Play

This book has provided numerous examples of games and activities that introduce the practice of mindfulness to clients. These playful and engaging methods make mindfulness accessible to children, helping them develop essential skills such as emotional regulation, self-awareness, and focused attention. By integrating mindfulness into play therapy, therapists can foster a therapeutic environment that supports holistic healing and growth.

Examples of mindfulness-based play activities include mindful breathing exercises using bubbles, guided imagery using storytelling, and sensory awareness activities with various textures and materials. These activities help children stay present, manage their emotions, and build a sense of calm and focus. By incorporating mindfulness into play, therapists can create a therapeutic experience that is both enjoyable and therapeutic for children.

### Family Involvement

Mindfulness practices can also be extended to family sessions, encouraging a cohesive and supportive home environment. Teaching mindfulness to caregivers and involving them in mindfulness activities enhances the therapeutic process and ensures that the benefits of mindfulness extend beyond the therapy room.

Family involvement in mindfulness practices can improve communication, reduce stress, and foster a sense of connection and support within the family unit. Activities such as family meditation sessions, mindful listening exercises, and collaborative mindfulness projects can help families develop a shared practice that enhances their relationships and overall well-being.

## Conclusion

By embracing Mindfulness-based Play Therapy®, therapists can profoundly impact their clients' mental health and their own professional well-being. Integrating mindfulness into play therapy offers a transformative approach that enhances therapeutic effectiveness, fosters deep empathy, and promotes sustainable practice. Mindfulness is not just an add-on but a foundational element that enriches the therapeutic experience for both clients and therapists. By continuing to cultivate mindfulness, we can create more compassionate, effective, and resilient therapeutic practices that support the well-being of children and families for generations to come. This final chapter serves as a reminder of the transformative power of mindfulness in play therapy and the profound impact it can have on the lives of those we serve.

# References

Hölzel, B. K., Carmody, J. F., Evans, K. C., Hoge, E. A., Dusek, J., Morgan, L., Pitman, R. K., & Lazar, S. W. (2010). Stress reduction correlates with structural changes in the amygdala. *Social Cognitive and Affective Neuroscience, 5*(1), 11–17. https://doi.org/10.1093/scan/nsp034

Taren, A. A., Gianaros, P. J., Greco, C. M., Lindsay, E. K., Fairgrieve, A., Brown, K. W., Rosen, R. K., Ferris, J. L., Julson, E., Marsland, A. L., Bursley, J. K., Ramsburg, J., & Creswell, J. D. (2015). Mindfulness meditation training alters stress-related amygdala resting state functional connectivity: A randomized controlled trial. *Social Cognitive and Affective Neuroscience, 10*(12), 1758–1768. https://doi.org/10.1093/scan/nsv066

Tomasino, B., & Fabbro, F. (2016). Increases in the right dorsolateral prefrontal cortex and decreases the rostral prefrontal cortex activation after-8 weeks of focused attention based mindfulness meditation. *Brain and Cognition, 102*, 46–54.

# INDEX